RESOURCES FOR NURSING RESEARCH

An annotated bibliography

RESOURCES FOR NURSING RESEARCH

An annotated bibliography

Cynthia G. L. Clamp
Honorary Research Fellow, Birmingham Polytechnic

With contributions from

Marie P. Ballard
Matron/Nursing Director, St Giles Hospice, Lichfield

and

Stephen Gough
Learning Resources Manager, Queen Elizabeth College of Nursing and Health Studies, Birmingham

Foreword by Lisbeth Hockey OBE

Library Association Publishing
London

Supported by the English National Board for Nursing, Midwifery and Health Visiting

© The Library Association 1991

Published by
Library Association Publishing Ltd
7 Ridgmount Street
London WC1E 7AE

First published 1991

British Library Cataloguing in Publication Data

Clamp, Cynthia G. L.
  Resources for nursing research: an annotated bibliography.
  I. Title II. Ballard, Marie P. III. Gough, Stephen
  610.73016

  ISBN 1-85604-028-3

Typeset in 10/11pt Times from author's disks by Library Association Publishing Limited
Printed and made in Great Britain by Bookcraft (Bath) Ltd

IN LOVING MEMORY OF

GWENDOLINE NORAH CLAMP

1903 – 1990

WHO GAVE SO MUCH

CONTENTS

DESIGNING NURSING RESEARCH

Experimental Designs

Non-experimental Designs/Approaches

COMMUNICATING NURSING RESEARCH

PART 3   THE BACKGROUND TO RESEARCH IN NURSING

DEVELOPMENT OF NURSING RESEARCH

A PROFESSION'S RESPONSIBILITY

THE ROLE OF GOVERNMENT

FUNDING FOR RESEARCH

NURSING RESEARCH UNITS/CENTRES/DEPARTMENTS

ACKNOWLEDGEMENTS

Many relatives, friends and colleagues have assisted in the development of this resource book and we would like to record our sincere thanks to them all.

A particular debt of gratitude is due to Professor David Cox, Head of the Department of Health Sciences at Birmingham Polytechnic, whose idea it was and who has maintained a keen interest in its development.

The Faculty of Health and Social Sciences at the Polytechnic have given generously by providing photocopying facilities and funding the numerous requests made to the British Library, without which this book could not have been compiled.

We are particularly grateful to Lisbeth Hockey who has written the foreword. She is probably the most distinguished nurse researcher in the United Kingdom and retirement has given her further opportunities to share her many skills.

Ian Martin of Birmingham Polytechnic, Computer Services Department, taught one of the authors patiently and skilfully how to use her computer.

Representatives of many government, statutory, publishing, professional and other organizations in the United Kingdom, North America and Europe have given generously of their time in providing information for this book, together with many librarians and individuals.

Rita Le Var and Jean Heath of the English National Board have given valuable assistance during the book's developmental stages, as has Barbara Jover of Library Association Publishing.

Permission has been given by Debra Unsworth, the Librarian responsible for maintaining the Index of Nursing Research at the Department of Health in London, to include the entries on *Nursing research abstracts*.

All the following people have also contributed to the book in various ways: Phyllis Archer, Philip Ballard, Conall Boyle, Peter Bradshaw, Chris Brannigan, George Castledine, Anna Cavill, Lyn Copcutt, Jean Davies, Ann Edney, Jane Fox, Jean Gardner, David Gill, Emma Griffiths, Chris Lester, John and Hazel Lloyd, Rosemary Morris, Peter Nolan, Carolyn Orme, Grace Poland, Jane Richards, Sarah Robinson, Elizabeth Scott, Charles Shute, Tomasi Tawake, John Taylor, Glenda Winson.

FOREWORD

It is a pleasure and an honour to write a foreword to this important book. My first reaction to it was amazement tinged with an element of jealousy – amazement at the richness of this new resource, jealousy of those who will be able to make use of it. I could not help wishing that it had been available when I needed it.

The volume breaks entirely new ground and is an impressive achievement. In bringing together literature relating to all aspects of research it fulfills a wide variety of purposes. A cursory glance at the contents pages and the authors' introduction will provide evidence for this statement.

Reflecting on the whole range of research-related activities, it is easy to see the contribution of this book to all of them. Although the literature related to the actual methods of inquiry forms the major part, many other topics, such as professional responsibility and education for research are given due attention. Research is now an accepted topic in nursing education and is by no means restricted to academic enterprises. It is presented in most basic and post-basic courses at various levels. Teachers in such courses will find this book invaluable in designing their curricula and in the directions to the available literature. It is so much simpler to have one source for the identification of the rapidly increasing literary sources instead of many. In addition, the reader is guided not only to the titles of publications, which are so often bland and unhelpful, but the authors' annotations allow a much more efficient selection of material.

Current nursing education encourages students to read around topics themselves instead of being presented with pre-selected photocopies. This new resource gives teachers badly needed help in this important activity with the least time consumption.

I am glad the authors opted for breadth rather than depth in their coverage of the literature. Depth tends to be dictated by individual need and the reader, following the given references, will be able to attain his or her own appropriate level or depth. Although the discipline of nursing appropriately provides the bulk of the literature other relevant sources are not excluded. Moreover, the references are by no means confined to the British literature. North American sources feature prominently, in line with their major contribution to nursing research, and literature is also included from Europe and Australia.

The authors of this book have rendered a tremendously helpful service, not only to nurse researchers, but to the whole nursing profession. I cannot see any role in nursing where research-related literature has no part to play. If the research basis to our profession, so often quoted today, is to become a reality, *Resources for nursing research* will become indispensible, perhaps not in its entirety and all of the time, but selectively and at different career stages.

I am pleased to know that the authors and publishers are already considering ways of adding to and updating this publication.

Lisbeth Hockey

INTRODUCTION

'Research is ... not a luxury for the academic, but a tool for developing the quality of nursing decisions, prescriptions and actions. Whether as clinicians, educators, managers or researchers we have a research responsibility: neglect of that responsibility could be classed as professional negligence' (McFarlane of Llandaff 1984)

Nurses are increasingly recognizing the importance of nursing research as the basis for professional practice and the subject is now included in most basic, post-basic and advanced level courses. In addition, it is a required component in many senior nurses' roles as the profession strives to improve the care it gives.

The volume of nursing research literature now available is considerable and increasing, and this resource book, in the form of an annotated bibliography, is designed to assist in its location. The book gives guidance on sources of literature; it identifies methodological literature, and that which enables nursing research to be seen in a wider context.

The book has been particularly designed with teachers in mind, as research is now part of most nursing curricula, but it will also be of value to researchers, practitioners, advanced level students and college librarians.

Three authors have been involved in its preparation, a librarian, nurse manager and a nurse researcher.

It is envisaged that this book will be of value in all English-speaking countries, and may be used as the first step in identifying literature relating to nursing research. Just under 50% of the annotations are from North American literature, a few from Europe and Australasia and the rest from the United Kingdom.

In Part 2 reference has been made to all the major areas of research processes from the discipline's own literature, sociological sources, and from others where appropriate.

There are over 1,300 entries in this book, of which 95% have been annotated, and although the number varies considerably within each section, this does not necessarily reflect the volume of literature available. Breadth rather than depth has been the aim in selection of materials, and the authors have identified some of the most important from which each reader will be able to follow up their own areas of interest.

There are three extensive sections, 2.1 on research texts, 2.17 on ethical issues in research and 3.18 on teaching nursing research. In most cases the annotations are non-evaluative, and are intended to give an idea of what the article or book contains. A few entries have not been annotated and this is where the whole issue of a journal is devoted to a particular topic but not all articles are about methodology. In addition to the annotations, lists of suggested textbook readings are included which will guide teachers and students towards appropriate sections, and entries in *Nursing research abstracts* are also identified.

Wherever possible, literature has been selected from 1980 onwards, unless there is only a relatively small amount related to the particular topic, it is a key text or article, or the work is acknowledged to be of major importance.

The arrangement of the book can best be seen by examining the expanded contents list at the beginning, and the author index at the end. Part 1 covers research resources which are available in the UK and overseas and via computer networks. Part 2 includes references to all aspects of research processes and Part 3 outlines background literature essential for seeing nursing research in its widest context. Details of the book's structure, format and numbering system may be found on page xix in 'How to use this book'.

Creating the index has been a difficult task and it has been through many drafts. This is partly because there is a lack of consistency in terms of order in the methodological textbooks. Classification of material has also given problems, even though all headings are derived from the literature. Readers are therefore advised to look carefully at the headings and consult others, if the material does not appear to be what is required.

There is some confusion and difference of opinion as to the meaning of words and phrases. In order to assist the reader, one definition, obtained from existing glossaries, literature or dictionaries, is included for each word or phrase as appropriate. A list of sources of these definitions may be found in Appendix E.

The level of methodology texts in section 2.1 differs, with some intended for students, undergraduates and postgraduates, and others for practitioners. The emphasis given to particular elements also differs considerably, so it may be necessary to consult more than one text.

Obtaining the literature cited has involved the use of many libraries, in particular the resources of the British Library, and a list of journals from which articles have been obtained is in Appendix C. As colleges of nursing are now being established and Project 2000 courses coming on stream, there will need to be close co-operation between teachers and librarians in terms of purchasing policies so that the major sources are available for all students.

The order within this bibliography may indicate that all matters relating to research are 'neat and tidy'. In fact this is not so and there are many areas of discord, debate and controversy. These have not been specifically identified, as this is not the purpose of the book, but readers will find them covered in the respective sections.

All nurses have an obligation to learn about research, whether it be to read the literature, create the climate in which utilisation becomes possible, implement findings or undertake projects. The authors hope that this book will contribute towards the teaching and learning of research in all places where nurses work and that as a consequence patient/client care will be improved as practice becomes increasingly based on firm foundations.

HOW TO USE THIS BOOK

INDEXES
There are two indexes in this book, a subject and an author index. The subject index also serves as the expanded contents list and is found at the beginning of the book. The author index is at the end.

STRUCTURE OF THE BOOK
The book is divided into three major parts:

Part 1 Sources of literature
Part 2 Methods of inquiry
Part 3 The background to research in nursing

FORMAT OF SECTIONS
The format of each section follows a similar pattern, although not all sections will include all items. Entries are listed in alphabetical order.

Title
Introductory statement
Definition
Example
Major text/article [specific to sub-section]
Annotations
Suggested textbook readings
Entries in *Nursing research abstracts*
Notes

NUMBERING SYSTEM
The numbering system used in the book should enable any item to be found without difficulty.

Part 1 items are numbered 1.1 − 1.12
Part 2 items are numbered 2.1 − 2.105
Part 3 items are numbered 3.1 − 3.28

Within each section entries have individual numbers e.g. 1.1.1, 2.1.2 or 3.1.3 and this number is also used in the cross-referencing system.

CROSS-REFERENCING SYSTEM
Many books and articles contain information which comes under several headings in the book. Where this occurs the item reference number is given at the end of the annotation so that other relevant entries can easily be found. The number may indicate a whole section e.g. 2.15 or a particular annotation e.g. 2.15.6.

SUGGESTED TEXTBOOK READINGS

In Parts 2 and 3 suggested textbook readings have been included. As there are now so many textbooks available on research methodology this information is included to give readers some idea of their content, and will be helpful when used together with their annotations in section 2.1. Although the page numbers given relate to a particular edition, they will nevertheless assist in the choice of texts.

The author(s) name, (plus initials if there are several with the same name), is given together with the page numbers which relate to each section. These are the major references within each text but readers will also need to consult the book's own index. Each entry is cross-referenced to its annotation. For example

Abdellah & Levine   382–396   2.1.1

NURSING RESEARCH ABSTRACTS

Because of the importance of *Nursing research abstracts* as a source of British research, reference to these is also made. Again the author(s) name is listed, together with the reference number in the *Abstracts*. For example

Phillips L.R.F.   86/451

'86' indicates the year of publication and '451' is the item number within that particular volume. Users will then need to read the abstract to see if the article or book is relevant to their needs.

Notes

Every effort has been made to ensure the accuracy of entries, but the authors will be pleased to know of any errors.

Inevitably in such a complex book there will be omissions. The authors will therefore be pleased to receive copies of papers, updated reports and other material, which would not normally be identified from the usual sources, so that these may be included in subsequent editions.

English spelling has been used throughout the text, except in journal titles, in order to achieve consistency.

International Standard Book Numbers (ISBNs) have been included for most books. Occasionally it has not been possible to find this number, or the book does not have one.

PROFILE OF AUTHORS

Cynthia G. L. Clamp MPhil BA SRN RSCN RNT
Honorary Research Fellow, Birmingham Polytechnic

Cynthia Clamp has had wide experience in teaching research to nurses on many basic and post-basic courses in four major schools of nursing in the United Kingdom. She recently held the post of Research Associate in Nursing Studies at Birmingham Polytechnic where she lectured on research methodology to students taking initial training and those taking diplomas and degrees. Her research experience included working on several projects at the Joint Board of Clinical Nursing Studies. These were on aspects of curriculum development, courses in action, assessment tools, the process of continuous assessment, course evaluation and group discussion as a method of learning. A number of reports have been written in this field. The development of attitude awareness and interpersonal communication skills in nursing was the subject of her MPhil degree. She now works as a research consultant.

Marie Ballard SRN
Matron/Nursing Director, St Giles Hospice, Whittington, Lichfield, Staffordshire

Marie Ballard's background is that of a ward sister and nursing officer in a district general hospital in Birmingham. She became the Matron of St Giles Hospice in 1983 and remains in this post. Whilst undertaking the English National Board course No. 870, an Introduction to the Understanding and Application of Research at Birmingham Polytechnic she compiled an annotated bibliography on 'Breaking Bad News' to patients with cancer or those who are dying.

Stephen Gough BA (Hons)
Learning Resources Manager, Queen Elizabeth College of Nursing and Health Studies, Birmingham

Stephen Gough's work includes the teaching of literature-searching skills to students on basic and post-basic courses, and on the English National Board course No. 870, an Introduction to the Understanding and Application of Research. In addition to his formal teaching commitments, he regularly assists nurse researchers within the South Birmingham and Solihull Health Authorities in identifying and exploring the literature of their subject. Publications include contributing a chapter on literature searching skills in *Nursing research: a skills based introduction* published in 1990 by Prentice Hall (CR 2.1.18)

Part 1

SOURCES OF LITERATURE

PROCESS OF LITERATURE SEARCHING

1.1 PROCESS OF LITERATURE SEARCHING

The purpose of this section is to highlight material which will be helpful in identifying sources of research methodology and other literature. It is not an exhaustive list, and where there are no guides the sources themselves have been documented.

Annotations

1.1.1 Berge, P. & Saffioti, C.L. (1987) *Basic college research*. New York: Neal-Schuman   ISBN 0555700187

Book is intended for teachers and students. Each chapter is completed by a set of assignments, some of which would need amending for use outside North America. Gives introduction to types and sources in the social sciences and humanities. Chapters are included on preparing final reports and note taking (CR 2.100).

1.1.2 DaRosa, D.A., Ross, D. & Folse, R. (1985) The way we teach information skills. *Medical teacher* 7(3/4) 297-300   2 References

A description of a problem-based approach to teaching information-seeking skills to medical students.

1.1.3 Gash, S. (1989) *Effective literature searching for students*. Aldershot: Gower   ISBN 0566057492

A general guide to the principles and practice of literature searching. It is not applied to any particular subject area and covers preparation, searching, online searching, keeping records, writing references and citing references in the text.

1.1.4 Grogan, D. (1982) *Science and technology: an introduction to the literature*. 4th edition London: Library Association   ISBN 0851573401

A guide to the structure of scientific literature. Chapter 1 provides definitions of primary, secondary and tertiary sources. (New edition in preparation).

1.1.5 Kilby, S.A., Fischel, C.C. & Gupta, A.D. (1989) Access to nursing information sources. *Image: the journal of nursing scholarship* 21(1) 26-30

Gives a brief overview of literature searching sources with some evaluative comment.

1.1.6 Kwater, E. (1987) Literature searching for starters. *Nurse education today* 7(2) 132-134

Article illustrates the basic principles and decision-making processes prior to starting a literature search.

3

1.1.7 O'Brien, D., Procter, S. & Walton, G. (1990) Towards a strategy for teaching information skills to student nurses. *Nurse education today* 10(2) 125-129

Describes a comprehensive information skills package developed for use in the Newcastle Polytechnic Library in conjunction with a Diploma in Nursing Science/Registered General Nursing course.

1.1.8 Polytechnic of the South Bank Library (1984) *Guide to searching the literature of nursing, community health and social services.* 3rd edition London: Polytechnic of the South Bank ISBN 0905267370

This guide is based on the resources and services of the Polytechnic of the South Bank and other services within the London area. Contents include basic steps in searching, writing your project and sources of information. The section on sources of information lists many of the currently available services with annotations.

1.1.9 Roddham, M. (1989) *Searching the literature.* Research Awareness, Module 4, London: Distance Learning Centre, South Bank Polytechnic ISBN 0948250399 References

This is number 4 in a series of 13 modules, each of which deals with a different aspect of nursing research. It was developed to assist nurses, midwives and health visitors in understanding research in terms of their own professional practice. Modules can be used separately or as part of a programme. The reader is encouraged to work through a number of activities, self-assessment questions and answers and progress summaries. Some articles/book extracts referred to in the text are reproduced in full.

This module stresses the importance of searching the literature as a preliminary stage of the research process. Comprehensive information is given about making the best use of libraries, and describes the wide range of materials available to trained and learner nurses. Clear explanations describe how to use the resources and frequent examples are given from the literature. A chapter is devoted to references and citations and another on planning and organising a literature search. A demonstration search is conducted to show how all the steps fit together. How to obtain access to inter-library networks is described, and addresses, opening times and other information are given for some larger and specialised libraries (CR 2.12, Appendix D).

1.1.10 Strauch, K., Linton, R. & Cohen, C. (1989) *Library research guide to nursing: illustrated search strategy and sources.* Ann Arbor, Michigan: Pieran Press ISBN 18006782435

Book explains certain key sources which will assist in searching the literature. Detailed information is given on defining a topic, locating books and current information. Advice is given on evaluating sources, computerised literature searches and using other libraries and their resources. Illustrations are given throughout the text from the cited sources. Appendices contain a library skills test, additional selected sources and how to develop a care plan.

1.1.11 **Wilson, M.E.** (1988) How to do a literature search. *Nursing standard* 2(3) October 8 39 No references

Briefly covers the use of abstracts and indexes.

1.2 LIBRARIES

Details are given here on general guides to using libraries together with information on specific national and specialist collections.

Annotations

General guides
1.2.1 Adkins, R.T. (ed) (1988) *Guide to government department and other libraries*. London: British Library   ISBN 071230746X

Provides basic information, addresses, telephone numbers, library hours, stock and subject coverage. Also included are availability, services and publications.

1.2.2 British Medical Association (1987) *Medical libraries: a user guide*. London: British Medical Association   ISBN 0727902156

A comprehensive guide to medical library services, facilities and the tools of medical literature searching. Excludes nursing and allied health professions although many of the services detailed are equally useful for nursing research subjects.

1.2.3 Gann, R. (1986) Information services and health promotion: what libraries can do. *Health education journal* 45(2) 112-115   26 References

A general introduction to library services related particularly to health promotion.

1.2.4 Harrold, A. (ed) (1990) *Libraries in the UK and Republic of Ireland*. 16th edition London: Library Association   ISBN 0853655995

Gives names and addresses of all public, university, polytechnic, selected government, national and specialised libraries. It also includes departments of librarianship and information science.

1.2.5 Morton, L.T. & Wright, D.J. (1989) *How to use a medical library*. 7th edition London: Library Association   ISBN 0851574661

Provides an introduction to medical libraries for practitioners, research workers and specialist librarians. The main sources of bibliographic data are given together with information on the catalogues, classification schemes, periodicals, indexes and abstracting services, manual and computer literature searching and audio-visual aids.

1.2.6 Strauch, K.P. & Brundage, D.J. (1980) *Guide to library resources for nursing.* New York: Appleton-Century-Crofts   ISBN 0838535283

This book is designed to identify a variety of current materials in nursing, how to locate and evaluate them easily and quickly. Features include: comprehensive listings of general reference sources, annotated lists of nursing literature organised by subject, separate listings of periodicals related to nursing, a list of audio-visual material and names and addresses of publishers.

National libraries

1.2.7 Sparks, S.M. (1986) The US National Library of Medicine: a worldwide nursing resource. *International nursing review* 33(2) 47-49

The National Library of Medicine materials and information services available to nurses are described.

Special collections

1.2.8 Akinsanya, J. (1984) Learning about nursing research. *Nursing times* 80(16) August 29   59-61   10 References Occasional paper

Describes a small scale survey of theses and dissertations in the Steinberg Collection at the Royal College of Nursing, London. The study, carried out by Diploma in Nursing Students, aimed to show the range and scope of nursing literature in this collection (CR 1.2.10).

1.2.9 Fairman, J.A. (1987) Sources and references for research in nursing history. *Nursing research* 36(1) 56-59

Lists the principal collections of nursing history material in North America together with a selected bibliography of publications.

1.2.10 Smith, J.P. (1983) Steinberg Collection of Nursing Research. *Journal of advanced nursing* 8(5) 357   Editorial

Outlines the history and background of this internationally important collection.

THE TOOLS FOR LITERATURE SEARCHING

1.3 SOURCEBOOKS/GUIDES

Sourcebooks and guides give information about primary (original) information and secondary sources: indexes, information centres, libraries.

Annotations
1.3.1 Association for Information Management (1990) *Forthcoming international scientific and technical conferences.* London: Aslib August 1990 List No. 67 Supplement 2

Gives details of forthcoming conferences, both national and international in the fields of science and technology, and nursing is included. Issues quarterly with the main issue in February and supplements in May, August and November (CR 1.9.3).

1.3.2 Bunch, A.J. (1979) *Health care administration: an information sourcebook.* London: Capitol Planning Information ISBN 0906011051

Makes reference to mainly British sources under the following headings: reference books; basic books and reports; statistical sources; periodicals; abstracting, indexing and current awareness services; bibliographies; current research and theses and libraries. Appendices include: directory of organisations, author/title index and subject index.

1.3.3 Cook, A., Bailey, P. & Ramsay, A. (1981) *Health studies: a guide to sources of information.* Newcastle upon Tyne: Newcastle upon Tyne Polytechnic ISBN 0906471044

In need of updating, but shows the range of information sources available in the health sciences.

1.3.4 Davinson, D. (1977) *Theses and dissertations as information sources.* London: Clive Bingley ISBN 0851572278 (Published in USA by Linnet Books ISBN 0208015396)

A general guide to theses and dissertations. Contents include: history of the thesis medium; nature and purposes of theses; bibliographic control; access and research in progress. An additional section lists guides to thesis preparation.

1.3.5 Interagency Council on Library Sources for Nursing (1988) Reference sources for nursing: a guide to the essential tools for research. *Nursing outlook* 36(5) 246-248

A comprehensive listing of sources for literature searching in the USA.

1.3.6 Lancaster, A. (1979) *Nursing and midwifery sourcebook.* London: Allen & Unwin   ISBN 004610013X

In need of updating but still a useful tool for identifying sources of nursing information.

1.3.7 Pantry, S. (1986) *Information sources for occupational health nurses.* Sheffield: SCP   ISBN 0951179403

Aims to provide a quick route to the various sources of information which anyone working in occupational health and safety nursing may need.

1.3.8 Thomson, I. (1989) *The documentation of the European Communities: a guide.* London: Mansell   ISBN 0720120225

Describes the range of printed information which is publicly available. This includes primary and secondary legislation through working documents and research reports, together with explanatory and background sources. References to health care are included.

1.4   DIRECTORIES

Directories are a useful source for identifying sources of information, people and possible assistance. However not all are truly comprehensive, as questionnaire returns are often the method used for compilation.

Annotations

1.4.1 *Councils, committees and boards: a handbook of advisory, executive and similar bodies in British public life.* (1984) 6th edition Edited by Sellar, L. Beckenham: CBD Research   ISBN 090024643X

Arranged alphabetically, each entry gives details of structure and purpose.

1.4.2 *Current British directories.* 11th edition (1988) Edited by Henderson, C.A.P. Beckenham: CBD Research   ISBN 0900246502

A guide to major directories covering Great Britain. Sections include: local directories, specialised directories, publishers and subject indexes.

1.4.3 *Current British journals: a bibliographic guide.* (1989) 5th edition Edited by Woodworth, D.P. & Goodair, C.M. Boston Spa: British Library Document Supply Centre   ISBN 0712320539

Arranged in 10 sections including social sciences, humanities and science, including nursing.

1.4.4 *Current research in Britain* (1989) *Social sciences.* Boston Spa: British Library   ISBN 0712320571

A national register of current research being carried out in universities, polytechnics, colleges and other institutions in the UK. The series is divided into four areas:

physical sciences	annual − 2 parts
biological sciences	annual − 2 parts
social sciences	annual
humanities	biennial.

Contains a department index, lists research in progress and has name, study area and keyword indexes. Social sciences covers nursing and medicine.

1.4.5 *Directory of British associations and associations in Ireland.* (1986) 8th Edition Edited by Henderson, G.P. & Henderson, S.P.A. Beckenham: CBD Research   ISBN 0900246456

Arranged alphabetically; each entry includes a statement of purpose, publications and whether there is a library. A subject index is also included (CR 1.4.7).

1.4.6 *Directory of British official publications: a guide to sources.* (1984) 2nd edition Compiled by Richard, S. London: Mansell   ISBN 0720117062

Directory identifies the full range of publications by official organisations and sources of supply. The book's introduction describes the pattern of official publications, bibliographical sources, HMSO and its services, cataloguing and information services, forthcoming publications and bookselling services. It also outlines the types of material published. The publications of the Department of Health and other bodies concerned with health and nursing are included.

1.4.7 *Directory of European professional and learned societies.* (1989) Beckenham: CBD Research   ISBN 1900246510

Directory is a complimentary volume to the *Directory of British Associations.* Arrangement is by subject (CR 1.4.5).

1.4.8 *Directory of hospitals* (1990) Harlow: Longman   ISBN 0582068339

Lists National Health Service hospitals. For each one there is a list of specialities and the consultants.

1.4.9 *Directory of medical and health care libraries in the United Kingdom and Republic of Ireland.* (1990) 7th edition Compiled by Wright, D.R. London: The Library Association   ISBN 0853657793

Each entry includes the name, address and telephone number, type of library, opening hours, stock policy, holdings, classification system, publications and network membership.

1.4.10 *Martindale: the extra pharmacopoeia.* (1989) Edited by Reynolds, J.E.F. London: The Pharmaceutical Press   ISBN 0853692106

Provides unbiased, concise reports on the actions and uses of most of the worlds drugs and medicines (CR 1.10.13).

1.4.11 *The Mental Health Foundation's someone to talk to directory 1985: a directory of self-help and community support agencies – national and local in the United Kingdom and Republic of Ireland.* (1985) Compiled by Webb, P. London: Mental Health Foundation   ISBN 0901944084

Arranged by broad subject sections, with national organisations listed first, followed by local. Details include a statement of purpose and type of service provided.

1.4.12 *Research centres directory.* (1990) 14th edition Edited by Dresser, P.D. & Hill, K. Detroit: Gale Research   ISBN 0810348616

This directory lists research centres in the United States and Canada together with their research activities. Entries are listed in subject categories, including one on the life sciences. It assists researchers in contacting one another in similar fields.

1.4.13 *Ulrich's international periodicals directory 1990-1991.* (1990) 29th edition New York: Bowker   ISBN 3 volume set 0835229858; Volume 1 0835229866; Volume 2 0835229874; Volume 3 0835229882

Arranged by subject, each entry includes title, publisher, year first published, frequency, special features, where indexed, online availability, title changes and a brief description of typical contents.

1.5   STATISTICS

This section gives details of guides to official statistics.

Annotations

1.5.1   Central Statistical Office *Guide to official statistics.* London: HMSO

Enables one to trace sources of official statistical data. There are periodic updates.

1.5.2 *Eurostat catalogue: publications and electronic services.* (1988) Luxembourg: Office for Official Publications of the European Communities   Catalogue No. CA-50-87-647-EN-C

Lists publications under themes and is produced annually. These are: 1. general statistics, 2. economy and finance, 3. population and social conditions, 4. energy and industry, 5. agriculture and fisheries, 6. foreign trade, 7. services and transport and 9. miscellaneous.

1.5.3 *Eurostat index: a detailed subject index to the series published by the statistics office of the European Communities.* (1986) 3rd edition Compiled by Ramsay, A. Stamford, Lincs: Capital Planning Information Ltd   ISBN 0906011353

A detailed keyword subject index to assist the layman in finding European Community statistics. Online access is publicly available via the Euronet DIANE network. It also contains a bibliography enabling Eurostat titles to be traced, lists other published titles, European documentation centres and depository libraries.

1.5.4 Radical Statistics Health Group (1980) *Unofficial guide to official health statistics.* London: Radical Statistics Health Group ISBN 0906081033

Outlines the types of official health statistics collected and where they may be found. Reliability of these data are questioned as they are collected and used for political purposes.

1.5.5 *Statistic sources* (1991) 14th Edition Edited by O'Brien, J.W. & Wasserman, S.R. Detroit: Gale Research Inc. ISBN set 0810373750; Volume 1 0810373769; Volume 2 0810373777

Content includes a selected bibliography of key statistical sources and a dictionary of statistics sources. The bibliography includes statistical databases online, almanacs and international sources as well as United States statistical sources. Topics covered include financial, business, social, educational and health.

1.5.6 *World Health statistics quarterly.* (1990) Geneva: World Health Organisation

Published quarterly and provides health guidance based on what can be learned from statistical data. Each issue focuses on a selected theme or topic of current public health interest which will be a prime source for health planners.

1.6 CORE JOURNALS

A number of journals regularly report on, or present research findings. These can be grouped into three principal categories: clinical and other specialities, general management and research. Standards vary between titles, especially in the general section where the title's principal aim may not be to present research findings. This listing is not comprehensive; rather it should be seen as an indicator of the breadth of specialist journals.

Clinical speciality

Critical Care/Emergency Care
Critical care nurse (USA)
Dimensions of critical care nursing (USA)
Emergency care nursing quarterly (USA)
Focus on critical care (USA)
Heart and lung (USA)
Intensive care nursing (UK)
Journal of emergency nursing (USA)

General
Clinical care specialist (USA)
Journal of clinical nursing (UK) (bi-monthly from January 1992)

Midwifery
Midwife, health visitor & community nurse (UK)
Midwifery (UK)
Midwives chronicle (UK)

Nephrology
American Nephrology Nurses Association journal

Oncology
Cancer nursing (USA)
Oncology nursing forum (USA)
Seminars in oncology nursing (USA)

Operating department
AORN — Association of Operating Room Nurses journal (USA)
NATN news — British journal of theatre nursing

Orthopaedics
Orthopaedic nursing (USA)

Paediatrics
American journal of maternal child nursing
Journal of paediatric nursing (USA)
Maternal child nursing journal (USA)
Paediatric nursing (UK)
Paediatrics (USA)
Pediatric nursing (USA)

Plastic surgery
Plastic surgical nursing (USA)

Primary care
Community outlook (UK)
Health visitor (UK)

Psychiatry/Psychology
Issues in mental health nursing (USA)
Journal of child and adolescent psychiatric and mental health nursing (USA)
Journal of psychosocial nursing and mental health services (USA)

Education
Journal of continuing education in nursing (USA)
Journal of nursing education (USA)
Nurse education today (UK)
Nurse educator (USA)
Patient education and counselling (USA)

Ethics
Bulletin of medical ethics (UK)
Hastings Center report (USA)
Journal of medical ethics (UK)

General
American journal of nursing (USA)
Canadian nurse
Chinese journal of nursing (Chung Hua Hu Li Tsa Chih)
International nursing review (Switzerland)
Journal of professional nursing (USA)
Nursing (UK)
Nursing (USA)
Nursing and health care (USA)
Nursing forum (USA)
Nursing outlook (USA)
Nursing practitioner (USA)
Nursing review (UK)
Nursing times (UK)
Professional nurse (UK)
Senior nurse (UK)
Sogo kango (Comprehensive Nursing Quarterly – Japan)

Information technology
Information technology in nursing (UK)

Management
Canadian journal of nursing administration
Journal of nursing administration (USA)
Nurse manager (USA)
Nursing administration quarterly (USA)

Research
Advances in nursing science (USA)
Applied nursing research (USA)
Australian journal of advanced nursing
Behaviour research methods, instruments and computers (USA)
Canadian journal of nursing research (Nursing papers)
Communicating nursing research: collaboration and competition (USA)
Health services research (USA)
Hospital topics (USA)
Image: the journal of nursing scholarship (USA)
International journal of nursing studies (UK)
Journal of advanced nursing (UK)
Nursing clinics of North America
Nursing research (USA)
Nursing science quarterly (USA)
Recent advances in nursing (ceased publication October 1990) (UK)
Research in nursing and health (USA)
Scandinavian journal of caring sciences
Western journal of nursing research (USA)

1.7 BIBLIOGRAPHIES

Bibliographies are listings of books and other materials which can be grouped by a common factor, hence the *British national bibliography* is based primarily on items received by the Copyright Receipt Office of the British Library. Two articles are also included in this section.

Annotations

1.7.1 *Bibliography of nursing literature 1859-1960: with an historical introduction.* (1968) Edited by Thompson, A.M.C. London: Library Association ISBN 0853654700

AND

1.7.2 *Bibliography of nursing literature 1961-1970.* (1974) Edited by Thompson, A.M.C. London: Library Association ISBN 085365316X

AND

1.7.3 *Bibliography of nursing literature 1971-1975.* (1985) Edited by Walsh, F. London: Library Association ISBN 0853656231

AND

1.7.4 *Bibliography of nursing literature 1976-1980.* (1986) Edited by Walsh, F. London: Library Association ISBN 0853657467

These bibliographies are of value to anyone researching the history of nursing. The entries include journal articles as well as books. The listings are, however, not comprehensive.

1.7.5 *Books in print*
Publisher: Bowker – Saur
Frequency: Monthly

Available on microfiche and CD-ROM. Contains author, title and publisher indexes. Covers books published in North America only.

1.7.6 *British national bibliography*
Publisher: British Library
Frequency: Weekly with four monthly and annual cumulations

BNB is a subject catalogue of all the titles published in Britain, received by the Copyright Receipt Office of the British Library. Published since 1950 it forms a reasonably comprehensive listing of nursing titles, but caution is needed as not all titles listed actually reach the booksellers' shelves.

1.7.7 *International books in print.*
Publisher: Saur, München
Frequency: Annual

Contains author and title indexes. Lists English language titles published in Canada, Continental Europe, Latin America, Oceania, Africa, Asia and the Republic of Ireland.

1.7.8 *Library of Congress catalogue (National Union Catalogue)*
Publisher: Library of Congress, Washington
Frequency: Monthly

Available on microfiche since 1983 and covers books and audio-visual materials. Includes the following indexes: name, title, subject and series (i.e. monographs, symposia, reports, periodicals, papers, occasional papers, intermittent publications and conference proceedings).

1.7.9 *Nursing data search*
Publisher: Bridge Medical Books, Whittakers Way, Loughton, Essex
Frequency: Quarterly or biannual

Currently only available on floppy disc for IBM compatible microcomputers. Entries are from approximately 130 publishers (British bias) for titles currently in print. Includes HMSO and WHO publications.

1.7.10 *Whitakers books in print* (formerly British Books in Print)
Publisher: Whitaker
Frequency: Monthly

Available on microfiche and has author, title and subject indexes. Also contains forthcoming books.

Articles
1.7.11 Sharp, D. (1986) Searching health education literature: bibliographic and indexing tools. *Health education journal* 45(5) 239-242   2 References

A general description of access services available in the field of health education in the UK.

1.7.12 South West Thames Regional Library Service (1984) Checklists for nursing libraries: checklist 2, indexes and bibliographies. *Health libraries review* 1   204-206

Lists the core printed services.

1.8 CURRENT AWARENESS SERVICES

Current awareness services are produced to provide up to date listings, sometimes annotated, of items usually of interest to a specific group.

Annotations
1.8.1 *Ethnic minorities health: a current awareness bulletin*
Publisher: Bradford Health Authority
Frequency: Quarterly with annual subject index

Arranged by broad subject categories, each entry includes a brief annotation where the item's title does not make the content clear.

1.8.2 *Health Visitors Association current awareness bulletin*
Publisher: Health Visitors Association
Frequency: Quarterly

Lists articles of interest to health visitors and their managers. Each entry includes a brief annotation. Journals indexed in the bulletin are listed.

1.8.3 *Midwives Information and Resource Service (MIDIRS)*
Publisher: MIDIRS
Frequency: Three times a year

An unusual service in that it includes original source material. Would be useful to teachers of midwifery, midwives, health visitors and students (CR 1.12.4).

1.8.4 *Nursing bibliography*
Publisher: Royal College of Nursing
Frequency: Monthly

A useful source of information but the lack of an annual cumulation makes searching slow.

1.8.5 *Royal College of Midwives current awareness service*
Publisher: Royal College of Midwives
Frequency: Quarterly

Gives lists of journals and available bibliographies. Also included are book reviews of items in current awareness service, information on books, reports, press releases, useful addresses and journal holdings of the library (CR 1.9.11).

Article
1.8.6 South West Thames Regional Library Service (1985) Checklists for nursing libraries: checklist 3, Current awareness services. *Health libraries review* 2   39-40

Lists the core printed services.

1.9 INDEXING SERVICES

Indexing services give brief details of items, most often periodicals, published during a specified period and are usually arranged by subject.

Annotations
1.9.1 *British education index*
Publisher: Leeds University Press
Frequency: Quarterly with annual cumulation

Issues are divided into two sections: author list and subject list. Entries in the author list include subject descriptor terms and the type of document. Subject list entries are more brief. Lists all periodicals indexed.

1.9.2 British humanities index
Publisher: Bowker – Saur
Frequency: Quarterly with annual cumulations

Covers a wide range of social science subjects and is particularly useful for community subjects.

1.9.3 British Library monthly index of conference proceedings
Publisher: British Library
Frequency: Monthly with annual cumulations

Covers all types of conference proceedings including those published in serial and book form. Nursing conferences are also included (CR 1.3.1, 3.26).

1.9.4 Cumulative index of nursing and allied health literature
Publisher: CINAHL
Frequency: Bimonthly with annual cumulations

Subject headings follow a very similar pattern to Medical subject headings (MeSH). Entries are similar to the *International nursing index* but are expanded to include qualifiers for the title and subject descriptors. A good service of its type, but because it is produced separately from other services, search strategies have to be devised only for use with *CINAHL.*

1.9.5 Current technology index (replaces *British technology index*)
Publisher: Bowker – Saur
Frequency: Monthly with annual cumulation

Covers all branches of engineering and chemical technology. Some subjects related to medicine are included e.g. health foods, health hazards, hearing, heart, medical equipment and medical photography.

1.9.6 Index medicus
Publisher: National Library of Medicine (USA)
Frequency: Monthly with annual cumulations

The major service in the field of health sciences. A good alternative to *INI* and *CINAHL* if these are unavailable. Fits well with *INI* as they both use Medical Subject Headings.

1.9.7 Index to social sciences and humanities proceedings
Publisher: Institute for Scientific Information Inc. Philadelphia
Frequency: 3 quarterly issues with an annual cumulation

Index publishes the most significant proceedings world wide in a range of disciplines in the social sciences and humanities. Nursing is included.

1.9.8 *Index to theses: with abstracts accepted for higher degrees by the universities of Britain including the Council for National Academic Awards (CNAA)*
Publisher: Aslib
Frequency: Each volume covers a calendar year

Contains abstracts of all theses accepted for higher degrees in the UK (CR 1.12.2).

1.9.9 *International nursing index*
Publisher: American Journal of Nursing Company
Frequency: Quarterly with annual cumulation

International nursing index (INI) uses Medical Subject Headings (MeSH), the authoritative list of terms produced by the United States National Library of Medicine. Because of its origin it uses American terminology and reflects American styles, needs and patterns of health care in the subject terms and arrangement. Entries are limited to title, author, journal title, date, volume/issue and page numbers. Where the original is not in English the language is noted. One or two major UK titles are not included but it generally gives worldwide coverage to the nursing journal literature.

1.9.10 *Popular medical index*
Publisher: Mede Publishing
Frequency: 3 issues per year plus cumulation

An index to articles on medical subjects written specifically for the lay person, appearing in popular magazines. Arranged alphabetically by subject headings.

1.9.11 *Royal College of Midwives* (1987) *Midwifery index: a source of journal references on midwifery and related topics 1980-1986.* (With selective coverage of 1976-1979) Edited and compiled by Ayres, J. London: Royal College of Midwives ISBN 1870822005

A cumulation of the main sections of the Royal College of Midwives Library's Current Awareness Service. A list of subject headings is given together with an author index. Journals only are covered and these are not listed (CR 1.8.5).

1.9.12 *Social sciences citation index*
Publisher: ISI
Frequency: Three times per year with an annual cumulation

Social sciences citation index comprises a citation index, source index, permuterm subject index and a corporate index. Citation services rely on the citations given by authors and are of particular use in establishing a body of literature on a subject and identifying key authors or seminal works. Nursing journals are covered by this service.

Guide
1.9.13 **Strickland-Hodge, B.** (1986) *How to use Index medicus and Excerpta medica.* Gower: Aldershot ISBN 0566035321

Manual aims to improve search techniques of students and others needing to use medical literature. It discusses all aids to searching *Index medicus* and *Excerpta medica*, and gives guidance on the use of Medical sub Headings (MeSH), both public and annotated, permuted MeSH and supplementary Chemical Records.

1.10 ONLINE DATABASES

Introduction

Online databases are increasingly becoming the major, albeit expensive way, of identifying relevant literature. Some of the most important health science sources are outlined here, together with articles describing the basic principles of online searching.

Annotations

1.10.1 *Biosis previews*
Period covered: 1970 –

Covers biosciences, particularly biomedical.

1.10.2 *British Medical Association press cuttings*
Period covered: 1984 –

Provides current awareness service on media coverage of health related issues.

1.10.3 *Cancerlit*
Period covered: 1963 –

Covers the treatment of cancer and includes information on epidemiology, pathogenesis and immunology.

1.10.4 *Clinical notes online*
Period covered: 1984 –

Gives concise accounts of notable clinical case notes.

1.10.5 *DHSS-DATA*
Period covered: 1983 –
Printed equivalent: (*Health service abstracts, Social service abstracts, Nursing research abstracts*)

Database based on Department of Health Library's published abstracting and current awareness services.

1.10.6 *English National Board health care database*
Period covered: 1988 –

Covers clinical aspects for all types of nursing, midwifery and health visiting. Education, management, communication and health education topics provide support materials for teachers. Database is searchable via the Campus 2000 network and by telephone or letter. This is a new, but developing service.

1.10.7 Excerpta medica
Period covered: 1974 —

Covers biomedical literature. Excludes nursing and dentistry.

1.10.8 F-D-C reports
Period covered: 1988 —
Printed equivalent: The Pink Sheet, the Gray Sheet and the Rose Sheet

Provides information on companies, products, markets, personnel, regulatory and legislative activities, financial performances and financial and legal news on those involved in the health care industry.

1.10.9 General practitioner
Period covered: 1987 —
Printed equivalent: *General practitioner, Mims magazine, Medeconomics*

Contains full online equivalent of the journals.

1.10.10 Hseline
Period covered: 1977 —
Printed equivalent: (published output of the Health and Safety Executive)

Produced by the Health and Safety Executive library and covers all aspects of occupational health and safety.

1.10.11 IDIS drug file
Period covered: 1966 —
Printed equivalent: (IDIS drug literature microfilm)

Index of articles on drug therapy.

1.10.12 IRCS medical science database
Period covered: 1981 —
Printed equivalent: IRCS medical science series

Current medical and biomedical research papers of clinical significance.

1.10.13 Martindale online
Period covered: 5 year cycle of updating
Printed equivalent: *Martindale: the extra pharmacopoeia*

Includes information on compounds used to treat disease; contra-indications, adverse effects, treatment precautions, interactions, dosage and administration (CR 1.4.10).

1.10.14 Medline
Period covered: 1966 —
Printed equivalent: *Index medicus, Index to dental literature, International nursing index*

The most comprehensive medical database. Entries mainly relate to American journals but does include most key UK titles.

1.10.15   *Nursing and allied health database*
Period covered: 1983 –
Printed equivalent: *Cumulative index of nursing and allied health literature (CINAHL)*

The major purely nursing database. Indexes all major United States, United Kingdom and English language nursing titles.

1.10.16   *Pre-med*
Period covered: Current 3-5 months
Printed equivalent: (abridged *Index medicus*)

Covers the same subjects as *Medline* but fewer journals and all English language. References appear within days of publication of source but only stay on the database for up to 5 months.

1.10.17   *Psych info – Psychological abstracts*
Period covered: 1967 –
Printed equivalent: *Psychological abstracts*

Subject content includes psychology, behavioural treatment of disease, drug therapy, drug addiction, developmental psychology, linguistics, social processes and management.

1.10.18   *Sedbase*
Period covered: Current information updated twice yearly
Printed equivalent: *Meyler's side effects of drugs* (side effects of drug annuals, pharmacological and chemical synonyms)

Contains synopses of clinically relevant drug reactions and interactions.

1.10.19   *Sociological abstracts*
Period covered: 1963 –
Printed equivalent: *Sociological abstracts*

Covers social sciences, especially family studies, urban and rural sociology and feminist studies.

1.10.20   *Toxline*
Period covered: 1965 –

Covers the toxicological effects of drugs, taken from published sources and research in progress reports. Based on US sources.

1.10.21   *Wiley medical research directory*
Period covered: Research currently in progress or just completed.

Gives details of research in British institutions related to the field of health care, currently in progress or just completed.

Articles/Report

1.10.22 Hannah, K.J. (1987) Uses for computers in nursing. *Recent advances in nursing* 17: 186-202   8 References

Article includes a list of databases of particular interest to nurse researchers when literature searching (CR 2.88.5).

1.10.23 *Midwifery research database (MIRAID)* (1990) First annual report. Oxford: National Perinatal Epidemiology Unit (No ISBN number)

Describes the development of MIRAID, gives the criteria for an entry and outlines future developments. The main part of the report comprises summary information on studies entered in MIRAID which cover clinical, educational and management topics. This information is incomplete and not all details have been checked. Additions are ongoing and entries will be updated regularly. Contact addresses and telephone numbers are given. Key words are listed (CR 1.12.4).

1.10.24 Shannon, M.D. & Arundel, K.F. (1988) ERIC: a resource for nursing education. *Journal of nursing education* 27(7) 328-329   4 References

Describes the database ERIC (Educational Resources Information Centre) and search methods.

1.10.25 Stoan, S.K. (1982) Computer searching: a primer for the uninformed scholar. *Academe* 68: 10-15

Describes the problems and advantages of online searching.

1.11   CD-ROM

CD-ROM (Compact Disc-Read only Memory) is a recent innovation for literature searching. It combines the great storage capacity of optical compact discs with computer database software to give those searching the literature a fast and efficient method of compiling a list of references. It offers the ability to use the search strategies of online searching but without the concerns of cost and possible delays in obtaining the results.

Currently available databases on CD-ROM include Medline, Nursing and Allied Health Database and ERIC (CR 1.10.14, 1.10.15, 1.10.23). Others include:

Health encyclopaedia
Health education bibliography
Health for all − primary care and consumer information
Health index
Health PLAN − CD
The nurse library
Nursing indisc

Annotation

1.11.1 *The CD-ROM Directory 1990* (1989) 4th edition London: TFPL Publishers   ISBN 1870889177

Lists title, publisher, information provided and distributor, present availability, update frequency, recommended hardware and CD-ROM drives, software used, price and content description. Also contains company information, guide books to CD-ROM, specialist journals, conferences and exhibitions.

[NB   New databases are being added to the list of CD-ROMs all the time so it is important to consult the most up to date directory]

1.12   ABSTRACTING SERVICES

Abstracting services provide a source for identifying relevant material in a literature search. They tend to be less comprehensive as an index but the abstracts (summaries) give details of item content which can save time in checking original sources.

Annotations
1.12.1   *ASSIA – Applied Social Sciences Index and Abstracts*
Publisher: Bowker – Saur
Frequency: Bi-monthly with an annual cumulation

Arrangement is by subject and author with the abstracts appearing in the subject listings. Includes nursing and newspapers. Of particular interest to the researcher who requires current or past coverage of issues.

1.12.2   *Dissertation abstracts international*
Publisher: University Microfilms Inc.
Frequency: Monthly

Contains abstracts of doctoral dissertations submitted by institutions. It is divided into three major sections:

A Humanities and Social Sciences
B Science and Engineering
C Worldwide

Each entry contains title, author, degree, date, name of institution, number of pages, location adviser and order number. Author's abstract is included. Theses related to all aspects of health sciences are included in section B. Abstracts are online on DIALOG or BRS. They are also available on CD-ROM (CR 1.9.8).

1.12.3   *Health service abstracts*
Publisher: Department of Health Library
Frequency: Monthly

Covers a broad range of subjects of interest in the health service.

1.12.4   *Midwifery research database (MIRAID)* (1990)
Publisher: National Perinatal Epidemiology Unit, Oxford
Frequency: Annual

A new national register, in the form of a computerised database, of all completed and ongoing research in midwifery in the UK. Information will be published 3 times a year from mid 1990 and includes an abstract, key words, details of the researchers, funding and publications. Future plans include the setting up of a telephone service (CR 1.10.22). (Source: Information leaflet, National Perinatal Epidemiology Unit, Radcliffe Infirmary, Oxford)

1.12.5 Nursing abstracts
Publisher: Nursing Abstracts Company
Frequency: Bi-monthly with annual author, subject and publication indexes

Individual issues are arranged by subject. Entries include bibliographic data and a concise abstract. Exclusively uses North American journal sources.

1.12.6 Nursing research abstracts
Publisher: Department of Health Index of Nursing Research
Frequency: Quarterly with an annual index

Enables one to trace completed and ongoing research in the UK, but relies on the authors or interested organisations for its information on unpublished and published projects. The abstracts are precise, making judgements on the source materials of the users' work more accurately than is the case with indexing services.

1.12.7 Psychological abstracts
Publisher: American Psychological Association
Frequency: Monthly with an expanded annual cumulation of the indexes

The monthly issues are divided into subject index, author index and abstracts. The abstracts are divided into 16 major categories with sub-categories where appropriate. As well as the standard bibliographic material the entries include the affiliation of the first named author, the number of references and the abstract source. This is the major abstracting service in the field of psychology.

1.12.8 Quality assurance abstracts
Publisher: Department of Health Library and the Quality Information Service of the King's Fund
Frequency: 6 per year

Contains information on quality assurance in the health service.

1.12.9 Social science abstracts
Publisher: Department of Social Security Library
Frequency: Monthly

Uses the same system of abstracts and indexes as *Nursing research abstracts*. Includes a broad range of subjects of particular interest to community nurses and service managers.

1.12.10 *Sociological abstracts*
Publisher: Sociological Abstracts
Frequency: Six issues per year, published in April, June, August, October and two in December

Divided into four sections: subject, author and source indexes and a main section of abstract entries. *Sociological abstracts* is the major abstracting service in the social sciences.

1.12.11 *Sociology of education abstracts*
Publisher: Carfax Publishing
Frequency: Quarterly with annual subject and author indexes

The quarterly issues are divided into five sections: journal abstracts, book abstracts, journals covered, author index and subject index. This service will be of particular interest to educational researchers but it should be noted that no nursing journals are covered.

Article
1.12.12 **Stodulski, A.H. & Stafford, S.M.** (1982) Disseminating nursing research information in the UK: 'Nursing Research Abstracts' from the 'Index of Nursing Research'. *International journal of nursing studies* 19(4) 231-236 4 References

Describes the development of the *Index of nursing research* and the resultant *Nursing research abstracts*.

Part 2
METHODS OF INQUIRY

AN INTRODUCTION TO RESEARCH

2.1 RESEARCH TEXTS

Two major categories of research methodology texts are included in this section, those written for nurses, which are mainly American, and both British and American general texts suitable for use by any discipline. The number of American texts written for nurses reflects the length of their experience in nursing research and the fact that more nurses have received research training.

Full bibliographical details of each text together with their annotations are included here. Subsequently in Part 2 under the heading 'suggested textbook reading' authors names only, are listed in alphabetical order, together with the main section page numbers. Readers will also need to consult the detailed index of the books selected. Each entry is cross-referenced to the original text.

Annotations

2.1.1 Abdellah, F.G. & Levine, E. (1986) *Better patient care through nursing research.* 3rd edition New York: Macmillan   ISBN 0023000805   References

Book focuses on the processes and techniques used in conducting nursing research. Each chapter contains objectives, extensive references and suggestions for further study. Part 1 is an introduction to nursing research, Part 2 discusses the steps in the research process and Part 3 identifies strategies and future directions for nursing research. (CR 2.2, 3.9 & 3.11).

2.1.2 Adams, G.R. & Schvaneveldt, J.D. (1985) *Understanding research methods.* New York: Longman   ISBN 0582284856   References

Text focuses on helping students to understand as well as conduct research. It emphasises how individuals may become more knowledgeable consumers of research.

2.1.3 Arkava, M.L. & Lane, T.A. (1983) *Beginning social work research.* Boston: Allyn & Bacon   ISBN 020507815   References

Primarily written for undergraduates in social work research and focuses on practical methods useful in day to day practice. Many examples of research design are used and each chapter is summarised to provide a study aid.

2.1.4 Bell, C. & Newby, H. (eds) (1977) *Doing sociological research.* London: Allen & Unwin   ISBN 0043000703   References

Eight British sociologists recount in detail the history of major research projects in which they have been involved. They show how the context of research, personal relationships of the researchers and the reactions of readers influence the findings no less than the methodological choices made by the researcher (2.16).

2.1.5   Bell, C. & Roberts, H. (eds) (1984) *Social researching, politics, problems, practice.* London: Routledge & Kegan Paul   ISBN 0710098847   References

A collection of essays related to methodological aspects of social science research which also reflects current interests.

2.1.6   Berger, R.M. & Patchner, M.A. (1988) *Planning for research: a guide for the helping professions.* Beverly Hills: Sage   ISBN 080393033X   References

Book aims to guide practitioners through the initial stages of the research process.

2.1.7   Brink, P.J. & Wood, M.J. (1988) *Basic steps in planning nursing research: from question to proposal.* 3rd edition Boston: Jones & Bartlett ISBN 0867204044   References

Book is intended for students undertaking a first course in research methods and deals solely with the beginning phase, the research plan. It begins with identifying a research topic and ends with the written proposal. There is recommended reading at the end of each chapter with four sample research proposals as appendices (CR 2.99).

2.1.8   Bulmer, M. (ed) (1984) *Sociological research methods: an introduction.* 2nd edition London: Macmillan   ISBN 0333373464   References

Purpose of the book is to examine ways in which sociologists gain systematic, reliable and valid knowledge about the real world. A variety of approaches are emphasised in order to highlight the central issues and complexities: these are social survey research, unobtrusive measures, historical sociology and interpretive procedures.

2.1.9   Burgess, R.G. (ed) (1982) *Field research: a source book and field manual.* London: Allen & Unwin   ISBN 004312013X   References

The text is a collection of readings of British and American material which aims to show the diversity of approaches used in fieldwork; it examines a range of research techniques and the problems which may ensue. Annotated suggestions for further reading are included. The book makes a contribution to research methodology by demonstrating how qualitative research can be scientifically credible.

2.1.10   Burgess, R.G. (1984) *In the field: an introduction to field research.* London: Allen & Unwin   ISBN 0043120180   References

Complements author's earlier anthology (2.1.9) and provides further detail on the major topics in field research, combined with information on data collection and data analysis.

2.1.11   Burnard, P. & Morrison, P. (1990) *Nursing research in action.* Basingstoke: Macmillan Education   ISBN 0333495632   References

Book aimed at beginners wishing to develop basic research skills. Each chapter is in the format of a 'Do it yourself' manual and comprises suggested reading, aims, information boxes, exercises and learning checks.

2.1.12 Burns, N. & Grove, S.K. (1987) *The practice of nursing research: conduct, critique and utilisation.* Philadelphia: Saunders   ISBN 0721610951   References

Text is intended for undergraduates, graduates and those practising in the field. It is organised into four units: an introduction to nursing research which includes discussion on quantitative and qualitative research; the research process; the pragmatics of research and the implications of research for nursing. Examples are given throughout the text.

2.1.13 Bynner, J. & Stribly, K.M. (eds) (1979) *Social research: principles and procedures.* London: Longman in association with the Open University Press   ISBN 0582295017   References

Book is a course reader for the Open University Course 'Research Methods in Education and the Social Sciences', (DE 304). It comprises critical writings on different aspects of social research. Three broad styles of research are studied – experimental, survey and ethnographic. The book is structured under the following headings: the language of social research, design, data collection, measurement, data analysis and report (CR 2.29, 2.43, 2.55).

2.1.14 Cahoon, M.C. (ed) (1987) *Research methodology.* Edinburgh: Churchill Livingstone *Recent advances in nursing* **17**   ISBN 0443039445   References/Bibliographies

This issue of the *Recent advances in nursing* series is designed to stimulate debate about advances in research methodology, and is intended to support existing texts. The three parts cover research designs, procedures and bibliographies which include literature published since 1980.

2.1.15 Castles, M.R. (1987) *Primer of nursing research.* Philadelphia: Saunders   ISBN 0721617131   References

Text written for nurses who are expecting to assume only one research role, that of utilisers of research findings. It concentrates on the essential elements of the research process enabling students to evaluate the technical soundness of research designs. Learning and terminal objectives are included in each chapter together with references and study activities.

2.1.16 Chisnall, P.M. (1986) *Marketing research.* 3rd edition London: McGraw Hill   ISBN 0070841551   References

Provides a comprehensive and authoritative text on marketing research. Part 1 covers the methodologies used in this type of research; part 2 covers the basic techniques; part 3 specific applications and part 4 discusses data handling and interpretation.

2.1.17 Christensen, L.B. (1980) *Experimental methodology.* 2nd edition Boston: Allyn & Bacon   ISBN 0205069606   References

Book focuses on experimental methodologies. Two topic areas, quasi-experimental and single subject designs have undergone change and development so separate chapters are included in this edition. Evaluation research is also explored in depth. Although intended mainly for students of psychology, nurses will readily identify with the examples given (CR 2.34, 2.35, 2.44).

2.1.18 Clifford, C. & Gough, S. (1990) *Nursing research: a skills based introduction.* Hemel Hempstead: Prentice Hall ISBN 0136291147 References

Book provides a practical introduction for those embarking on their first research-based study and it would also be useful to practitioners who wish to increase their skills in reading research reports. Many points about the practicalities of doing research are included which are sometimes omitted from other texts. In addition to discussing the research process in differing levels of detail, chapters are included on finding information, research in nursing, research awareness, presenting results and change theory (CR 2.16).

2.1.19 Cohen, L. & Manion, L. (1989) *Research methods in education.* 3rd edition London: Routledge ISBN 0415036488 References

Book will serve both researchers and consumers of research evidence. A wide range of traditional and more recent approaches are included together with many examples of British research reported since 1980. Additional material has been added to this edition and references have been updated.

2.1.20 Cormack, D.F.S. (ed) (1984) *The research process in nursing.* Oxford: Blackwell Scientific ISBN 0632010134 References

Text includes writings by a group of research specialists to guide nurses step by step through the research process. References and resources are largely British.

2.1.21 Couchman, W. & Dawson, J. (1990) *Nursing and health care research: a practical guide.* London: Scutari ISBN 1871364221 References

A self instruction workbook, designed to introduce research to nurses who are in the initial stages of learning, and would also be useful for updating and professional development. An extended fictitious nursing research project is used to illustrate each step in the process and chapters contain exercises and references.

2.1.22 Darling, V.H. & Rogers, J. (1986) *Research for practising nurses.* Basingstoke: Macmillan Education ISBN 0333367316 References

Written for practising nurses this book provides a set of guidelines to the processes involved in research. Difficulties are identified together with appropriate routes to enquiry. Recommended reading is given together with some sources of information.

2.1.23 Denzin, N.K. (1970) *Sociological methods: a sourcebook.* London: Butterworths ISBN 0408701250 References

A comprehensive collection of readings on sociological methods which provides analyses of the major strategies employed in social research. Its thirteen sections cover theory and its development, issues of sampling units, problems in developing new measurement techniques, the difficulties of interviewing, the nature of causation and a review of the major methods of proof available to the sociologist (CR 2.7, 2.22, 2.56, 2.70).

2.1.24 Field, P.A. & Morse, J.M. (1985) *Nursing research: the application of qualitative approaches.* Rockville, Maryland: Aspen   ISBN 0709910460   References/Bibliography

Book aims to assist nurses undertaking qualitative research for the first time. The types of problems best approached by qualitative methods are outlined and chapters cover the major schools of thought of ethnography, ethnology and phenomenology. Participant observation, interviewing and case studies are described and methods of analysis presented. All themes are illustrated mainly by American studies. (CR 2.2).

2.1.25 Fox, D.J. (1982) *Fundamentals of research in nursing.* 4th edition Norwalk, Connecticut: Appleton-Century-Crofts   ISBN 0838527973   References

Readers of all levels of experience will be provided with the conceptual background to execute research programmes and critically evaluate the literature of nursing and other disciplines.

2.1.26 Holm, K. & Llewellyn, J.G. (1986) *Nursing research for nursing practice.* Philadelphia: Saunders   ISBN 0721611788   References

Book aims to provide the reader with an understanding of the research process, a rationale for deciding if a study is relevant to clinical practice and to highlight issues in clinical research. It is intended to complement existing research texts. The practical aspects of research implementation are discussed in chapters 13, 14 and 15. Each chapter contains objectives, questions, activities and a bibliography. There are ten appendices (CR 2.1.34, 2.105).

2.1.27 Isaac, S. & Michael, W.B. (1981) *Handbook in research and evaluation.* 2nd edition San Diego, California: Edits   ISBN 0912736259   References

A collection of principles, methods and strategies useful in the planning, design and evaluation of studies in education and the behavioural sciences.

2.1.28 Johnson, J.M. (1975) *Doing field research.* New York: The Free Press ISBN 0029166004   References

Book discusses the major arguments in the traditional methodological literature about the problems of conducting field research. The research situations which occurred in the author's observations in social welfare offices are described, as these highlight many of the practical problems likely to be encountered. These are gaining access, developing trust, personal relationships and the fusion of thinking and feeling. Final chapters examine report writing and objectivity in sociology (CR 2.16).

2.1.29   Kane, E. (1985) *Doing your own research: basic descriptive research in the social sciences and humanities.* London: Marion Boyars   ISBN 0714528439   References

Book is intended for those undertaking research for the first time. All stages necessary to conduct a research project are included.

2.1.30   Kidder, L.H. & Judd, C.M. (1986) *Research methods in social relations.* 5th edition New York: CBS Publishing Japan Ltd   ISBN 0039107140   References

Provides information on multiple research strategies, methods of measurement and techniques of analysis. The methods examined are applicable across many disciplines and the social issues addressed are also cross-disciplinary (CR 2.2).

2.1.31   Kovacs, A.R. (1985) *The research process: essentials of skill development.* Philadelphia: Davis   ISBN 0803654456   References

A basic text or reference for nurses with little or no experience in research. Its five sections include basic concepts, planning a study, presentation, analysis and interpretation of data, statistical analysis, assessment of findings and communication of results. Learning activities include assigned readings, questions for study and exercises. Appendix B provides an index to research content in various American research texts (CR 2.2).

2.1.32   Krampitz, S.D. & Pavlovich, N. (1981) *Readings for nursing research.* St Louis: Mosby   ISBN 0801627478   References

A series of readings designed to assist undergraduates, faculty and teachers in developing research skills and learning programmes. The needs of clinical practitioners are also considered. Book contains in-depth chapters on the research process and a collection of previously unpublished original research.

2.1.33   Krathwohl, D.R. (1985) *Social and behavioural science research: a new framework for conceptualising, implementing and evaluating research studies.* San Francisco: Jossey-Bass   ISBN 0875896375   References

Book is an adjunct to research methodology textbooks and aims to develop understanding of how social and behavioural research proceeds. The process by which findings become knowledge is conceptualised, the type of decisions necessary for different orientations, and the implications for implementing and evaluating research are discussed. The examination of qualitative, quantitative and statistical methods provides the 'conceptual cement' integrating the three.

2.1.34   Leach, A.K. (1986) *Using the knowledge base in Holm, K. & Llewellyn, J.G. Instructors manual to accompany nursing research for nursing practice.* Philadelphia: Saunders   ISBN 0721621101   References

Each chapter is linked with the main text and provides new terms, student exercises, teaching strategies, series of questions, quizzes and multiple choice with answers (CR 2.1.26).

2.1.35 Leedy, P.D. (1989) *Practical research: planning and design.* 4th edition New York: Macmillan ISBN 0023692413 References

A practical text which encourages learning by doing, with assignments linked to each chapter. Book is suitable for all courses in basic research methodology and references are given from different disciplines, including nursing. Examples of research are given in each chapter, and a series of discussions on the computer as a tool of research. Appendix contains an annotated research proposal (CR 2.99).

2.1.36 Leininger, M.M. (ed) (1985) *Qualitative research methods in nursing.* Orlando: Grune & Stratton ISBN 0808916769 References

Book aims to introduce nurses to the nature, purposes and different types of approaches to qualitative research. The author contends that examining human care requires different methods and modes of analysis than quantitative research approaches. Original articles are included which illustrate the wide variety of methods available − ethnographic, ethnonursing, ethnoscience, life history, historical, phenomenological and many others (CR 2.43, 2.47, 2.52).

2.1.37 Lin, N. (1976) *Foundations of social research.* New York: McGraw Hill ISBN 0070378673 References

Identifies ways in which social researchers construct theories about social activities. The procedures used in conducting research are discussed and problems which may be encountered are identified. The final chapter considers the implications of social research for policy (CR 3.10).

2.1.38 LoBiondo-Wood, G. & Haber, J. (1990) *Nursing research: methods, critical appraisal and utilisation.* 2nd edition St Louis: Mosby ISBN 0801630304 References

Text prepares nursing students and practitioners to become knowledgeable research consumers. It addresses the role of the research consumer, teaches the fundamentals of the research process as well as critical appraisal. Each chapter relating to the research process includes lists of critiquing criteria and examples to illustrate each stage. An accomanying study guide, instructor's manual and questbank complement the textbook (CR 2.1.60).

2.1.39 Luck, M., Lawrence, B., Pocock, B. & Ruth, K. (1988) *Consumer and market research in health care.* London: Chapman & Hall ISBN 0412328003 References

Book addresses evaluation and accountability in the health service. The use of market research is discussed and surveys on coronary risk factors, satisfaction of elderly people and their carers, and carers of the mentally handicapped are reported. Part three discusses how results could be used and sets out a framework for developing market research in health authorities.

2.1.40 McNeill, P. (1985) *Research methods.* London: Tavistock ISBN 0442795402 References

Written for the non-specialist, but introduces all the central issues of social research. Examples are taken from British, American and European literature and student activities are included. There are chapters on surveys, ethnographic methods, secondary sources and discussion on science and values in social research (CR 2.43, 2.55, 2.94).

2.1.41 Miller, B.C. (1986) *Family research methods.* Beverly Hills: Sage ISBN 0803921446 References

An elementary research methods text which uses marriage and the family for illustrative purposes. Its intended readership is both graduates and undergraduates.

2.1.42 Munhall, P.L. & Oiler, C.J. (1986) *Nursing research: a qualitative perspective.* Norwalk, Connecticut: Appleton-Century-Crofts ISBN 0838570488 References

A text and reference work for researchers and nursing students. Part 1 of the book gives a rationale for the choice of qualitative method in nursing research; Part 2 includes selected approaches which are described and a research study presented to illustrate each one. These are phenomenology, grounded theory, ethnography, historical research and foundational inquiry. Part 3 provides an overall summary of qualitative research and problems related to assessing the value of and difficulties in reporting such studies (CR 2.43, 2.46, 2.47, 2.52).

2.1.43 Nieswiadomy, R.M. (1987) *Foundations of nursing research.* Norwalk, Connecticut: Appleton & Lange ISBN 0838526926 References

Primary goal is to create interest in nursing research and enable students to develop research skills. Readers will also be able to evaluate studies and use findings in clinical settings. Each chapter includes a list of objectives, new terms introduced and a self-test. (CR 2.2).

2.1.44 Notter, L.E. & Hott, J.R. (1988) *Essentials of nursing research.* 4th edition New York: Springer ISBN 0826115977 References

A concise introductory guide for nurses embarking on a research project or attempting to evaluate published research. The text makes reference to many American clinical nursing studies to illustrate each step of the research process. (CR 2.2).

2.1.45 to 2.1.54 Open University (1979) (DE 304) *Research methods in education and the social sciences.* Milton Keynes: Open University Press

[NB The format of this entry differs from the previous ones. Each unit within this Open University course is given an individual number but they all form part of the total. The code preceding each entry indicates the course unit number.]

2.1.45 DE 304 1 **Wilson, M.J. & Bynner, J.** (1979) *Variety in social science research.* ISBN 0335074359

2.1.46 DE 304 2A **Bulmer, M., Atkinson, P., Brook, C., Drake, M., Peacock, R., Pollard, A. & Sapsford, R.J.** (1979) *Beginning research.* ISBN 0335074367

2.1.47 DE 304 2B **Lewis, R.W.** (1979) *Beginning research.* ISBN 0335074375

2.1.48 DE 304 3A **Evans, J., Greene, J. & Swift, B.** (1979) *Research design.* ISBN 0335074383

2.1.49 DE 304 3B **Calder, J., Atkinson, P., & Evans, J.** (1979) *Research design.* ISBN 0335074235

2.1.50 DE 304 4 **Bynner, J., Oppenheim, R.N. & Hammersley, M.** (1979) *Data collection procedures.* ISBN 0335074391

2.1.51 DE 304 5 **Bynner, J., Nuttall, D.L., Romney, D. & Thomas, A.** (1979) *Classification and measurement.* ISBN 0335074405

2.1.52 DE 304 6 **Hammersley, M., Marsh, C., Bynner, J., Murphy, J. & Sapsford, R.J.** (1979) *Making sense of data.* ISBN 0335074405

2.1.53 DE 304 7 **Pillener, A.E.G., Coxhead, P. & Atkins, E.** (1979) *Modelling relationships in data.* ISBN 0335074421

2.1.54 DE 304 8 **Sapsford, R.J. & Evans, J.** (1979) *Evaluation of research.* ISBN 0335074286

Two main aims of this course are to equip students with the information and skills needed to evaluate research in the social sciences and to provide a grounding for those who wish to conduct research. The course concentrates on three broad research styles − ethnography, survey and experiment. Part 1 uses case studies to introduce the theory and practice of social science research. Part 2 concentrates on the origin of research ideas, the use of existing data sources and descriptive data analysis. Part 3 considers research design including surveys and sampling techniques. Parts 4 and 5 discuss problems and methods of data collection. Parts 6 and 7 are concerned with data analysis and statistical inference, and Part 8 concentrates on evaluation of research reports.

2.1.55 Polgar, S. & Thomas, S.A. (1988) *Introduction to research in the health sciences.* Melbourne: Churchill Livingstone ISBN 0443036071 References

This book introduces the concepts and basic techniques of research and statistics. It draws on situations commonly encountered by health professionals, gives an understanding of how research affects their work and provides a grounding in practical research skills. Each chapter concludes with self-assessment tests.

2.1.56 Polit, D.F. & Hungler, B.P. (1987) *Nursing research: principles and methods.* 3rd edition Philadelphia: Lippincott ISBN 0397546319 References

A comprehensive text covering the fundamentals of research methods. Liberal use is made of actual and hypothetical research studies to illustrate each concept. Six major sections cover the scientific research process, preliminary research steps, designs for nursing research, measurement and data collection, the analysis of research data and communication in the research process (CR 2.2).

2.1.57 Polit, D.F. & Hungler, B.P. (1989) *Essentials of nursing research: methods, appraisal and utilisation.* 2nd edition Philadelphia: Lippincott ISBN 0397547129 References

Text written for consumers of nursing research to assist in evaluating the adequacy of research findings in terms of their scientific merit and utilisation potential. It does not include a 'how to do it' approach as this is in another text (CR 2.1.56). Each chapter contains guidelines for conducting a critique and two types of research examples, the first fictitious and the other real. Final chapters discuss the utilisation of nursing research (CR 2.98, 2.104).

2.1.58 Reid, N.G. & Boore, J.R.P. (1987) *Research methods and statistics in health care.* London: Edward Arnold ISBN 0713145226 References

Text written for nurses discusses research in the practice context and illustrates the practical aspects of conducting such studies. Statistical tests are used, clearly explained and again applied to practice.

2.1.59 Roberts, C.A. & Burke, S.O. (1989) *Nursing research: a quantitative and qualitative approach.* Boston: Jones & Bartlett ISBN 086720415X References

Book will enable nurses to evaluate research findings and use them in clinical practice. Each step in the research process is covered and points to look for are outlined. Flowcharts are included in many chapters which identify the research element, scientific adequacy with both quantitative and qualitative criteria, implications for clinical applicability and concepts for review. Objectives are given for each chapter, a list of new terms, exercises and references. Examples are given throughout from quantitative and qualitative studies.

2.1.60 Rose-Grippa, K. & Gorney-Fadiman, M.J. (1986) *Study guide to accompany Nursing research: critical appraisal and utilisation.* St Louis: Mosby ISBN 0801618916 References

Keyed to the text *Nursing research* (CR 2.1.38) the study guide includes in each chapter an introduction, learning objectives, pre-test, learning activities, post-test, checkpoints, answers and references.

2.1.61 Sarter, B. (ed) (1989) *Paths to knowledge: innovative research methods for nursing.* New York: National League for Nursing ISBN 0887374158 Publication number 15-2233

A collection of original articles which introduces several research methods largely unexplored by nurses and provides new insights into others. The history and philosophical foundations of each are given, together with implementation and applications. The five major sections cover the empirical, personal, aesthetic, ethical and intellectual/interpretive paths to nursing knowledge.

2.1.62   Seaman, C.H. (1987) *Research methods: principles, practice and theory for nursing.* 3rd edition Norwalk, Connecticut: Appleton and Lange   ISBN 083852753   References

Written for undergraduates and graduates this provides readers with skills to design and carry out research and evaluate their own and others literature. Each chapter includes a set of objectives and study questions (CR 2.2).

2.1.63   Sweeney, M.A. & Olivieri, P. (1981) *An introduction to nursing research: research, measurement and computers in nursing.* Philadelphia: Lippincott   ISBN 0397542631   References

Textbook aims to provide a basis for the study of nursing problems by enabling the language of research to be understood; giving concepts needed to read research publications and demonstrate some of the steps of the research process. Aspects of statistics and computer science are also included. Each chapter contains objectives and research studies are used for illustration throughout.

2.1.64   Thomas, B.S. (1990) *Nursing research: an experiential approach.* St Louis: Mosby   ISBN 0801660610   References

Book encourages active involvement in the process of learning about research by including problems and exercises throughout the text. It is intended for undergraduate and post-graduate nursing students and covers all elements of the research process. Both quantitative and qualitative approaches are included.

2.1.65   Treece, E.W. & Treece, J.W. Jr. (1986) *Elements of research in nursing.* 4th edition St Louis: Mosby   ISBN 0801651050   References

A comprehensive text for undergraduates and graduates learning research methods particularly using quantitative techniques. Each chapter is summarised and contains discussion questions, class activities and suggested readings (CR 2.2).

2.1.66   Walker, R. (ed) (1985) *Applied qualitative research.* Aldershot: Gower   ISBN 056600898X   References

Comprehensive guide to qualitative research methods. Its origins are traced, strengths and weaknesses examined, practical examples given together with criteria for evaluating qualitative research. Four key methods of data collection are described, depth interviews, group discussions, participant observation and projective techniques (CR 2.70, 2.71, 2.73, 2.74).

2.1.67   Williamson, Y.M. (ed) (1981) *Research methodology and its application to nursing.* New York: Wiley   ISBN 0471033138   References

Book is intended for nursing students and aims to provide a comprehensive overview of the entire research process. It aims to prepare students to carry out research as well as develop critiquing skills.

2.1.68   Wilson, H.S. (1987) *Introducing research in nursing.* Menlo Park, California: Addison-Wesley   ISBN 0201088649   References

This book, based on the first edition of 'Research in nursing' (Wilson H.S. 1987) covers similar ground but is intended particularly for the beginning researcher. Objectives are given for each chapter together with suggestions for further reading.

2.1.69   Wilson, H.S. (1989) *Research in nursing.* 2nd edition Menlo Park, California: Addison-Wesley   ISBN 020159460   References

A comprehensive introductory text which is an innovative application and resource workbook for students at various levels. It contains action orientated assessment tools, exercises and practical opportunities to use the skills of research. The book's four parts focus on the research process as a tool of science, the skills of research consumership, the steps involved in conducting both quantitative and qualitative research, together with guidelines and strategies for communicating research findings through written and oral media. In the new edition the relationship of nursing theory to practice is expanded and updated; the chapter on qualitative analysis includes phenomenological techniques; a new chapter on advanced statistics is included and the examples and references have been updated (CR 2.2).

2.1.70   Wilson, M. (ed) (1979) *Social and educational research in action: a book of readings.* London: Longman in association with the Open University Press   ISBN 058229004X   References

Book is a course reader for the Open University course 'Research methods in education and the social sciences' (DE 304). It contains articles showing social science research in action. Section 1 discusses aspects of the Plowden Report on Primary Education. Section 2 is on problem formulation and Sections 3,4 & 5 cover research design, data collection and data analysis. Stress is placed on the diversity of methods – experimental, survey and ethnographic (CR 2.18, 2.29, 2.43, 2.55).

2.1.71   Woods, N.F. (1988a) *Nursing research: a learning resource.* St Louis: Mosby   ISBN 0801657059

A companion volume to Woods & Catanzaro (2.1.72) which gives practical exercises related to the learning objectives in each section. This learning resource places emphasis on the linking of research issues to nursing practice rather than the acquisition of facts.

2.1.72   Woods, N.F. & Catanzaro, M. (1988b) *Nursing research: theory and practice.* St Louis: Mosby   ISBN 0801657032   References

Text is primarily for undergraduates, graduates and clinicians who are preparing to conduct research or utilise findings. Aspects covered are conceptualising nursing research, designing nursing studies, measuring phenomena of interest to nurses, analysing and interpreting findings and communicating information about research. Two appendices provide up to date resource information – one on software useful for managing bibliographical citations, text, numerical data and statistical analysis.

The second is an annotated listing of source books that provide reviews and critiques of available research instruments (CR 2.1.71, 2.2).

2.2 THE LANGUAGE OF RESEARCH

Research, as with any other discipline, has its own terminology which can sometimes hinder understanding of reported research. Researchers are often urged to write in language which is readily understandable but inevitably there are technical words to be learnt.

This section contains references to published glossaries. Not all textbooks contain such lists but those which do usually include both research and statistical terms. Suggested textbook readings in section 2.84 gives texts which contain only statistical terms.

Annotations

2.2.1 Berger, R.M. & Patchner, M.A. (1988) Research vocabulary. IN Authors *Planning for research: a guide for helping professions.* Beverly Hills: Sage ISBN 080393033X Chapter 2 29-47

Chapter defines some research terms using a narrative format.

2.2.2 Davitz, J.R. & Davitz, L.L. (1977) The language of research: definitions and applications. IN Authors *Evaluating research proposals in the behavioural sciences: a guide.* 2nd edition, New York: Teachers College Press ISBN 0807725447 References

Research and some statistical terms and concepts used in the behavioural sciences are defined and an example of use is given for each one.

2.2.3 Miller, P.McC. & Wilson, M.J. (1983) *A dictionary of social science methods.* Chichester: Wiley ISBN 0471900362

Collects in one source accounts of current methods of inquiry which the empirical social sciences share in common. Definitions and explanations are also given and a cross-referencing system leads to other relevant items. Many statistical terms are also included (CR 2.84).

2.2.4 Powers, B.A. & Knapp, T.R. (1990) *A dictionary of nursing theory and research.* Newbury Park: Sage ISBN 0803934122 References

A compilation of definitions, and discussion of both research and statistical terms likely to be encountered in the nursing scientific literature. Examples of where terms are used are included and citations provided to books and articles where they are more fully explained. The book is intended for nurses at all levels of learning (CR 2.84).

2.2.5 Presly, A. (1984) Common terms and concepts in nursing Research. IN Cormack, D.F.S. (ed) *The research process in nursing.* Oxford: Blackwell Scientific ISBN 0632010134 References Chapter 4 30-36

Chapter explains some of the terms commonly used in research (CR 2.1.20).

2.2.6 Sweeney, M.A. & Olivieri, P. (1981) *An introduction to nursing research: research, measurement and computing in nursing.* Philadelphia: Lippincott   ISBN 0397542631   References   Chapter 2   32-42

Chapter explains the use of research terms by describing the research process in a general way (CR 2.1.63).

Textbooks containing glossaries

	Pages	*Cross Reference*
Abdellah & Levine	382-396	2.1.1
Burns & Grove	741-755	2.1.12
Field & Morse	137-139	2.1.24
Holm & Llewellyn	261-275	2.1.26
Katzer, Cook & Crouch	195-231	2.98.8
Kidder & Judd	511-520	2.1.30
Kovacs	339-349	2.1.31
LoBiondo-Wood & Haber	415-424	2.1.38
Nieswiadomy	405-421	2.1.43
Notter & Hott	175-183	2.1.44
Phillips L.R.F.	453-465	2.98.11
Polit & Hungler (1987)	525-538	2.1.56
Roberts & Burke	355-372	2.1.59
Seaman	425-441	2.1.62
Thomas	286-292	2.1.64
Treece & Treece	510-512	2.1.65
Wilson H.S. (1989)	724-730	2.1.69
Wilson M.J. (DE 304)	77-135	2.1.70
Woods & Catanzaro	552-568	2.1.72

2.3   THE NATURE AND PURPOSE OF RESEARCH IN NURSING

The knowledge base for nursing practice is generated through research and it must be the goal of every professional nurse to provide patients and clients with the most up to date care. Research is the link between practice, education and theory and it is therefore essential for all nurses to become knowledgeable consumers or, for the minority, research doers.

Annotations
2.3.1 Hockey, L. (1981) Knowledge is a precious possession. *Nursing mirror* 152(13) September 23   46−49   1 Reference

Examines what nursing research is and what it is not. The scepticism and enthusiasm of some nurses for research is contrasted and the value of and necessity for research as a basis for practice is discussed.

2.3.2 Montgomery Robinson, K.M., Montgomery Robinson, H.M., Hilton, A. & Clark, E. (1991) *What is research?* Research Awareness, Module 3. London: Distance Learning Centre, South Bank Polytechnic ISBN 094825047X References

This is number 3 in a series of 13 modules, each of which deals with a different aspect of nursing research. It was developed to assist nurses, midwives and health visitors in understanding research in terms of their own professional practice. Modules can be used separately or as part of a programme. The reader is encouraged to work through a number of activities, self-assessment questions and answers and progress summaries. Some articles/book extracts referred to in the text are reproduced in full.

This module examines the role science can play within nursing. Included are definitions of research, reasons why nurses should know more about science and their relationships with other researchers, scientific method and an introduction to the research process. Issues, such as how science can reflect society in general, and is open to criticism, are explored (CR Appendix D).

Suggested textbook readings

	Pages	*Cross reference*
Abdellah & Levine	3-27	2.1.1
Burns & Grove	3-27	2.1.12
Castles	3-9	2.1.15
Hockey L. IN Cormack	3-10	2.1.20
Holm & Llewellyn	3-18	2.1.26
Kovacs	9-13	2.1.31
Leedy	3-13	2.1.35
LoBiondo-Wood & Haber	3-18	2.1.38
Nieswiadomy	3-21	2.1.43
Notter & Hott	19-42	2.1.44
Polit & Hungler (1987)	3-12	2.1.56
Seaman	3-20	2.1.62
Treece & Treece	3-33	2.1.65
Williamson	3-11	2.1.67
Wilson H.S. (1989)	3-33	2.1.69
Woods & Catanzaro	530-539	2.1.72

Nursing research abstracts

Castledine G.	84/133
Rampton Hospital Conference	88/193

2.4 RESEARCH PROCESSES – AN OVERVIEW

Although the phrase 'research process' is frequently used the practice of research often involves a series of processes. Science does not occur in stages or, follow a linear path, but instead consists of overlapping processes in all parts of the investigation. Literature in this section provides brief overviews of these processes.

Definition
A process of using quantitative and qualitative methods to collect and analyse data for the purpose of prediction and explanation

Annotations
2.4.1 Hawkins, C. & Sorgi, M. (1985) *Research: how to plan, speak and write about it.* Berlin: Springer-Verlag   ISBN 3540139923

A practical text covering several aspects of the research process. It also includes guidance on speaking at meetings and aspects of publication processes (CR 2.102, 2.103).

2.4.2 Parahoo, K. & Reid, N. (1988) Research skills series 1-5 *Nursing times* 84 (39-43)

No 1   28.9.1988   Getting started: the language of research 67-70   2 References
No 2   5.10.1988   The research process 67-70   5 References
No 3   12.10 1988   Writing a research proposal 49-52   7 References
No 4   19.10 1988   Writing up a research report 63-67   2 References
No 5   26.10 1988   Critical reading of research 69-72   3 References

Series covers various aspects of undertaking research and practical exercises are included to facilitate learning.

2.4.3 Sheehan, J. (1985) Research series 1-6 *Nursing mirror* 160 (18-23)

No 1   1.5.1985   Starting the study 17-18   2 References
No 2   8.5.1985   Reviewing the literature 29-30   2 References
No 3   15.5.1985   Selecting the right method 19-20   2 References
No 4   22.5.1985   Collecting the data 25-26   1 Reference
No 5   29.5.1985   Analysing the data 25-26   2 References
No 6   5.6.1985   Presenting the report 36-37   1 Reference

Series covers some of the basic elements to be considered when undertaking research.

Suggested textbook readings

	Pages	Cross reference
Abdellah & Levine	75-85	2.1.1
Castles	13-19	2.1.15
Cormack (1984)	37-44	2.1.20
Cormack (1990)	110-129	3.16.4
Fox	26-50	2.1.25
Polit & Hungler (1987)	27-46	2.1.56
Seaman	37-62	2.1.62
Sweeney & Olivieri	43-49	2.1.63
Williamson	43-63	2.1.67
Wilson H.S. (1989)	16-21	2.1.69

Nursing research abstracts

Behi, R.	90/112
Hunt, J.	84/400
Lancaster, A.	R27 (Retrospective volume 1968-1976)

CONCEPTUALISING NURSING RESEARCH

2.5 PHILOSOPHICAL BASES FOR RESEARCH

'Research focused on philosophical questions is difficult to design and pursue . . . yet for nurses some issues loom large such as euthanasia, organ transplantation and genetic engineering. These demand investigation and interpretation so that nurses can make clinical decisions which are rational and defensible' (Brophy, E.B. IN Krampitz & Pavlovich 1981).

Definition
A love or pursuit of wisdom: a search for the underlying causes and principles of reality

Annotations
2.5.1   Dzurec, L.C. (1989) The necessity for and evolution of multiple paradigms for nursing research: a post-structuralist perspective. *Advances in nursing science* 11(4)   69-77   19 References

Author examines logical positivism and phenomenology/hermeneutics* from a perspective beyond both i.e. post- structuralism using the ideas of Foucault. This is explored as a background to nursing's significant and growing acceptance of multiple paradigms for the conduct of research (CR 2.52).

*Hermeneutics − the theory of textual interpretation

2.5.2   Flew, A. (1985) *Thinking about social thinking: the philosophy of the social sciences.* Oxford: Blackwell   ISBN 063114191X   References

Book challenges the methodology of social science and its applications in the form of contemporary social policies. Illustrative material is provided from recent and classical literature.

2.5.3   Gortner, S.R. (1983) The history and philosophy of nursing science and research. *Advances in nursing science* 5(2) 1-8   21 References

A general discussion on the development of nursing research in the USA over the last 150 years. Particular reference is made to the choice of research ideas, education of nurses and nursing research's philosophical and scientific basis (CR 2.8).

2.5.4 Hindess, B. (1977) *Philosophy and methodology in the social sciences.* Hassocks, Sussex: Harvester Press ISBN 0855273445 References

Book provides a systematic critique of epistemological and philosophical interventions in the social sciences and of prescriptive methodology in general. The works of Weber, Schutz, Husserl, Mills and Popper are analysed and discussed (CR 2.6).

2.5.5 Holmes, C.A. (1990) Alternatives to natural science foundations for nursing. *International journal of nursing studies* 27(3) 187-198 68 References

Paper discusses some of the philosophical assumptions associated with humanistic and holistic approaches to nursing and outlines their impact on nursing theory, education and practice. Author believes nursing should concentrate on phenomenological and humanistic methodologies.

2.5.6 Hughes, J. (1980) *The philosophy of social research.* London: Longman ISBN 0582490324 References

An introductory text which examines some philosophical views arising from social research practices. Ways of evaluating both current and historical research in the social sciences are discussed.

2.5.7 Lanara, V. (1984) *Values in nursing research – a philosophical commentary.* Proceedings of the 7th Workgroup Meeting and 2nd Open Conference of the Workgroup of European Nurse Researchers 10-13 April London: Royal College of Nursing ISBN 0902606891 158-175 25 References

The philosophical underpinning of nursing is described. How nursing theory can and should become the basis for practice is discussed as are ethical issues in nursing research. The paper asks whether nurses undertaking research are aware of the ethical codes and guidelines promulgated by many professional bodies. Suggestions are made for the teaching of nursing research stressing the values involved. It is suggested that nurses, collectively and individually must ensure that nursing research in the future must be imbued with humanistic principles (CR 3.26).

2.5.8 Manchester, P. (1986) Analytical philosophy and foundational inquiry: the method. IN Munhall, P.L. & Oiler, C.J. (eds) *Nursing research: a qualitative perspective.* Norwalk, Connecticut: Appleton-Century-Crofts ISBN 0838570488 References Chapter 12 229-249

Discusses ways in which analytical philosophy can contribute to the development of scientific methods in nursing. Sections are included on rational reconstruction and theory generation i.e. the conditions whereby a developing science can generate knowledge and methods according to its own goals; implications for the idea on nursing, science and philosophical analysis (CR 2.1.42).

2.5.9 Munhall, P.L. (1982) Nursing philosophy and nursing research: in apposition or opposition? *Nursing research* 31(3) 176-177, 181 3 References

Discusses the problem of relating nursing philosophy and the scientific method, to nursing research (CR 2.8).

2.5.10 Munhall, P.L. & Oiler, C.J. (eds) (1986) Philosophical foundations of qualitative research. IN Authors *Nursing research: a qualitative perspective.* Norwalk, Connecticut: Appleton-Century-Crofts ISBN 0838570488 References Chapter 3 47-63

Chapter presents a broad philosophical framework for qualitative research (CR 2.1.42).

2.5.11 Outhwaite, W. (1987) *New philosophies of social science realism, hermeneutics and critical theory.* Basingstoke: Macmillan Education ISBN 0333363159 References

Outlines earlier positivist orthodoxy and its effects on the social sciences. The realist alternative is discussed with its implications for social theory and the contribution which hermeneutics and critical theory can make to an overall framework.

2.5.12 Phillips, D.C. (1987) *Philosophy, science and social inquiry: contemporary methodological controversies in social science and related applied fields of research.* Oxford: Pergamon ISBN 0080334113 References

Discusses the contemporary debates concerning the scientific status of research in the social and human sciences. It provides a clear exposition of the relevant developments in philosophy against which research needs to be seen: the works of Kuhn, Winch, Lakatos, Feyerband and especially Popper; the demise of positivism; the rise in interest in hermeneutical approaches, relativism and holism. A detailed case study illustrates the main ideas. (Contains a glossary).

2.5.13 Popper, K.R. (1961) *The poverty of historicism.* London: Routledge & Kegan Paul ISBN 0710046162 References

Historicism as an approach to the social sciences assumes that historical prediction is the principal aim. It is exposed in this book in order to account for the unsatisfactory state of the theoretical social sciences. This is contrasted with scientific empiricism and suggestions made as to what the character and methods of social science should be.

2.5.14 Ryan, A. (1970) *The philosophy of the social sciences.* London: Macmillan SBN 333109724 References

Explores many of the major philosophical issues within the social sciences. The scientific basis of social inquiry is discussed together with problems raised by the application of scientific explanations to human behaviour. The role of theory in science, functionalism, social sciences as ideologies, and objectivity in the description and analysis of social facts are all discussed.

2.5.15 Smith, J.A. (1986) The idea of health: doing foundational inquiry. IN Munhall, P.L. & Oiler, C.J. (eds) *Nursing research: a qualitative perspective.* Norwalk, Connecticut: Appleton-Century-Crofts ISBN 0838570488 References Chapter 13 251-262

Outlines a process for foundational inquiry based around the idea of health. Chapter includes ideas about design, its implications for nursing and future directions (CR 2.1.42).

2.5.16   Trigg, R. (1985) *Understanding social science: a philosophical introduction to the social sciences.* Oxford: Blackwell   ISBN 0631141618   References

Book examines the scientific basis of social science and the philosophical controversies are illustrated by examples from sociology, economics, anthropology and psychology.

Suggested textbook readings

	Pages	*Cross reference*
Carter M.A. IN Leininger	27-32	2.1.36
Gaut D.A. IN Leininger	73-80	2.1.36
Wilson, H.S. (1989)	16-21	2.1.69

2.6   EPISTEMOLOGY

'Knowledge progresses not by absolute establishment of conclusions, but by the exposing of conjectures or hypotheses to criticism and to the possibility of refutation. However not even this process yields certainty, for a position that is soundly criticisable today might undergo resuscitation tomorrow. Progress follows a tentative and meandering course' (Phillips DC 1987).

Definition
The division of philosophy that investigates the nature and origin of knowledge.

Annotations
2.6.1   Aggleton, P. & Chalmers, H. (1986) Nursing research, nursing theory and the nursing process. *Journal of advanced nursing* 11(2) 197-202   38 References

The development of nursing research, nursing theories and models and their interrelationship is discussed. The inductive and hypothetico-deductive approaches to developing theory are compared. The possible use of the nursing process to facilitate the development of nursing is described.

2.6.2   Bloch, D. (1985) A conceptualisation of nursing research and nursing science. IN McCloskey, J.C. & Grace, H.K. (eds) *Current issues in nursing.* 2nd edition Boston: Blackwell Scientific   ISBN 086542019X   Part 2   10   124-138   47 References

Chapter discusses nursing research and nursing science and suggests how they may be conceptualised and linked with nursing practice. Author highlights the existence of a vast communal pool of knowledge upon which all health professionals can draw and which is relevant to nursing practice. Studies are reviewed which demonstrate the links between theory and practice.

2.6.3 Burnard, P. (1987) Towards an epistemological basis for experiential learning in nurse education. *Journal of advanced nursing* 12(2) 189-193   24 References

Experiential learning is being recommended for psychiatric nursing students but there is not a sound theory of knowledge to underpin the concepts involved. Paper offers an epistemological theory divided into three domains − propositional, practical and experiential knowledge as a basis for a theory of experiential learning. This is then re-defined and practical issues discussed.

2.6.4 Chenitz, W.C. & Swanson, J.M. (1984) Surfacing nursing process: a method for generating nursing theory from practice. *Journal of advanced nursing* 9(2) 205-215   32 References

Authors contend that lack of knowledge about processes in nursing has consequences for professional development and nursing theory. A method for generating theory from systematic observation, description, identification and analysis of nursing practice is presented.

2.6.5 Clark, E. (1987) *Sources of nursing knowledge.* Research Awareness, Module 2. London: Distance Learning Centre, South Bank Polytechnic   ISBN 0948250259 References

This is number 2 in a series of 13 modules, each of which deals with a different aspect of nursing research. It was developed to assist nurses, midwives and health visitors in understanding research in terms of their own professional practice. Modules can be used separately or as part of a programme. The reader is encouraged to work through a number of activities, self-assessment questions and answers and progress summaries. Some articles/book extracts referred to in the text are reproduced in full.
   This module compares and contrasts tradition, trial and error, and science as the knowledge base for nursing practice, and considers the role of authority, common sense and experience in nursing. Nurses are encouraged to question their practice and examples are given where this has been changed following research findings, for example the use of shaving, and enemata, in midwifery (CR Appendix D).

2.6.6 Crow, R. (1981)   Research and the standards of nursing care: what is the relationship? *Journal of advanced nursing* 6(6) 491-496   18 References

Author suggests that research can provide a scientific knowledge base for practising nurses and can contribute to the setting of standards albeit with some limitations.

2.6.7 Dunlop, M.J. (1986) Is a science of caring possible? *Journal of advanced nursing* 11(6) 661-670   26 References

A socio-historical view of caring is discussed and some of the problems of conceptualising and developing a science of caring are explored. The recognition of nursing skills, knowledge and values is linked to the struggles of the feminist movement (CR 2.10).

2.6.8 Fawcett, J. (1983) Contemporary nursing research: its relevance for nursing practice. IN Chaska, N.L. *The nursing profession: a time to speak.* New York: McGraw Hill ISBN 0070106967 References Chapter 14 169-182

Examines whether nursing research is generating and validating the knowledge necessary for underpinning practice. Four types of nursing knowledge are explored – scientific, ethical, aesthetic and personal knowledge of the therapeutic use of self, and the author asks if nursing researchers are focusing on these. Not all research can be applied to practice, and criteria are discussed which identify the necessary conditions for this transfer (CR 3.6.2).

2.6.9 Gortner, S.R. (1980) Nursing science in transition. *Nursing research* 29(3) 180-183 19 References

Nursing science, the bases of knowledge underlying human behaviour and social interaction is distinguished from its inquiry. Inquiry and especially methodology have been afforded greater attention than science. The requirements for increasing science are noted: communality, colleagueship and competition among scientists and continuity and confirmation of scientific activity and evidence.

2.6.10 Harvey, L. (1990) *Critical social research.* London: Unwin Hyman ISBN 0044453604 References

This methodology textbook provides all involved in social research a perspective which transcends divisions between quantitative and qualitative approaches. At the heart of critical social research is the idea that knowledge is structured by existing sets of social relations; its aim is to provide knowledge that engages with and challenges prevailing, oppressive social structures. Case studies, based on class, gender and race are used extensively to illustrate how critical social research has been done and show the epistemological underpinnings to practical techniques (author annotation) (CR 2.4, 2.5, 2.10, 2.37, 2.47).

2.6.11 Howard, M.J. & Knafl, K.A. (1985) Generating nursing knowledge: whose work? IN McCloskey, J.C. & Grace, H.K. (eds) *Current issues in nursing.* 2nd edition Boston: Blackwell Scientific ISBN 086542019X Part 2 12 149-160 10 References

Nursing authorship was examined in a survey of 353 articles from four American nursing journals. Articles were also classified into eleven coding categories in order to report on their content. The review showed a clear predominance of nurse authors with about half doctorally prepared. Compared with previous surveys there is less reliance on members of other disciplines but increasing collaboration.

2.6.12 Johnson, M. (1986) Models of perfection. *Nursing times* 82(6) February 5 42,44 15 References

Concern is expressed that researchers do not publicly criticise each others work and therefore do not advance nursing knowledge by opening up the debate to public and professional scrutiny.

2.6.13 Kuhn, T.S. (1970) *The structure of scientific revolutions.* 2nd edition Chicago: University of Chicago Press   ISBN 0226458040   References

Author argues that science is not a gradual accumulation of knowledge, but a series of developments interrupted by 'intellectually violent revolutions'. He believes science is often influenced in apparently non-rational ways and new theories develop which may appear more complex but are not any nearer to the truth.

2.6.14 Loomis, M.E. (1985) Emerging nursing knowledge. IN McCloskey, J.C. & Grace, H.K. (eds) *Current issues in nursing.* 2nd edition Boston: Blackwell Scientific   ISBN 086542019X   Part 2   Chapter 14   171-181   4 References

An analysis of the content of 319 nursing doctoral dissertations completed between 1976 and 1982. Broad categories were developed with studies of clinical nursing and social issues identified. The majority were clinically orientated studies.

2.6.15 Meleis, A.I. (1985) *Theoretical nursing: development and progress.* Philadelphia: Lippincott   ISBN 0397544553   References

A comprehensive text which explores, discusses, analyses, critiques, compares and contrasts different epistemologies, theories of truth and nursing theories. Although the focus is on nursing theories it is emphasised that nursing is based on philosophy, theory, practice and research. The theory-research/theory-strategy is explained, abstracts of theoretical writing in nursing are given and there is an extensive bibliography on theory and meta-theory (CR 2.5).

2.6.16 Munhall, P.L. & Oiler, C.J. (1986) Epistemology in nursing. IN Authors *Nursing research: a qualitative perspective.* Norwalk, Connecticut: Appleton-Century-Crofts   ISBN 0838570488   References   Chapter 2   27-45

Chapter proposes an epistemology for nursing research which includes both quantitative and qualitative methods of research. It explores paths to knowledge, the purpose of science, epistemological interests of nursing and methods (CR 2.1.42).

2.6.17 Schultz, P.R. & Meleis, A.I. (1988) Nursing epistemology: traditions, insights, questions. *Image: the journal of nursing scholarship* 20(4)   217-221   27 References

Three types of knowledge specific to the discipline of nursing are described: clinical, conceptual and empirical. Criteria for evaluating each type are suggested.

2.6.18 Sheehan, J. (1986) Aspects of research methodology. *Nurse education today* 6(5) 193-203   45 References

Discusses the creation of knowledge and its relationship to research. Six research methods are summarised: historical, developmental, survey, correlational, experimental and action research (CR 2.29, 2.37, 2.40, 2.47, 2.49, 2.55).

2.6.19 Smith, M.C. (1984) Research methodology: epistemological considerations. *Image: the journal of nursing scholarship* 16(2) 42-46   44 References

Article poses four questions derived from epistemological origins for consideration in the selection of appropriate research methodologies in nursing. These are, where does the source of the problem reside?, what is the appropriate mode of inquiry to acquire knowledge?, what subject matter is sought? and what are the desired ends of the research? The implications of these are discussed.

2.6.20 Styles, M.M. (1990) A common sense approach to nursing research. *International nursing review* 37(1) Issue 289 203-206, 218   9 References

Article aims to start a debate about the political significance of knowledge, appropriate paradigms, the presentation of knowledge, power brokers, professional priorities and evaluation.

2.6.21 Tripp-Reimer, T. (1985) Expanding four essential concepts in nursing theory: the contribution of anthropology. IN McCloskey, J.C. & Grace. H.K. (eds) *Current issues in nursing.* 2nd edition Boston: Blackwell Scientific   ISBN 086542019X   References   Part 1   Chapter 8   91-103

Discusses the contribution of anthropology to nursing knowledge through examination of the environment, human interactions, health and nursing.

2.6.22 Visintainer, M.A. (1986) The nature of knowledge and theory in nursing. *Image: the journal of nursing scholarship* 18(2) 32-38   6 References

Examines the characteristics of theoretical constructs as they apply to the practice of nursing, the use of theory in that practice and its limitations.

Suggested textbook readings

	Pages	Cross reference
Aamodt A.M. IN Morse (1989)	29-40	2.36.8
Burns & Grove	19-29	2.1.12
Castles	25-26	2.1.15
Christensen	10-13	2.1.17
Field & Morse	1-18	2.1.24
Kidder & Judd	4-19	2.1.30
Krathwohl	6-29/156-210	2.1.33
Munhall & Oiler	27-45	2.1.42
Wilson H.S. (1989)	7-13	2.1.69

Nursing research abstracts

Crow R.	82/1
Fawcett J. & Downs F.S.	87/108
Hockey L.	82/288
Pollock L.	85/0237

2.7 THEORETICAL FRAMEWORKS

The nature of nursing as a science and an art requires a strong theoretical basis which needs translating into practice. Nurse researchers are now developing this base which will inform all subsequent studies.

Definition
A systematic vision of reality: a set of inter-related concepts that is useful for prediction and control.

Annotations
2.7.1 Camilleri, S.F. (1970) Theory, probability and induction in social research. IN Denzin, N.K. *Sociological methods: a sourcebook.* London: Butterworths   ISBN 0408701250   References   Part 2 Chapter 4 70-83

Includes discussion on some aspects of scientific theory, sampling and experimentation and the verification of hypotheses (CR 2.1.23).

2.7.2 Chinn, P.L. (ed) (1986) *Nursing research methodology: issues and implementation.* Rockville, Maryland: Aspen   ISBN 0871893738   References

Addresses fundamental philosophical issues, those concerning theory development, and aspects of research methodology in quantitative and qualitative approaches. Examples are given which use selected methodological approaches (CR 2.9).

2.7.3 Chinn, P.L. & Jacobs, M.K. (1987) *Theory and nursing: a systematic approach.* St Louis: Mosby   ISBN 0801609836   References   Chapter 7   149-166

Chapter examines the relationship between theory and research and identifies ways in which a research study can be designed or be judged to be theoretically sound.

2.7.4 Fawcett, J. & Downs, F.S. (1986) *The relationship of theory and research.* Norwalk, Connecticut: Appleton-Century-Crofts   ISBN 0838583652   References

Book fills a major gap in the literature and presents a detailed discussion of the relationship between theory and research. The types and functions of theory and research are discussed together with a format for analysing the theoretical elements of research reports, formal procedures for integrating results from different studies, and the influence of conceptual models. Appendices contain three studies, descriptive, correlational and experimental and their theoretical elements are analysed.

2.7.5 Hockey, L. (1982) Some methodological issues in nursing research. IN Redfern, S.J., Sisson, A.R., Walker, J.F. & Walsh, P.A. (eds) *Issues in nursing research.* Papers from the 22nd annual conference of the Royal College of Nursing Research Society. London: Macmillan   ISBN 0333324501   References 433-437

Author seeks to explain her view that research in nursing may require a mix of theoretical frameworks, designs and methods. There is discussion of the problem of building a body of knowledge when most research is done for higher degrees and replication is not generally encouraged (CR 2.7, 2.13, 3.26.3).

2.7.6 Johnson, M. (1983) Some aspects of the relation between theory and research in nursing. *Journal of advanced nursing* 8(1) 21-28   46 References

The theoretical approaches of induction, deduction, and speculation are discussed in relation to nursing research. Some theorists' claims for scientific status are questioned and the author believes that these methods are complementary rather than mutually exclusive.

2.7.7 Kim, H.S. (1989) Theoretical thinking in nursing: problems and prospects. *Recent advances in nursing* 24: 106-122   59 References

Paper examines the nature of theoretical thinking and the status, problems and prospects of its development in nursing.

2.7.8 Newman, M.A. (1979) *Theory development in nursing.* Philadelphia: Davis   ISBN 0803665202   References

Discusses the process of theory development in the context of nursing and nursing research. Author urges the execution of studies which examine as many relationships as possible about a particular concept. Researchers should systematically consider how their findings inter-relate and could be developed into a theory.

2.7.9 Silva, M.C. (1986) Research testing nursing theory: the state of the art. *Advances in nursing science* 9(1) 1-11   20 References

62 studies in which the nursing models of Johnson, Roy, Orem, Rogers and Newman had been used, were utilised as a framework to examine the extent to which nursing theories had been examined through empirical research. Nine of the studies specified evaluation criteria for the explicit testing of nursing theory. The implication of this is discussed.

2.7.10 Suppe, F. & Jacox, A.K. (1985) Philosophy of science and the development of nursing theory. IN Werley, H.H. & Fitzpatrick, J.J. (eds) *Annual review of nursing research.* Volume 3 New York: Springer   ISBN 0836143520   Chapter 11 241-267   100 References

Chapter reviews the literature on the philosophy of science in the development of nursing theory over the past 30 years. Concepts, theories, conceptual frameworks, approaches to nursing theory development and their evaluation are all discussed. Suggestions are made for developing nursing theories and frameworks (CR 2.12).

2.7.11   Walker, L.O. (1983a) Theory and research in the development of nursing as a discipline: retrospect and prospect. IN Chaska, N.L. *The nursing profession: a time to speak.* New York: McGraw Hill   ISBN 0070106967   References   Chapter 30   406-415

Chapter examines three movements – metatheoretical, theoretical and practice theory and their influence on nursing as a scholarly discipline. The author believes that innovation in nursing practice will be enhanced through using a theoretical perspective (CR 3.6.2).

2.7.12   Walker, L.O. & Avant, K.C. (1983b) *Strategies for theory construction in nursing.* Norwalk, Connecticut: Appleton-Century-Crofts   ISBN 0838586864   References

Aims to provide a developmental approach to theory. A general overview of the state of the art is given followed by concept, statement and theory development using three approaches: analysis, synthesis and derivation. Finally the nature of theory in nursing is discussed. Actual and hypothetical examples are used for illustration and the links between theory development and research are explored. Chapters contain practice exercises.

2.7.13 to 2.7.19   *Advances in nursing science* (1986) 9(1) Edited by Chinn, P.L. Theory testing research.

[NB   The following two entries differ in format as they document two special issues of the journal *Advances in nursing science*. These articles have not been annotated]

2.7.13   Burbank, P.M. Psychosocial theories of ageing: a critical evaluation. 73-86   50 References

2.7.14   Clarke, P.N. Theoretical and measurement issues in the study of field phenomena. 29-39   40 References

2.7.15   Cox, C.L. The interactions model of client health behaviour: application to the study of community based elders. 40-57   18 References

2.7.16   Davis-Sharts, J. An empirical test of Maslow's theory of need heirarchy using hologeistic comparison by statistical sampling. 58-72   30 References

2.7.17   Mentzer, C.A. & Schorr, J.A. Perceived situational control and perceived duration of time: expressions of life patterns. 12-20   20 References

2.7.18   Silva, M.C. Research testing nursing theory: state of the art. 1-11   20 References (CR 2.7.9)

2.7.19   Smith, M.J. Human-environment process: a test of Roger's principle of integratility. 21-28   26 References

2.7.20 to 2.7.26 *Advances in nursing science* (1978) Edited by Chinn, P.L. Theory generating research.

2.7.20 Bowers, B.B. Intergenerational caregiving: adult caregivers and their ageing parents. 20-31 26 References

2.7.21 Haase, J.E. Components of courage in chronically ill adolescents; a phenomenological study. 64-80 28 References

2.7.22 Ketefian, S. A case study of theory development: moral behaviour in nursing. 10-19 31 References

2.7.23 Olshansky, E.F. Identity of self as infertile: an example of theory generating research. 54-63 30 References

2.7.24 Rigdon, I., Clayton, B.C. & Dimond, M. Toward a theory of helpfulness for the elderly bereaved: an invitation to a new life. 32-43 30 References

2.7.25 Sarter, B. Evolutionary idealism: a philosophical foundation for holistic nursing theory. 1-9 40 References

2.7.26 Wewers, M.E. & Lenz, E.R. Relapse among smokers: an example of theory derivation. 44-53 29 References

Suggested textbook readings

	Pages	*Cross reference*
Abdellah & Levine	50-72/106-113	2.1.1
Burns & Grove	155-180	2.1.12
Castles	21-27	2.1.15
Fox	7-25	2.1.25
Lin	15-70	2.1.37
Feldman H.R. IN LoBiondo-Wood & Haber	91-106	2.1.38
Nieswiadomy	39-54/91-106	2.1.43
Phillips L.R.F. (critique)	135-202	2.98.11
Polit & Hungler (1987)	80-101	2.1.56
Seaman	65-103	2.1.62
Silva M.C. IN Krampitz & Pavlovich	17-28	2.1.32
Smith H.W.	21-53	2.98.14
Sweeney & Olivieri	93-100	2.1.63
Treece & Treece	72-88	2.1.65
Williamson	19-24	2.1.67
Wilson H.S. (1989)	275-332	2.1.69
Woods & Catanzaro	18-34/66-76	2.1.72

2.8 SCIENTIFIC METHOD

The major components of the scientific method are asking questions, defining problems, obtaining and interpreting data and drawing conclusions. These allow researchers to complete work according to a set of rules and a series of workable ideas is generated. Over time, better ideas and theories emerge, which is the ultimate goal of science.

Definitions
Science is a systematically organised body of knowledge which consists of:

(a) statements which record and clarify observations that are relevant for the solution of a problem in the most accurate and definite way possible
(b) general statements, laws and hypotheses which assert regularities among certain classes of observed or observable phenomena
(c) theoretical statements which connect and account for the largest possible number of laws
(d) other general or specific statements which are deducible from the initial descriptors and from laws and theories which are confirmed by further observations and testing. As a process science is a means by which a body of knowledge evolves and progresses. As an outcome, it represents the ever-growing, ever-changing, accumulated knowledge of a particular discipline.

deductive — reasoning from the general abstraction to the particular case
inductive — reasoning from the particular case to the more general abstraction

Annotations
2.8.1 Chalmers, A.F. (1982) *What is this thing called science: an assessment of the nature and status of science and its methods.* 2nd edition. Milton Keynes: Open University Press   ISBN 0335101070   References

Provides an introduction to the new philosophy of science. The shortcomings of the empiricist accounts of science are explored and modern writings which replace these are discussed.

2.8.2 Crow, R. (1981) Scientific nursing research: art and science. IN Smith, J.P. *Nursing science in nursing practice.* London: Butterworths   ISBN 0407002022 References   Chapter 4   29-42

Discusses the nature of scientific research, strategies adopted and its inherent problems. Author points out that application of knowledge to nursing practice is never straightforward and clinical judgement will determine the ultimate success with which it is done.

2.8.3 DeGroot, H.A. (1988) Scientific inquiry in nursing: a model for a new age. *Advances in nursing science* 10(3) 1-21   58 References

Discusses the nature of scientific inquiry and its fundamental role in research practice. The importance of the individual investigator's beliefs are explored and the implications this has for nursing science.

2.8.4 Law, J. & Lodge, P. (1984) *Science for social scientists.* London: Macmillan   ISBN 0333351010   References

Fundamental questions are asked about learning, knowledge and the 'scientific method', and many examples are used from different disciplines to illustrate these themes. Authors believe there is no such thing as a special scientific method, but that all knowledge is constitutively social. Social scientists are urged to solve more limited intellectual problems and study empirical findings, rather than concentrate on philosophical arguments.

2.8.5 Medawar, P. (1984) *The limits of science.* Oxford: Oxford University Press   ISBN 019283048   References

Comprises three essays which discuss the limitations of science. Author believes that science is unable to answer those ultimate questions which are 'beyond its explanatory competence'.

2.8.6 Morgan, G. (ed) (1983) *Beyond method: strategies for social research.* Beverly Hills: Sage   ISBN 0803920784   References

Editor believes that understanding and debate about research should be reframed in a way that goes beyond considerations of method alone. 21 different approaches are addressed to illustrate the diversity and contradictions which make the selection of a research strategy such a problematic and value-laden affair.

2.8.7 Phillips, D.L. (1973) *Abandoning method: sociological studies in methodology.* San Francisco: Jossey-Bass   ISBN 0875891659   References

Challenges conventional views of methodology in the social sciences and presents evidence which shows bias and invalidity in large scale survey studies. Assumptions underlying the practice of sociology are questioned and the author believes that such questioning is essential so that methodological progress can be achieved (CR 2.55).

Suggested textbook readings

	Pages	*Cross reference*
Abdellah & Levine	38-49	2.1.1
Adams & Schvaneveldt	7-23	2.1.2
Christensen	1-21	2.1.17
Cohen & Manion	1-46	2.1.19
LoBiondo-Wood & Haber	18-28	2.1.38
Phillips D.C.	21-22	2.5.12
Polgar & Thomas	7-21	2.1.55

	Pages	*Cross reference*
Polit & Hungler (1987)	13-26	2.1.56
Rowan J. IN Reason & Rowan	37-41/83-91	2.11.5
Silverman D.	29-49	2.16.13
Treece & Treece	37-55	2.1.65

2.9   QUANTITATIVE/QUALITATIVE DEBATE

The debate about quantitative and qualitative research took root in the 1960's although many of the central themes go back centuries. These two approaches are more than just differences between research strategies and data collection procedures. They represent fundamentally different epistemological frameworks for conceptualising the nature of knowing, social reality and procedures for comprehending these phenomena.

Definitions

Qualitative research − this is usually inductively derived and seeks to name and describe the categories into which observations belong e.g. grounded theory or ethnomethodology

Quantitative research − this mode of research is often deductively derived and seeks to confirm the construct validity and internal structure of a research instrument designed to measure a particular concept

---

Major text

Bryman, A. (1988) *Quantity and quality in social research.* London: Unwin Hyman   ISBN 0043120407   References (CR 2.9.1).

Annotations

2.9.1   Bryman, A. (1988) *Quantity and quality in social research.* London: Unwin Hyman   ISBN 0043120407   References

Book focuses on the debate about quantitative and qualitative research and the nature and relative virtues of each perspective. Underlying philosophical positions are also discussed. Research from a wide range of the social sciences is used for illustrative purposes, and the book is intended for the graduate and undergraduate studying research methods.

2.9.2   Duffy, M.E. (1985) Designing nursing research: the qualitative/quantitative debate. *Journal of advanced nursing* 10(3) 225-232   18 References

Issues relating to the use of quantitative/qualitative methodologies in nursing research are discussed. The two approaches are contrasted in terms of their origins, sampling techniques, reliability, validity and ethics. Researchers are encouraged to debate the issues so that nursing may select appropriately along the continuum.

2.9.3   Goodwin, L.D. & Goodwin, W.L. (1984) Qualitative versus quantitative research or qualitative and quantitative research? *Nursing research* 33(6) 378-380   28 References

Article describes three myths about the differences of the two approaches (a) quantitative/qualitative strategies represent clearly different, mutually exclusive paradigmatic perspectives (b) qualitative methods are always naturalistic, unobtrusive and subjective whereas quantitative methods are always controlled, obtrusive and objective (c) measurement-related validity and reliability are irrelevant in qualitative research. Authors discuss the use of both strategies in a single study.

2.9.4   Harré, R. (1981) The positivist-empiricist approach and its alternative. IN Reason, P. & Rowan, J. (eds) *Human inquiry : a sourcebook of new paradigm research.* Chichester: Wiley   ISBN 0471279358   References   Chapter 1   3-17

Author discusses the meaning and problems related to the positivist-empiricist approach to research and suggests an alternative which acknowledges the humanity and contribution of those being used as research subjects (CR 2.11.5).

2.9.5   Leach, M. (1990) Philosophical choices. *Nursing* 4(3) 15.1.1990/7.2.1990 16-18   10 References

Discusses the differences between quantitative and qualitative research and the implications for nursing studies.

2.9.6   Moccia, P. (1988) A critique of compromise: beyond the methods debate. *Advances in nursing science* 10(4) 1-9   35 References

Fundamental differences between quantitative and qualitative research methods which go beyond techniques are identified. These are the nature of reality, knowledge and science. The implications for nursing, nurses and practice are discussed.

2.9.7   Phillips, J.R. (1988) Research blenders. *Nursing science quarterly* 1(1) 4-5   8 References

Author believes that quantitative and qualitative research methods are incompatible and discusses their essential differences. Scholars are urged to develop new modes of inquiry.

2.9.8   Porter, E.J. (1989) The qualitative-quantitative dualism. *Image: the journal of nursing scholarship* 21(2) 98-102   51 References

The characteristics of both research approaches are described and suggestions made as to how to decide which may be the most appropriate in particular circumstances. Author advocates ways of overcoming the dichotomy which exists.

2.9.9   Powell, D. (1982) *Learning to relate.* London: Royal College of Nursing ISBN 0902606697   References   Chapter 3   33-41

Chapter discusses the decisions taken about the methods used in this study and more generally, together with the problems a nurse-researcher may encounter in attempting to apply qualitative research methods to nursing.

2.9.10   Smith, J.K. (1983) Quantitative versus qualitative research : an attempt to clarify the issue. *Educational researcher* 12(3) 6-13   21 References

Provides an overview of the quantitative/qualitative debate. The subject is approached by examining historical origins, the relationship between investigator and what is to be investigated, and that between facts and values in the process of the investigation. Author urges that the subject should continue to be debated in order for judgements to be made about what is good research.

Suggested textbook readings

	Pages	Cross reference
Brophy E.B. IN Krampitz & Pavlovich	41-42	2.1.32
Polgar & Thomas	94-102	2.1.55
Seaman	165-180	2.1.62
Tripp-Reimer T. IN Leininger	179-194	2.1.36
Watson J. IN Leininger	343-349	2.1.36

Nursing research abstracts

Myers S.T. & Haase J.E.	90/012
Spencer J.	84/7

2.10   FEMINIST RESEARCH

'Not only do men and women view a common world from different perspectives, they view different worlds as well' (Bernard 1973). Feminist research is multidisciplinary in nature and is in the process of defining knowledge, knowledge gathering and making. It is rigorous because gender is taken into consideration and the experiences of women are deemed to be as important as those of men. As such it has much to offer the predominantly female nursing profession.

Definition

Feminist research involves a new way of classifying the world from the perspective of women's experiences (adapted from Spender 1978)

Example

MacPherson, K.I. (1985) Osteoporosis and menopause: a feminist analysis of the social construction of a syndrome. *Advances in nursing science* 7(4) 11-22   47 References

Using a feminist framework the roles of science, medicine, pharmaceutical companies, government and the media are analysed in the social construction of menopause as a syndrome that includes osteoporosis. Debates over who defines osteoporosis and controls its treatment are discussed. Alternative therapies are suggested and nurses urged to protect themselves and others from osteoporosis and hormone treatment.

Annotations

2.10.1 Callaway, H. (1981) Women's perspectives: research as re-vision. IN Reason, P. & Rowan, J. (eds) *Human inquiry: a sourcebook of new paradigm research*. Chichester: Wiley ISBN 0471279358 References Chapter 39 457-471

Chapter traces the development of research on women and by women and shows how it has led to new approaches in methodology, theory construction and modes of expression (CR 2.11.5).

2.10.2 Easterday, L., Papademas, D., Schorr, L. & Valentine, C. (1982) The making of a female researcher: role problems in fieldwork. IN Burgess, R.G. (ed) *Field research: a sourcebook and field manual*. London: Allen & Unwin ISBN 0043120148 References Chapter 9 62-67

Specific problems of being a female field researcher are related to general methodological issues. Suggestions are made as to how they may be overcome (CR 2.1.9).

2.10.3 Eichler, M. (1988) *Nonsexist research methods: a practical guide*. Boston: Allen & Unwin ISBN 0044970455 References

Book, written for students in many disciplines, provides a systematic approach to identifying, eliminating and preventing sexist bias in social science research. Each chapter is illustrated from recent literature. A non-sexist research checklist is included which may be used when evaluating or carrying out research.

2.10.4 Harding, S. (ed) (1987) *Feminism and methodology: social science issues*. Milton Keynes: Open University Press ISBN 033515560X References

A collection of essays which provide an introduction to the crucial methodological and epistemological issues feminist inquiry raises for scholars in all fields.

2.10.5 MacPherson, K.I. (1983) Feminist methods: a new paradigm for nursing research. *Advances in nursing science* 5(2) 17-25 35 References

Discusses the origins and development of feminist research, its components, methods and its future.

2.10.6 Roberts, H. (ed) (1981) *Doing feminist research*. London: Routledge & Kegan Paul ISBN 0710007728 References

Volume presents accounts of research where practical, methodological, theoretical and ethical issues are raised where the sociologist adopts or is aware of a feminist perspective.

2.10.7   Webb, C. (1984) Feminist methodology in nursing research. *Journal of advanced nursing* 9(3) 249-256   24 References

Author discusses her experiences as a feminist, nurse and sociologist when carrying out a study of patients undergoing hysterectomy. The difficulties encountered in carrying out interviews and publishing reports which resulted from the constraints of masculine research models, and the context of medical domination are described. An analysis is made of these experiences in terms of feminist methodology and a case made for the value of a feminist perspective.

Suggested textbook reading

	Pages	*Cross reference*
Glennon L.M. IN Morgan G.	260-271	2.8.6

2.11   NEW PARADIGM RESEARCH

New paradigm research is another way of doing research. It puts forward alternatives to 'orthodox' research methods and capitalises on the contributions of those who are normally just subjects. It is an approach to inquiry which is a systematic, rigorous search for truth but which does not kill off all it touches. It is a synthesis of naive inquiry and orthodox research (Reason & Rowan 1981)

Definition
Research which is done with people rather than on people. It involves working with people so that they may discover some truth about themselves.

Example
Collin, A. (1981) Mid-career change: reflections upon the development of a piece of research and the part it played in the development of the researcher. IN Reason, P. & Rowan, J. (eds) *Human inquiry: a sourcebook of new paradigm research.* Chichester: Wiley   ISBN 0471279358   References

Discusses the learning process of discovering a methodology while undertaking research on the changes various groups of men were experiencing in a new phase of their life or experience (CR 2.11.5).

Major text
Reason, P. & Rowan, J. (eds) (1981) *Human inquiry: a sourcebook of new paradigm research.* Chichester: Wiley   ISBN 0471279358   References (CR 2.11.5)

Annotations
2.11.1   Connors, D.D. (1988) A continuum of researcher − participant relationships: an analysis and critique. *Advances in nursing science* 10(4) 32-42   33 References

Explores the nature of researcher-practitioner relationships and discusses the importance of this as a central focus of nursing enquiry.

2.11.2 Hamilton, D., Jenkins, D., King, C., Macdonald, B. & Parlett, M. (eds) (1977) *Beyond the numbers game: a reader in educational evaluation.* Basingstoke: Macmillan Education   ISBN 0333198727   References

This reader on illuminative evaluation covers innovation in the school context or 'learning milieu'. Its methodological strategies are described, together with techniques of data collection and analysis, problems versus potential, range of applicability, validity and generalisability of evidence and the skills and obligations of the research worker.

2.11.3 Heron, J. (1981) Experiential research methodology IN Reason, P. & Rowan, J. (eds) *Human inquiry: a sourcebook of new paradigm research.* Chichester: Wiley   ISBN 0471279358   References   Chapter 12   153-166

Traditional and experiential research methodologies are contrasted. Contributions of the latter to the body of knowledge are explored (CR 2.11.5).

2.11.4 Parlett, M. (1981) Illuminative evaluation. IN Reason,P. & Rowan, J. (eds) *Human inquiry: a sourcebook of new paradigm research.* Chichester: Wiley   ISBN 0471279358   References   Chapter 19   219-226

Chapter summarises this approach, largely, although not exclusively used in education. Four perspectives are examined − definition of problems studied, its methodology, underlying conceptual framework and the values embodied in this approach (CR 2.11.5).

2.11.5 Reason, P. & Rowan, J. (eds) (1981) *Human inquiry: a sourcebook of new paradigm research.* Chichester: Wiley   ISBN 0471279358   References

Sourcebook suggests a new paradigm for the philosophy and practice of research which is collaborative and experiential. New paradigm research means doing research with people rather than on people and seeks to develop new insights into the actions and behaviours of diverse groups. The book covers the philosophy, methodology, practice and prospects of new paradigm research. Many examples are included to illustrate these new approaches.

2.11.6 Reinhart, S. (1981) Implementing new paradigm research: a model for training and practice. IN Reason, P. & Rowan, J. (eds) *Human inquiry: a sourcebook of new paradigm research.* Chichester: Wiley   ISBN 0471279358   Chapter 36 415-435

Chapter presents a model of the process by which individuals may develop a commitment and skills to carry out new paradigm research. An appendix suggests the elements needed in a training programme for researchers (CR 2.11.5).

2.12 SEARCHING THE LITERATURE

Once a preliminary working definition has been developed for the proposed research, the next step is to examine current knowledge about the concept under study by means of a literature review. This should be carried out carefully and critically with special attention being given to identifying inconsistencies, incompleteness and subtle differences of meaning. The reviewer should include, but not be confined to, the nursing literature and attempts made to trace the development of the concept under study. Both recent and past literature should be examined.

Definition

A . . . literature review is a carefully designed, logically developed discussion that provides the rationale for the problem statement, significance of the problem, theoretical perspective, research design and methodology

Annotations

[NB Included in this section are several examples of published literature reviews. They cover a variety of subjects and will help to show how literature reviews may be constructed. Further examples may be found in the International Journal of Nursing Studies and the Journal of Advanced Nursing. Two particular reviews, Choppin (1983) and Walton (1986) are major works commissioned by the Department of Health and Social Security (DHSS) (now the Department of Health). Other reviews may be found in research monographs and theses.]

2.12.1 Brearley, S. (1990) *Patient participation: the literature.* Harrow, Middlesex: Scutari   ISBN 1871364248   References

Reviews theoretical and descriptive literature from 1951-1989 on patient participation under headings of the active patient, chronic illness and patient participation re-examined. Final chapter discusses the research findings, implications and suggestions for further research of the project of which this review forms a part.

2.12.2 Choppin, R.G. (1983) *The role of the ward sister: a review of the British literature since 1967.* London: King's Fund Centre   KF Project Paper No 33

Report commissioned by the DHSS whose aim was to review the research literature relating to the role of ward sisters in the UK. It comprises 3 parts − Part I terms of reference, review of the area, the project's development, foci, methods and findings of the literature reviewed; Part II comprises summaries of the studies reviewed which are grouped under structure and management, teaching, job and professional attitudes and management training.

Each study includes aim(s), method, sample, findings, conclusions and comments. Part III is an extensive bibliography of the studies reviewed, references, and abstracts of research studies which were not reviewed, and a list of relevant non-research studies.

2.12.3 Cohen, S.A. (1981) Patient education: a review of the literature. *Journal of advanced nursing* 6(1) 11-18   75 References

Review of primarily North American Literature covers research and non-research material from 1957-1978. It seeks to provide a baseline of knowledge for those interested in beginning or re-evaluating patient education programmes and covers patient education in general. The non-research material covers principles methodology, content and barriers to patient education. Research based literature describes types of designs used by researchers or results of the studies. Comparisons between individual and group instruction are made.

2.12.4 Close, A. (1988) Patient education: a literature review. *Journal of advanced nursing* 13(2) 203-213   92   References

Covers British and American literature from 1940-1985 which examines the role of nurses as patient teachers. It covers the following aspects: the meaning of and necessity for patient education; reasons why nurses should be educators and the skills required; an examination of its present effectiveness and the barriers which exist to developing this aspect of the nurse's role.

2.12.5 Cooper, H.M. (1984) *The integrative research review: a systematic approach.* Beverly Hills: Sage   ISBN 0803920628   References

Book gives guidance on conducting an integrative research review in a systematic, objective way. The process of reviewing is carried out in five phases; problem formulation, data collection, data evaluation, analysis and interpretation and public presentation. This enables more rigorous reviews to be carried out with greater potential for creating consensus among scholars and focusing debate in a constructive fashion.

2.12.6 Goodman, C. (1986) Research on the informal carer: a selected literature review. *Journal of advanced nursing* 11(6) 705-712   24 References

A selected review of predominantly British literature from 1957-1985 on the role of the family in caring for elderly or handicapped relatives. Studies examine who the carers are, the nature of their responsibilities and the physical and mental costs involved. The paucity of research by nurses is highlighted.

2.12.7 Hurst, K. (1985) Traditional versus progressive nurse education: a review of the literature. *Nurse education today* 5(1) 30-36   42 References

Provides a summary of studies between 1965-1983 from Britain, the Commonwealth, European and American literature which examined the two categories of nurse education practices. These were traditional education which was teacher-centred and followed the medical model, and progressive methods characterised by student and patient predominance.

2.12.8 Kelly, M.P. & May, D. (1982) Good and bad patients: a review of the literature and a theoretical critique. *Journal of advanced nursing* 7(2) 147-156   102 References

British and American literature between 1950 and 1981 is reviewed to examine research into good and bad patients from the disciplines of nursing, psychology and sociology. Themes discussed include patient's diagnosis, behaviour, social background, attitudes and staff attitudes. Much of the literature was felt to be deficient on empirical, methodological, epistemological and theoretical grounds.

2.12.9 Myco, F. (1984) Stroke and its rehabilitation: the perceived role of the nurse in medical and nursing literature. *Journal of advanced nursing* 9(5) 429-439   146 References

Review covers nursing, medical and para-medical literature from English speaking countries and Scandinavia from 1951-1984 and aims to examine the perceived role of the nurse in the rehabilitation of stroke patients.

2.12.10 O'Kell, S.P. (1986) A literature search into the continuing education undertaken in nursing. *Nurse education today* 6(4) 152-157   36 References

Reviews British and American literature from 1954-1958 into continuing education. The provision made for doctors is noted and the various problems which seem to deter nurses from continuing this important aspect of professional development.

2.12.11 Sheehan, J. (1986) The professional standing of nurse teaching: a review of the literature. *Nurse education today* 6(1) 36-41   38 References

A review of predominantly British literature from 1906-1979 examining the concept of profession, professional status of nursing and teaching and the effect in terms of status of nurses who hold a teaching qualification.

2.12.12 Sims, S.E.R. (1987) Relaxation training as a technique for helping patients cope with the experience of cancer: a selective review of the literature. *Journal of advanced nursing* 12(5) 583-591   58 References

British and American literature from 1954-1985 is reviewed from the disciplines of nursing, medicine, psychology and psychiatry. It examines the use of relaxation training as a method of helping cancer patients together with progressive muscle relaxation and guided imagery. Summaries of some studies are included in table form.

2.12.13 Spencer, J.K. (1983) Nurses and cigarette smoking: a literature review. *Journal of advanced nursing* 8(3) 237-244   47 References

Review covers literature from the English speaking world from 1953-1982 and is concerned with three major areas: in what way are nurses heavy smokers, what particular aspects of nursing may cause nurses to smoke, and what influence does nurses' smoking behaviour have on the effectiveness of the use of nurses in health education campaigns.

2.12.14 Walton, I. (1986) *The nursing process in perspective: a literature review.* York: Department of Social Policy and Social Work, University of York   References (No ISBN number)

A review, commissioned by the Nursing Research Liason Group of the DHSS, of literature, both British and American, relating to the nursing process published between 1973 and 1983. It aimed to cover the vast anecdotal literature and the far less extensive but growing amount of research-based material. Part I comprises four sections − the emergence of the nursing process in the context of prevailing issues and concerns in British nursing; the confused and confusing way the process was often presented in the literature; an examination of reports of implementation in various areas of nursing and some evaluative research which has been attempted. Part 2 examines the nursing process in its wider theoretical and care contexts in a cross-disciplinary way. It reviews qualitative initiatives in medicine, developments in social work and some common strands between these disciplines and nursing. A postscript briefly reviews some relevant trends in the two years since the other surveys were completed.

2.12.15 Wright, D. (1984) An introduction to the evaluation of nursing care: a review of the literature. *Journal of advanced nursing* 9(5) 457-467   65 References

Review covers literature from the English-speaking world from 1957 to 1983 and examines ways of assessing the quality and consistency of nursing care and the maintenance of high standards. Three established methods are discussed − the Phaneuf audit, Slater Nursing Competencies Rating Scale and Quality Patient Care Scale (QUALPACS). Several management audit schemes are discussed together with the processes of peer review (CR 2.63.12, 2.63.19, 2.63.20).

Suggested textbook readings

	Pages	*Cross reference*
Abdellah & Levine	94-105	2.1.1
Adams & Schvaneveldt	49-75	2.1.2
Brink & Wood	57-65	2.1.7
Burns & Grove	127-153	2.1.12
Castles	45-53	2.1.15
Cormack (1990)	130-147	3.16.4
Fox	87-109	2.1.25
Grey M. IN LoBiondo-Wood & Haber	77-88	2.1.38
Gunter L. IN Krampitz & Pavlovich	11-16	2.1.32
Holm & Llewellyn	45-62	2.1.26
Howard & Sharp	67-96	3.21.5
Kovacs	41-48	2.1.31
Leedy	66-78	2.1.35
Nieswiadomy	73-89	2.1.43
Notter & Hott	54-62	2.1.44
Phillips L.R.F. (critique)	148-155	2.98.11
Polit & Hungler (1987)	62-79	2.1.56
Roberts & Burke	110-142	2.1.59
Seaman	141-152	2.1.62
Stodulski A.H. IN Cormack	60-73	2.1.20

2.13   REPLICATION RESEARCH

Replication of nursing research, particularly clinical studies, is an essential element of a sound empirically based body of knowledge fundamental to nursing practice. Replication studies are rarely found in the literature and the subject is largely ignored in many current research texts. Replication is a vital step in the development of nursing science and should therefore be supported and encouraged.

Definition
Replication means that researchers in other settings with different samples attempt to reproduce the research as closely as possible

Example
Ogier, M. (1986) An 'ideal' sister: seven years on. *Nursing times* 82(2) January 29   54-57   13 References   Occasional Paper

Describes the replication of a larger study conducted between 1977 and 1979 into the leadership style of ward sisters and its effect on nurse learners (Ogier 1982). The aim was to establish whether previous research findings were still relevant to a changing scene. Remarkably similar results were found.

Annotations
2.13.1   Collins, H.M. (1985) *Changing order: replication and induction in scientific practice.* London: Sage   ISBN 0803997574   References

Discusses the processes and outcomes of replication from a philosophical point of view and uses three field studies for illustration. These examined laser building, the detection of gravitational radiation and mind over matter. The complexities involved are explored.

2.13.2   Connelly, C.E. (1986) Replication research in nursing. *International journal of nursing studies* 23(1) 71-77   27 References

Discusses the importance and contribution of replication research in nursing to the development of nursing science. Factors which have deterred such studies are discussed together with various types and examples of replication research. Criteria for replicating a study are outlined.

2.13.3 Krueger, J.C., Fitzpatrick, J.J. & Kramer, M. (1981) Questions and answers: research replication. *Western journal of nursing research* 3(1) 94-97   5 References

Various points related to research replication are posed: ethical issues, a change of site and additional tools. Each question is answered by three experts.

2.13.4 Mulkay, M. & Gilbert, G.N. (1986) Replication and mere replication. *Philosophy of the social sciences* 16(1) 21-37   12 References

Documents some of the recurrent factors in scientists talk of replication. It identifies how scientists conceptions of research differ and ways in which these may be used to portray their own and others' reactions.

2.13.5 Neuliep, J.W. (ed) (1991) *Replication research in the social sciences.* Newbury Park: Sage   ISBN 0803940920   References

Discusses all aspects of replication research including the processes involved, its importance and editorial bias against it. Illustrative material is given from the literature of several disciplines.

2.13.6 Ryland, R.K. (1989) A plea for replication studies. *Journal of advanced nursing* 14(9) 699   Guest Editorial

Author argues that we cannot afford the luxury of allowing students in centres of higher education always to produce original work. More co-operation is needed within universities and research centres to concentrate on key issues and undergraduates should be encouraged to replicate other studies. In this way the body of nursing knowledge would grow and students would also receive the research training required.

Suggested textbook readings

	Pages	Cross reference
Barlow & Hersen	325-371	2.34.1
Burns & Grove	112-113	2.1.12
Bryman	37-38	2.9.1
Hakim	124-127	2.21.1
Kazdin	284-287	2.34.2
Kidder & Judd	26	2.1.30
Krathwohl	123-126/274-277/2 92-293	2.1.33
	Pages	Cross reference
Levin R.F. IN LoBiondo-Wood & Haber	371-372	2.1.38
Locke, Spirudoso & Silverman	49-52	2.99.6

Nursing research abstracts
Roper N.   78/2

2.14   RESEARCH PLANNING

There is no one design for research in nursing, just as there is no single design in any of its related sciences. Despite different philosophical origins, research methods and procedures are complementary. Studies of previous research in nursing reveal that many have had both quantitative and qualitative components, and to understand the complexity of nursing with its wide range of problems a variety of methods and procedures are required.

[Many textbooks do not include a section entitled 'Research Planning', rather a heading 'Research Processes'. In view of this please also refer to section 2.4.]

Annotations
2.14.1   Batey, M.V. (1990) Respect and appreciation for diversity in research. *Nursing science quarterly* 3(1) 4-5   No References

Nurse researchers are urged to respect and appreciate the diversity of methods which may be used to study nursing issues. Fixed philosophical or methodological positions may limit the value of the young field of nursing science.

2.14.2   Cormack, D.F.S. (1980) Obtaining access to data sources: an exploration of method, problems and possible solutions. *Journal of advanced nursing* 5(4) 357-370   18 References

The difficulties of gaining access to the field are discussed and some short and long term recommendations made to avoid problems in the future.

2.14.3   Herbert, M. (1990) *Planning a research project: a guide for practitioners and trainees in the helping professions.* London: Cassell Educational   ISBN 0304318469   References

A practical text covering all aspects of planning and executing a research project from generating ideas to the final report.

2.14.4   Sleep, J. (1985) Things I wish I'd known before I started. *Midwifery* 1(1) 54-57   7 References

Considers some points which need to be examined when embarking on any research project.

2.14.5   Vanetzian, E. (1987) Using PERT to keep a nursing research project humming. *Nursing research* 36(6) 388-392   2 References

Describes use of a tool Program Evaluation and Review Technique (PERT) for organising nursing research projects. It allows nurse researchers to estimate the time needed for each phase of the project and so increases efficiency.

2.14.6   Warren, M.D. (1985) Plan a research project. IN British Medical Association *How to do it.* London: BMA   ISBN 0727901869   117-121   14 References

A checklist of 13 items to be remembered when planning a research project. Each is elaborated upon.

Suggested textbook readings

	Pages	Cross references
Burgess R.G. (1984)	31-38	2.1.10
Fox	126-133	2.1.25
Leedy	14-42/79-102	2.1.35
Phillips L.R.F. (critique)	394-405	2.98.11
Polgar & Thomas	25-36	2.1.55
Smyth K. & Pavlovich N. IN Krampitz & Pavlovich	167-173/193-198	2.1.32
Sweeney & Olivieri	101-125	2.1.63
Wilson H.S. (1989)	227-274	2.1.69

2.15   COLLABORATIVE RESEARCH

This is an interdisciplinary approach to research where rights and responsibilities relating to the division of labour, ownership of ideas, publication rights and ethical issues are fully discussed before and during the project.

Definition
To work jointly, especially with one or a limited number of others, in a project involving composition or research

---

Example
Sweeney, M.A., Gulino, C., Lora, J.M. & Small, M.A. (1987) Collaboration in clinical research: bi-national projects shed new light on old issues. *Journal of professional nursing* 3(1) 28-38   38 References

Advantages and disadvantages of collaborative research cited in the literature are outlined and points are illustrated from a prospective study of 200 ante-partum patients in southern California and Mexico. The research team comprised 18 people and the issues arising were placed within a three-tiered framework covering technical, cultural and interpersonal dimensions.

Annotations

2.15.1 Chenger, P.L. (1988) Collaborative nursing research: advantages and obstacles. *International journal of nursing studies* 25(4) 295-300 12 References

Collaborative research in an academic and clinical setting are described. This provides one approach to developing the scientific base for nursing practice but also recognises economic realities. The advantages and obstacles of this type of research are highlighted.

2.15.2 Denyes, M.J., O'Connor, N.A., Oakley, D. & Ferguson, S. (1989) Integrating nursing theory, practice and research through collaborative research. *Journal of advanced nursing* 14(2) 141-145 16 References

One method for achieving the integration of theory, practice and research is described.

2.15.3 Engstrom, J.L. (1984) University, agency, and collaborative models for nursing research: an overview. *Image: the journal of nursing scholarship* 16(3) 76-80 25 References

Research based in academic institutions is compared with that of research agencies and the advantages and disadvantages of both are discussed. It is suggested that collaborative research might be advantageous as it combines the best of both worlds. Various types of collaborative research are described.

2.15.4 Hanson, S.M.H. (1988) Collaborative research and authorship credit: beginning guidelines. *Nursing research* 37(1) 49-52 14 References

Article outlines the advantages of collaborative research and discusses the issues and problems which can arise especially for inexperienced teams.

2.15.5 Hinshaw, A.S., Chance, H.C. & Atwood, J. (1981) Research in practice: a process of collaboration and negotiation. *Journal of nursing administration* 11(2) 33-38 6 References

A discussion of the problems encountered by undertaking research in a practice setting, using an actual study for illustration. Collaboration and negotiation between researcher and clinicians were found to be most important. Other issues discussed are the rights of research subjects, interpretation and use of results, risk taking, vested interest and contribution to scientific knowledge.

2.15.6 Keefe, M.R., Pepper, G. & Stoner, M. (1988) Towards research-based nursing practice: the Denver collaborative research network. *Applied nursing research* 1(3) 109-115 14 References

Describes the development of a network linking a centre for nursing research at the University of Colorado School of Nursing with three hospitals. Its research programmes are described and strategies offered for guiding the programme in the four critical stages of inititation, generation, incorporation and validation.

2.15.7 Lancaster. J. (1985) The perils and joys of collaborative research. *Nursing outlook* 33(5) 231-232, 238   3 References

The advantages and disadvantages of collaborative research are described and summed up by the author as the six *C*s: communication, commitment, consensus, compatibility, credit and contribution. The issues of project leadership, interpersonal relationships, organisational and funding difficulties and publication are discussed.

2.15.8 Thiele, J.E. (1989) Guidelines for collaborative research. *Applied nursing research* 2(4) 150-153   5 References

Study examined guidelines for collaborative research and the extent of agreement and disagreement within the research groups. Author suggests that written guidelines at the onset of a project may enable difficulties to be avoided.

Suggested textbook readings

	Pages	*Cross reference*
Boyle J.S. IN Morse (1989)	257-281	2.36.8
Grady & Wallston	20-35	3.11.2
Strasser J.A. IN Morse (1989)	95-113	2.36.8
Strauss A.L.	130-150	2.89.7

Nursing research abstracts

Lanara, V.	82/290
LeLean, S.R.	82/291
LeLean, S.R.	82/292
Lorenson, M.	81/133
McFarlane of Llandaff	82/293

2.16   THE REALITIES OF DOING RESEARCH

The conventions within research usually require authors to present their work in a particular order and format. In most instances this is of course most appropriate, but it tends to give the impression that research is more 'tidy' than it actually is, and the problems and difficulties encountered are not mentioned.

Annotations
2.16.1 Bell, C. (1978a) Studying the locally powerful: personal reflections on a research career. IN Bell, C. & Encel, S. (eds) *Inside the whale: ten personal accounts of social research.* Rushcutters Bay, New South Wales: Pergamon ISBN 0080222447   References 14-40

Author describes his development as a researcher, and summarises and criticises some of the studies in which he became involved. His changing views of sociology and the directions which were being pursued in the late 1960s and 1970s are outlined. There was a realisation that research was being commissioned by the locally powerful, often for political ends. The complexities of communities create almost insoluble problems for the social researcher, together with the surrounding political interests and issues which may limit access. The author recommends that sociological researchers should concentrate on the powerful so that the way they make decisions about the lives of others may be documented (CR 2.16.2).

2.16.2   Bell, C. & Encel, S .(eds) (1978b) *Inside the whale: ten personal accounts of social research.* Rushcutters Bay, New South Wales: Pergamon ISBN 0080222447   References

A collection of papers which allow a view into a normally closed world. They discuss many of the activities and factors which take place behind and around the methodology of research. The political and social issues which lie behind much research are highlighted and a wide range of styles are included to illustrate the problems, issues and constraints.

2.16.3   Bottomley, B. (1978) Words, deeds and post-graduate research. IN Bell, C. & Encel, S. (eds) *Inside the whale: ten personal accounts of social research.* Rushcutters Bay, New South Wales: Pergamon   ISBN 0080222447   References 216-237

Discusses the context, compromises made and restraints which occur in social research. Author highlights the inappropriateness of using quantitative methods in social situations, and claims that some academic departments pretend the problems do not exist and continue to teach students those particular methods. Some of the institutional problems and beliefs relating to post-graduate work are highlighted and the ensuing problems for the student are discussed (CR 2.16.2).

2.16.4   Bryman, A. (ed) (1988) *Doing research in organisations.* London: Routledge   ISBN 0415002583   References

Inside accounts are given of the processes involved in doing research in organisations.

2.16.5   Cannon, C. (1989) Social research in stressful settings: difficulties for the sociologist studying the treatment of breast cancer. *Sociology of health and illness* 11(1) 62-77   22 References

Author discusses some methodological and ethical issues arising in a three year study of breast cancer patients. Questions of involvement, detachment and personal responsibility are explored and the effects these had on the researcher (CR 2.17).

2.16.6   Gale, A. (1985) On doing research: the dream and the reality. *Journal of family therapy* 7(3) 187-211   17 References

Focuses on the experience of engaging in research and attempts to destroy some myths about researchers, research, the motives of research and those who become the subjects.

2.16.7 Georges, R.A. & Jones, M.O. (1980) *People studying people: the human element in fieldwork.* Berkeley, California: University of California Press ISBN 0520040678 References

Drawing on many researchers' experiences, authors discuss many of the difficulties inherent in conducting fieldwork.

2.16.8 Hockey, L. (1985) *Nursing research: mistakes and misconceptions.* Edinburgh: Churchill Livingstone ISBN 0443028621 References

Discusses in a light hearted way some of the pitfalls encountered by nurse researchers and how they might be avoided.

2.16.9 James, N. (1984) A postscript to nursing. IN Bell, C. & Roberts, H. (eds) *Social researching, politics, problems and practice.* London: Routledge & Kegan Paul ISBN 0710098847 References 7 125-146

Describes the experience of undertaking fieldwork in a continuing care unit (CR 2.1.5).

2.16.10 Lamb, G.S. (1989) Reflexivity in nursing research. *Western journal of nursing research* 11(6) 765-772 15 References

Highlights some problems which may arise when researchers become personally involved in the research process and discusses how objectivity may be sought. The philosophical content of reflexivity and the processes involved in quantitative and qualitative research are all discussed.

2.16.11 Morgan, D.H.J. (1982) The British Association scandal: the effect of publicity on a sociological investigation. IN Burgess, R.G. (ed) *Field research: a sourcebook and field manual.* London: Allen & Unwin ISBN 0043120148 References Section 9 34 254-263

Following the presentation of a paper to the British Association for the Advancement of Science about a workshop employing women workers, the author describes the ensuing publicity and the way in which this brought home some of the issues involved in any piece of sociological investigation (CR 2.1.9).

2.16.12 Roth, J. (1970) Hired hand research. IN Denzin, N.K. *Sociological methods: a sourcebook.* London: Butterworths ISBN 0408701250 References Part XIII Chapter 35 540-557

Section discusses some of the disadvantages and problems relating to the use of additional researchers in a project. Using three case studies of his own the author shows how observers may cheat in their record keeping; coders can be inconsistent in analysing questionnaire responses and how interviewers may fill in or fabricate answers for respondents (CR 2.1.23).

2.16.13 Silverman, D. (1987) *Communication and medical practice: social relations in the clinic.* London: Sage ISBN 0803981090 References

An account of several research studies which examined doctor-patient interactions in hospital clinics. Author believes that many research reports are too 'polished' and do not necessarily reflect reality, so the book includes detailed accounts of his feelings as a researcher, and how apparently disparate work can be woven into a whole.

Key themes are how doctor-patient talk varies according to the trajectory of the patients medical career, the method of payment for treatment, the problems implicit in paediatric medicine with children and parents as actors, and the intrinsic difficulties in reforming medical practice and making it more patient centred.

Suggested textbook reading

	Pages	Cross reference
Payne G. et al	181-210/211-235	2.36.10

Nursing research abstracts

Conneely F. & Badger F.	84/2
Fisher J.	85/530
Hockey L.	82/45 & 85/381
Luker K.A. & Box D.F.	86/074
Milne M.A.	80/7 & 81/283

2.17 ETHICAL ISSUES IN RESEARCH

Subjects in research studies have human rights that must be considered by investigators. Investigators also have rights, obligations and responsibilities to protect their subjects. There is a moral obligation to seek new knowledge, but it is never separate from the obligation to consider the rights of subjects who are expected to provide the new knowledge.

There are now many codes and regulations published by governments and professional organisations, but they are not enforceable, they have no legal sanction and documented instances show that they have a tendency to be ignored (Brandt 1978, Gray 1975, Pappworth 1967 & Rothman 1982). Neither has the setting up of ethical committees always provided the necessary safeguards, and examples of this are also cited in the literature (Anonymous 1988, Nicholson 1987 & Pappworth 1978).

Definition

A branch of philosophy concerned with what is good and bad and what one's moral obligations are.

Annotations

2.17.1 Anonymous (1988) Research without consent continues in the UK. London: *Institute of Medical Ethics bulletin* 40 July   Review 13-16

A patient describes feelings of outrage at discovering that she had been used in trials of breast cancer treatment without her knowledge or consent.

2.17.2 Association of American Medical Colleges (1982) The maintenance of high ethical standards in the conduct of research. *Journal of medical education* 57: November 895-902

Brief mention is made of the necessity for high ethical standards in research and reference is made to recent fraudulent misconduct in reporting of data. The need for the public to be protected and the maintenance of their confidence is stressed. Guidelines for the promotion of ethical standards within academic institutions are given, as is a detailed protocol for handling alleged fraud.

2.17.3 Besser, G.M. (1987) Portrait of an ethical committee. *Medical Research Council news* June No 35 21-24

Chairman of a District Health Authority Ethical Committee describes its nature and role.

2.17.4 British Sociological Association (1970) Statement of ethical principles and their application to sociological practice. *Sociology* 4(1) 114-117

Statement considers the responsibilities of the sociologist acting in a professional capacity to the discipline and subjects of study.

2.17.5 Bulmer, M. (ed) (1982) *Social research ethics*. London: Macmillan   ISBN 0333291980   References

This anthology re-examines the responsibilities of social researchers to their subjects in terms of privacy, confidentiality and ethical practice. The merits of covert participant observation are evaluated by experienced researchers in studies relating to mental patients, policemen, extremist political groups, pentecostal sects and homosexuals. The ethical and philosophical implications of covert research are discussed. Book contains a select bibliography.

2.17.6 Canadian Nurses Association (1972) Ethics of nursing research. *The Canadian nurse* 68(9) September 23-25

Provides guidelines for nurses relating to research subjects, the researcher and setting in which it takes place.

2.17.7 Clark, E. & Montgomery Robinson, K. (forthcoming) *Ethics in nursing and midwifery research*. Research Awareness, Module 6. London: Distance Learning Centre, South Bank Polytechnic   ISBN 0948250526   References

This is number 6 in a series of 13 modules, each of which deals with a different aspect of nursing research. It was developed to assist nurses, midwives and health visitors in understanding research in terms of their own professional practice. Modules can be used separately or as part of a programme. The reader is encouraged to work through a number of activities, self- assessment questions and answers and progress summaries. Some articles/book extracts referred to in the text are reproduced in full.

This module includes a general discussion about ethics in nursing and health care. The ethical issues involved in research and the rights of human subjects are explored in depth under five *C*s: caring, consent, confidentiality, codes and committees. Many examples of good and poor research practices are shown. It is stressed that this is not a text to prepare would-be researchers, but rather to assist nurses and midwives deal with the practical issues which may arise when a researcher asks for their assistance or access to patients, their records or staff (CR Appendix D).

2.17.8 Data Protection Registrar (1987) *Data Protection Act guidelines.* Wilmslow, Cheshire Office of the Data Protection Registrar   March

Guideline 1   *Introduction to the Act* Revision 1
             ISBN 1870466004
Guideline 2   *The definitions*
             ISBN 1870466012
Guideline 3   *The register and registration*
             ISBN 1870466020
Guideline 4   *The Data Protection principles*
             ISBN 1870466039
Guideline 5   *Individual rights*
             ISBN 1870466047
Guideline 6   *The exemptions*
             ISBN 1870466055
Guideline 7   *Enforcement and appeals*
             ISBN 1870466063
Guideline 8   *Summary for computer bureaux*
             ISBN 1870466071

Series of guidelines published by the Data Protection Registrar to inform individuals of their rights under the Act and help those who process personal data to understand their obligations.

[These guidelines will be revised from time to time. The Registrar's enquiry service will provide copies free and give advice re updating. Telephone no. Wilmslow (0625) 535777.]

2.17.9 Davis, A.J. & Krueger,J.C. (eds) (1980) *Patients, nurses and ethics.* New York: American Journal of Nursing Company   ISBN 0937126845   References

Book contains papers presented at a symposium of the Western Society of Nurse Researchers at Portland, Oregon in 1979, together with some additional material. Its aim was to discuss selected ethical issues central to nursing research. Major areas included are ethical concerns, background, federal regulations and institutional review boards, dimensions of informed consent, ethics of research with specific subject groups and research and professional dilemmas. Appendices include guidelines and a code for nurses, a manual of procedures, sample consent forms and an experimental subjects Bill of Rights.

2.17.10   Denham, M. (1984) Ethics of research. *Nursing mirror* 158(3) January 18 36-38   12 References

Author argues that research in the elderly should be subject to the same high ethical standards as in any other subject.

2.17.11   Duncan, A.S., Dunstan, G.R. & Welbourn, R.B. (eds) (1981) *Dictionary of medical ethics.* London: Darton, Longman & Todd   ISBN 0232514925

A source of information on all aspects of ethics.

2.17.12   Dworking, G. & Taylor, R.D. (1989) *Blackstone's guide to the Copyright, Designs and Patents Act 1988.* London: Blackstone Press   ISBN 1854310232 References

Gives coverage of copyright and related rights and is intended as a book of first reference. It explains the basic principles and rules so that decisions can be made as to whether further advice is necessary. A copy of the Act is included.

2.17.13   Erikson, K.T. (1971) A comment on disguised observation in sociology. IN Franklin, B.J. & Osborne, H.W. (eds) *Research methods: issues and insights.* Belmont: California, Wadsworth   (No ISBN number)   Chapter 8   66-75

Chapter discusses the question of the researcher in a covert or disguised role. Although rarely used by sociologists it raises ethical issues.

2.17.14   Ethical Committee, University College Hospital (1981) Experience at a clinical research ethical review committee. *British medical journal* 283(6302) November 14 1312-1314   10 References

One hospital ethical committee expresses some opinions about its functions.

2.17.15   Faulder, C. (1985) *Who's body is it?: the troubled issue of informed consent.* London: Virago   ISBN 0860686450   References

Book opens the debate about the ethical and medical issues raised for all health care consumers. Appendices contain some ethical codes/declarations, a Patient's Bill of Rights and a pro forma for informed consent to participate in a clinical trial.

2.17.16   Faulkner, A. (1980) Nursing as a research based profession: some ethical issues. *Nursing focus* August 476-479, 481   11 References

Article discusses nurses ethical responsibilities in gaining permission for research projects, the choice of data collection methods, confidentiality and the importance of honesty with subjects.

2.17.17 Fleetwood, J.E., Arnold, R.M. & Baron, R.J. (1989) Giving answers or raising questions: the problematic role of institutional ethics committees. *Journal of medical ethics* 15(3) 137-142   14 References

Discusses the growing phenomenon of institutional ethics committees in the American Health Care system, analyses the assumptions underlying their establishment and evaluates their strengths and weaknesses.

2.17.18 Fowler, M.D.M. (1988) Ethical issues in nursing research: a call for an international code of ethics for nursing research. *Western journal of nursing research* 10(3) 352-355   4 References

Following an international conference on nursing research in July 1987 in Edinburgh, Scotland it was proposed that nursing should develop an international code of ethics for nursing research, because of the problems highlighted by delegates from many parts of the world.

2.17.19 Fry, S.T. (1981) Accountability in research: the relationship of scientific and humanistic values. *Advances in nursing science* 4(1) 1-13   22 References

An overview of nurses' moral, ethical, professional and personal values. The potential conflict in moral values of the nurse as clinician and researcher are identified.

2.17.20 Great Britain. *Copyright, Designs and Patents Act 1988.* London HMSO   ISBN 0105448885

Act covers in Part 1 subsistence, ownership and duration of copyright, rights of copyright owners and acts permitted in relation to copyright works. It also includes remedies for infringement, copyright licensing, the copyright tribunal, qualification for and extent of protection, miscellaneous and general. Part 2 covers rights in performances, miscellaneous and general. Schedule 8 lists all related acts which have been repealed.

2.17.21 Great Britain. *Data Protection Act 1984.* London: HMSO   ISBN 0105435848

Act covers preliminary details, registration and supervision of data users and computer bureaux, rights of data subjects, exemptions and a general section.

2.17.22 Institute of Medical Ethics (1987a) Integrity of scientific literature questioned. *IME bulletin* No 26 May 4-6

Briefly describes an investigation into the integrity of scientific literature after a well known case involving fraud; errors and sloppiness had been identified. A primary cause was felt to be the pressure to publish to enhance career advancement.

2.17.23 Institute of Medical Ethics (1987b) The Lugano statements on controlled clinical trials. *IME bulletin* April 1-2

An attempt to create some general guidelines on controlled clinical trials.

2.17.24   Institute of Medical Ethics (1987c) Medicines Commission advice to health ministers on healthy volunteer studies. *IME bulletin* No 30 September 8-9

A summary of the conclusions and recommendations made to health ministers on healthy volunteer studies. The advice is said to be complementary to that given by the Royal College of Physicians (CR 2.17.45).

2.17.25   Institute of Medical Ethics (1987d) Research ethics committees and public responsibility. *IME bulletin* No 22 January 1 Editorial

Discusses whether a register of approved research projects should be available for public inspection. Guidelines from the Royal College of Physicians contain a dichotomy. An alternative approach used in the USA is outlined (CR 2.17.45).

2.17.26   Institute of Medical Ethics (1987e) Towards an international ethic for research involving human subjects. Boi-Ethics Summit Conference: Ottawa, Canada April 5-10 1987 *IME bulletin*   Supplement No 6 May 1-6

Summarises the main recommendations of the conference. Included in their deliberations were for example the development and implementation of national ethical standards, pilot studies and the introduction of novel therapies, industrial research, the selection of research topics, directed research and the improvement of ethical standards.

2.17.27   Institute of Medical Ethics (1987f) The use and abuse of confidentiality. *IME bulletin* No 31 1 Editorial

Editor of this bulletin gives an account of his removal from the ethics committee of a private hospital because it was said that he had broken the rule of confidentiality. There is full discussion about confidentiality and whether by maintaining this the committee is actually fulfilling its duty of protecting the public (CR 2.17.32).

2.17.28   Kelman, H.C. (1971) Deception in social research. IN Franklin, B.J. & Osborne, H.W. (eds) *Research methods: issues and insights*. Belmont: California, Wadsworth   (No ISBN Number)   Chapter 7   58-65

Discusses the potential and actual effects on subjects where full information about the research in which they are participating is not given. The ethical implications of this are explored.

2.17.29   Lawrence, J.A. & Farr, E.H. (1982) The nurse should consider critical care ethical issues. *Journal of advanced nursing* 7(3) 223-229   20 References

Nurses attending a workshop on the ethics of critical care nursing were asked to respond to the questions, What should you do and what would you do in a hypothetical dilemma relating to the resuscitation of an intensive care patient. They agreed that patients wishes and rights, the legal consequences and physician authority should be considered and peer influence should not. The nurses were divided in their attitudes to following procedures, personal moral beliefs and job risk. The most contentious issues related to the nurses role as a decision-making member of the health care team.

2.17.30   Leino-Kilpi, H. & Tuomaala, U. (1989) Research ethics and nursing science: an empirical example. *Journal of advanced nursing* 14(6) 451-458   13 References

Article identifies points in the research process where ethical considerations are of particular importance. The reporting of ethical problems in theses produced by Finnish nursing science graduates is used to illustrate the difficulties.

2.17.31   Macmillan, M. (1987) Research issues 4. informed consent. *Senior nurse* 7(3) 12   11 References

The elements which make up fully informed consent are discussed and nurses urged to become aware of the complexities involved.

2.17.32   Nicholson, R. (1987) Sickness of the secret society. *The Mail on Sunday*, November 15

Serious questions are raised about the medical profession's willingness to be frank with the public, after a leading member of an ethical committee was sacked for breaching confidentiality about test tube baby techniques which he considered raised serious ethical questions (CR 2.17.27).

2.17.33   Oddi, L.F. & Cassidy, V.R. (1990) Participation and perception of nurse members in the hospital ethics committee. *Western journal of nursing research* 12(3) 307-317   28 References

Describes a study, as part of a larger investigation, which explored the degree to which nurses are involved in the decision making of ethical committees. How they saw their role was examined together with the preparation they had received.

2.17.34   Pappworth, M.H. (1978) Medical ethical committees: a review of their functions. *World medicine* February 22 19-21,57,61,64,67-69,71-72,74,76,78

Examples of unethical practices are cited which happened despite the existence of ethical committees. The author believes entrenched attitudes and collusion between researchers is considerable.

2.17.35   Pearce, P., Parsloe, P., Francis, H., Macara, A. & Watson, D. (1988) *Personal data protection in health and social sciences.* London: Croom Helm   ISBN 0709936818   References

Book describes the implications of the 1984 Data Protection Act for students and professionals in the health and social services.

2.17.36   Pence, T. (1986) *Ethics in nursing: an annotated bibliography.* 2nd edition New York: National League for Nursing   ISBN 0887371922

Contains 1324 citations from 1965 to 1985. References are mainly to American literature but some British sources are also included. Several citations refer to the ethics of nursing research.

2.17.37   Phillips, M. & Dawson, J. (1985) *Doctors dilemmas, medical ethics and contemporary science*. Brighton: Harvester Press   ISBN 0710809832   References

Contains the Inter-Professional Working Group Code of Confidentiality of Personal Health Data; the Hippocratic Oath; International Code of Medical Ethics and other Declarations of the World Medical Association from 1948 to 1983. A doctor and a journalist explore and analyse the key ethical questions currently in the headlines. Book is written without jargon for the general public.

2.17.38   Pollock, L. & Tilley, S. (1988) Submitting for approval. *Senior nurse* 8(5) 24-25   3 References

Some novice researchers discuss their experiences when presenting their work to medical ethics committees.

2.17.39   Ramos, M.C. (1989) Some ethical implications of qualitative research. *Research in nursing and health* 12(1) 57-63   45 References

Briefly outlines ethical considerations in quantitative research and then discusses the research relationship, confidentiality issues, interpretation and reporting, informed consent and deception relating to qualitative research.

2.17.40   Renaud, M. (1980) The ethics of consumer protection research. *American journal of public health* 70(10) 1098-1099   4 References

Author puts one viewpoint about the appropriateness of using pseudo patients to evaluate the quality of care i.e. that information gathered is both necessary and ethically acceptable within certain limits (CR 2.17.52).

2.17.41   Reynolds, P.D. (1982) *Ethics and social science research.* Englewood Cliffs, New Jersey: Prentice Hall   ISBN 0132909650   References

Book discusses the decisions which sociologists need to make when undertaking research and the implications of these for making valid conclusions. It focuses on general methodological problems which are clarified by use of illustrative material. Basic issues are discussed, overt and covert research, cross-cultural research, studies of social systems, external control and applications of scientific knowledge.

2.17.42   Royal College of Nursing of the United Kingdom (1977) *Ethics related to research in nursing.* London: RCN

Outlines the responsibilities of nurses undertaking research, those in positions of authority where research is to be carried out and practising nurses who may need also to give permission or become involved.

2.17.43   Royal College of Physicians (1990a) *Guidelines on the practice of ethics committees in medical research involving human subjects.* 2nd edition London: RCP   ISBN 0900596902

A detailed and comprehensive guide to the role, functions and responsibilities of ethics committees is provided. The membership, terms of reference, scope, methods of working and of referral to the committee and its responsibilities in law are all examined. Issues of consent, therapeutic trials, research involving vulnerable groups, healthy volunteers and foetuses, payment for participation in trials and injuries due to clinical investigations are all fully explored.

2.17.44   Royal College of Physicians (1990b) *Research involving patients.* London: RCP   ISBN 0900596910

This report constitutes a detailed guide to the issues which need to be addressed prior to involving patients in research. These include definition of patient status and of research, justification for the research, the role of ethics committees, the quality of research and selection of patients. Much of the report is devoted to problems of consent, for example in children, the very ill and prisoners. Payments, contracts and inducements are examined as are problems surrounding controlled therapeutic trials. How research should be conducted and monitored, and the ownership of results are reviewed. Arrangements for compensation of patients injured by participation in research are clarified.

2.17.45   Royal College of Physicians of London (1984) *Guidelines on the practice of ethics committees in medical research.* London: RCP

Provides a source of information and opinion on a range of matters concerning the procedures of ethics committees. Contains a bibliography (CR 2.17.25).

2.17.46   Sawyer, L.M. (1989) Nursing code of ethics: an international comparison. *International nursing review* 36(5) Issue 287 145-148   17 References

Analyses the codes of selected national nurses associations.

2.17.47   Scott, D. (1982) Ethical issues in nursing research: access to human subjects. *Topics in clinical nursing* April: 74-83   8 References

The process of obtaining ethical approval for nursing research is described. Particular reference is made to the institutional review or ethics committee. Five stages in the process of recruiting are described, each one raising different ethical issues.

2.17.48   Sieber, J.E. (ed) (1982) *The ethics of social research: fieldwork, regulation and publication.* New York: Springer-Verlay   ISBN 0387906916   References

Identifies how ethical dilemmas arise in day to day conduct of social research and suggests how they may be resolved.

2.17.49   Tingle, J.H. (1988) Some recent court cases of interest to nurses. *Senior nurse* 8(6) 11-12

Some recent judicial decisions are outlined including a case relating to the legal position of a hospital's ethical committee and the discretion of a consultant.

2.17.50   Veatch, R.M. & Fry, S.T. (1987) *Case studies in nursing ethics.* Philadelphia: Lippincott   ISBN 0397544731   References

Volume contains a collection of cases focusing on the ethical problems faced by nurses. It is divided into three parts — ethics and values in nursing, ethical principles and special problem areas in nursing practice.

2.17.51   Wallis. R. (1977) The moral career of a research project. IN Bell, C. & Newby, H. (eds) *Doing sociological research.* London: Allen & Unwin References   ISBN 0043000711   Chapter 7   149-167

Chapter discusses the moral and political dilemmas posed when doing research on human subjects. A study of Scientology is used to illustrate these problems (CR 2.1.4).

2.17.52   Weiss, R.J. (1980) The use and abuse of deception. *American journal of public health* 70(10) 1097-1098   3 References

Paper refers to a research project where pseudo-patients are used to evaluate the quality of care. Author feels that such deception is unjustified and discusses some of the moral and ethical issues involved (CR 2.17.40).

Suggested textbook readings

	Pages	Cross reference
Abbott N.K. IN Krampitz & Pavlovich	98-102	2.1.32
Abdellah & Levine	314-317	2.1.1
Adams & Schvaneveldt	27-35	2.1.2
Brink & Wood	184-197	2.1.7
Burgess R.G. (1984)	38-52/185-208	2.1.10
Burns & Grove	335-359	2.1.12
Castles	126-137	2.1.15
Chenitz & Swanson	155-164	2.46.2
Christensen	329-350	2.1.17
Fowler M. & Fry S.T. IN Sarter	145-163	2.1.61
Fox	53-73	2.1.25
Holm & Llewellyn	229-245	2.1.26
Jackson B.S. IN LoBiondo-Wood & Haber	37-55	2.1.38
Kidder & Judd	452-510	2.1.30
Kovacs	15-28	2.1.31
Nieswiadomy	173-185	2.1.43
Notter & Hott	34-37	2.1.44
Phillips L.R.F. (critique)	272-303	2.98.11
Polgar & Thomas	30-31	2.1.55
Polit & Hungler (1987)	22-24	2.1.56
Roberts & Burke	184-210	2.1.59
Schrock R. IN Cormack	193-204	2.1.20
Seaman	21-35	2.1.62

	Pages	*Cross reference*
Smith H.W.	3-17	2.98.14
Sweeney & Olivieri	151-162	2.1.63
Thomas	63-66	2.1.64
Treece & Treece	126-142	2.1.65
Waltz, Strickland & Lenz	325-339	2.56.5
Wilson H.S. (1989)	65-102	2.1.69
Wilson-Barnett J. IN Cormack	74-80	2.1.20

Nursing research abstracts

Alderson, P.	81/116
Allen, P.A. & Walters, W.E.	83/1
Altschul, A.	82/47
Gutteridge, F.	82/446
Hockey, L.	83/5
Hurst, K.	85/527

2.18   DEFINING THE PROBLEM

The word 'problem' has several meanings and authors are not in agreement about this. They do all agree however that whatever the meaning the problem should be clearly formulated. This is important as it provides the frame of reference for the study, structures the ideas of the researcher and dictates the content of the literature review.

Definitions

The problem statement is a focused description of the area under investigation that presents the unanswered question and provides information about where specific answers are needed

An operational definition assigns meaning to a variable and describes the activities required to measure it

---

Annotations

2.18.1 Baldamus, W. (1979) Alienation, anomie and industrial accidents IN Wilson, M. (ed) *Social and educational research in action: a book of readings.* London: Longman in association with the Open University Press   ISBN 058229004X References   Section 2 Reading 6 104-140

This paper by a social scientist is rare in that it reports the very early stages of a major research project. It takes the reader to the position where an idea begins before it is known whether there is a problem worth researching or what the problem is. The focus is on the startling rise in industrial accidents reported to the Factory Inspectorate in the 1960s and the similarity between the variations by days of the week in the patterns of absenteeism and industrial accidents. More widely, methodological issues in studies on social change are explored and a preliminary assessment of the use and limitations of sociological time-series studies is made (CR 2.1.70).

2.18.2   Campbell, J.P., Daft, R.L. & Hulin, C.L. (1982) *What to study: generating and developing research questions.* Beverly Hills: Sage   ISBN 0803918720 References

A teaching device intended to examine what is being investigated versus what should be. Book discusses how research questions are developed, gives a list of ideas for consideration, suggests ways of reformulating research questions and how difficulties may be avoided. Some resource materials are also included.

2.18.3   Clark, E. (1987) *Identifying and defining questions for research.* Research Awareness, Module 5   London: Distance Learning Centre, South Bank Polytechnic ISBN 0948250275   References

This is number 5 in a series of 13 modules, each of which deals with a different aspect of nursing research. It was developed to assist nurses, midwives and health visitors to understand research in terms of their own professional practice. Modules can be used separately or as part of a programme. The reader is encouraged to work through a number of self-assessment questions and answers and progress summaries. Some articles/book extracts referred to in the text are reproduced in full.

This module looks at the identification and refining of questions which could be researched, formulating hypotheses if appropriate, and discusses the relationship between clinical nurses and the nurse researcher (CR 2.20, Appendix D).

2.18.4   Fleming, J.W. (1984) Selecting a clinical nursing problem for research. *Image: the journal of nursing scholarship* 16(2) 62-64   5 References

A series of questions are identified which will assist in the appropriate selection of problems.

2.18.5   Moody, L., Vera, H., Blanks, C. & Visscher, M. (1989) Developing questions of substance for nursing science. *Western journal of nursing research* 11(4) 393-404   15 References

Describes a study undertaken to establish from leading nurse researchers the sources and origins of their ideas, devices for finding and developing researchable questions or hypotheses and how they decided which were significant for the discipline.

Focused interviews were conducted by telephone and data analysed by computer. Data showed that significant questions are those aimed at nursing intervention and clinical research and that students need to be guided early to find those important to nursing (CR 2.72).

Suggested textbook readings

	Pages	Cross reference
Abdellah & Levine	86-93	2.1.1
Brink & Wood	1-56	2.1.7
Burns & Grove	109-125	2.1.12
Castles	29-33	2.1.15
Christensen	51-61	2.1.17
Eells M.A.W. IN Krampitz & Pavlovich	3-10	2.1.32
Fox	74-86	2.1.25
Grady & Wallston	36-47	3.11.2
Kovacs	29-39	2.1.31
Lin	133-144	2.1.37
LoBiondo-Wood & Haber	59-74	2.1.38
Leedy	45-65	2.1.35
Nieswiadomy	57-72	2.1.43
Notter & Hott	45-53	2.1.44
Phillips L.R.F. (critique)	135-148	2.98.11
Polit & Hungler (1987)	49-61	2.1.56
Roberts & Burke	80-108	2.1.59
Seaman	128-131	2.1.62
Sweeney & Olivieri	67-73	2.1.63
Thomas	38-48/56-57	2.1.64
Treece & Treece	65-71	2.1.65
Wilson H.S. (1989)	207-226	2.1.69
Woods & Catanzaro	35-45	2.1.72

2.19 IDENTIFICATION OF VARIABLES

Variables are those factors, events or behaviours about which information is desired, and they may be studied in isolation or in combination. They can be examined in their natural setting or manipulated to see if a particular response is evoked. During a study unknown variables may arise which may affect the data collected.

Definitions

Variable − factor within a situation which can change or be changed

Dependent variable − dependent upon or caused by another variable. It is NOT controlled by the researcher

Independent variable − believed to cause or influence the dependent variable. In experimental studies it IS manipulated by the researcher

---

Annotation

2.19.1 Burgess, R.G. (ed) (1986) *Key variables in social investigation.* London:
Routledge & Kegan Paul ISBN 0710206216 References

A series of papers which examine the relationship between theory and research, the
identification of concepts and their translation into variables. Health and illness are
two key variables explored.

Suggested textbook readings

	Pages	Cross reference
Abdellah & Levine	125-163	2.1.1
Brink & Wood	84-86	2.1.7
Burns & Grove	197-204	2.1.12
Castles	33-38	2.1.15
Christensen	66-100	2.1.17
Fox	239-240	2.1.25
Holm & Llewellyn	63-71	2.1.26
Kidder & Judd	70-72/83-84/ 319-321	2.1.30
Kovacs	147-148	2.1.31
Lin	73-109	2.1.37
Notter & Hott	70-71	2.1.44
Polit & Hungler (1987)	106-110	2.1.56
Treece & Treece	156-173	2.1.65
Williamson	103-104	2.1.67

2.20 FORMULATING HYPOTHESES OR RESEARCH QUESTIONS

A frequent goal in scientific research is to test a hypothesis which may be concerned
with explaining relationships between observations or differences between groups.
Some research projects do not have hypotheses because they have different objectives
and these may be guided by research questions and/or research objectives.

Definitions

Hypotheses — a statement of relationship between two or more variables
Null hypothesis — a statistical hypothesis claiming no difference between groups
Research objective — states the goal(s) of a study which is intended to describe rather
  than predict

Suggested textbook readings

2.21 SELECTING A RESEARCH DESIGN

The design is a blueprint for conducting the research. It contains plans for collecting, organising and analysing the data. The choice of design depends on the purposes of the study but it is generally approached from a descriptive or experimental perspective.

'Research is never as perfect as we would like; every type of design involves compromise and error' (Phillips L.R.F. 1986).

Definition

A set of instructions to the investigator for gathering and analysing data

---

Annotations

2.21.1 Hakim, C. (1987) *Research design: strategies and choices in the design of social research.* London: Allen & Unwin   ISBN 0043120326   References

Text deals with all aspects of the design of social research covering both theoretical and policy research. The key features, strengths and limitations of eight main types of design are discussed. These are literature reviews, secondary analysis and meta-analysis of existing data, qualitative research, analysis of administrative records, ad hoc sample surveys, regular surveys, case studies, longitudinal studies and experimental social research. The focus is not on how to do any type of research but when and why a particular design should be chosen. The second part of the book focuses on more general issues such as potential difficulties and possible solutions, obtaining research funding and designing and managing research programmes.

2.21.2 Leatt, P. (1986) Descriptive and experimental approaches to nursing problems: issues in design. IN Stinson, S.M. & Kerr, J.C. *International issues in nursing research.* Beckenham: Croom Helm   ISBN 07099443733   References   Part 1 Chapter 1   1-27

Chapter discusses the purposes, types and complexity of research designs appropriate for studying a practice discipline. The major types of research design are discussed using the concept of a continuum of control and each is illustrated by existing studies (CR 3.27.7).

2.21.3 Spector, P.E. (1981) *Research designs.* Beverly Hills: Sage   ISBN 0802917090   References

An introduction to the basic principles of experimental and non-experimental design in the social sciences.

2.21.4 Waltz, C.F. & Bausell, R.B. (1981) *Nursing research: design, statistics and computer analysis.* Philadelphia: Davis   ISBN 0803690401   References

Text designed for basic and advanced level students which will assist in the design, analysis and reporting of research. Little or no background knowledge is assumed so detailed explanations of concepts and principles are included. Examples are used throughout the text (CR 2.82, 2.88, 2.100).

Suggested textbook readings

	Pages	Cross reference
Abdellah & Levine	164-213	2.1.1
Adams & Schvaneveldt	101-118	2.1.2
Brink & Wood	94-117	2.1.7
Burns & Grove	227-280	2.1.12
Castles	55-59	2.1.15
Christensen	22-50	2.1.17
Cook and Campbell	341-386	2.35.1
Evans J. (DE 304) 3A/3B	5-44/83-111	2.1.48/49

	Pages	*Cross reference*
Fox	137-142	2.1.25
Grady & Wallston	48-65	3.11.2
Holm & Llewellyn	73-96	2.1.26
LoBiondo-Wood	127-144	2.1.38
Miller D.C.	1-61	2.56.3
Murdaugh C. IN Phillips L.R.F. (critique)	203-248	2.98.11
Polgar & Thomas	94-102	2.1.55
Polit & Hungler (1987)	117-205	2.1.56
Seaman	165-230	2.1.62
Stinson & Kerr	1-27	3.27.7
Treece & Treece	113-125/174-214	2.1.65
Williamson	113-121	2.1.67
Wilson H.S. (1989)	132-175	2.1.69
Woods & Catanzaro	117-132	2.1.72

2.22 POPULATIONS AND SAMPLES

Nursing research is usually concerned with populations of people and the intention of the researcher is to say something about them and their responses to a health care system. Careful identification and description of the population, together with appropriate sample selection techniques, are important steps in any research design.

Researchers are not entirely in agreement about the language used to define populations but the following set of definitions is listed in descending order of size.

Definitions
Universe − all possible respondents or measures of a certain kind
Population − the portion of the universe to which the researcher has access
Target population − all the cases that meet a designated set of criteria
Population stratum − a population contained within another population
Population element − a single member of a population

Sampling is the process of selecting a few elements from a population. These elements are expected to stand for all those within the population. The way in which this is done allows one to generalise the sample findings to a population, or does not allow one to do so. Sampling strategies are divided into two major groups:

1. Probability sampling techniques
2. Non-probability sampling techniques

Definitions
1. Probability sampling techniques

Cluster sample − groups of population elements with the same characteristics are chosen rather than individuals

Simple random sample −obtained using a table of random numbers, or some other means, and each population element has an equal probability of being selected

Stratified random sample − population divided into sub-groups called strata and then a simple random sample is obtained

Systematic random sample − obtained by taking every Kth (selection interval) name on a population list

2. Non-probability sampling techniques

Convenience (accidental) sample − sample obtained by accessing individuals who are easy to identify and contact

Purposive sample − cases to be included are handpicked for their experience or knowledge or some other characteristic of interest to the researcher

Quota sample − sample aimed at ensuring adequate representation of underlying groups e.g. age or ethnic groups

Snowball sample − selection is carried out by word of mouth. The first people contacted are asked to name others with similar characteristics

Annotations
2.22.1 Diekmann, J.M. & Smith, J.M. (1989) Strategies for accessing and recruiting of subjects for nursing research. *Western journal of nursing research* 11(4) 418-430   35 References

Discusses strategies for recruiting appropriate subjects into a study.

2.22.2 Honigmann, J.J. (1982) Sampling in ethnographic fieldwork. IN Burgess, R.G. (ed) *Field research: a sourcebook and field manual.* London: Allen & Unwin   ISBN 004312014   References 12: 79-90

Probability and non-probability sampling techniques as applied to ethnographic research are discussed (CR 2.1.9, 2.43).

2.22.3 Stewart, M.J. (1989) Target populations of nursing research on social support. *International journal of nursing studies* 26(2) 115-129   136 References

63 empirical studies carried out over the last decade were examined to ascertain their target populations. Nurses have tended to study populations central to their professional activities and those examined related to surgical patients, the chronically ill, expectant couples, parents of infants, the bereaved and lay care givers. Author

believes there are several groups which have been overlooked, for example children, males, native peoples, the poor, unemployed and the victims of child and elderly abuse.

Suggested textbook readings

	Pages	*Cross reference*
Abdellah & Levine	214-231	2.1.1
Adams & Schvaneveldt	173-195	2.1.2
Brink & Wood	120-136	2.1.7
Burgess (1982)	53-77	2.1.9
Burns & Grove	205-226	2.1.12
Calder J. (DE 304) 3B	3-40	2.1.49
Castles	71-85	2.1.15
Chisnall	47-103	2.1.16
Christensen	118-123	2.1.17
Fox	272-288	2.1.25
Grady & Wallston	66-83	3.11.2
Holm & Llewellyn	143-153	2.1.26
Kidder & Judd	143-167	2.1.30
Kovacs	99-108	2.1.31
Lin	145-165	2.1.37
LoBiondo-Wood & Haber	267-288	2.1.38
Miller D.C.	52-56	2.56.3
Morse (1989)	117-131	2.36.8
Nieswiadomy	155-172	2.1.43
Phillips L.R.F. (critique)	223-228	2.98.11
Polgar & Thomas	37-49	2.1.55
Polit & Hungler (1987)	206-223	2.1.56
Roberts & Burke	212-234	2.1.59
Seaman	223-249	2.1.62
Smith H.W.	105-131	2.98.14
Sweeney & Olivieri	137-147	2.1.63
Treece & Treece	215-236	2.1.65
Waltz & Bausell	31-38	2.21.4
Williamson	169-190	2.1.67
Wilson H.S. (1989)	256-270	2.1.69
Woods & Catanzaro	97-116	2.1.72

Nursing research abstracts

Hardy, L.K.	83/364
Wilson, K.J.W.	R 29 (Retrospective volume 1968-1976)

2.23   PILOT STUDIES

Pilot studies are undertaken to assess the feasibility of a planned study, adequacy of the instrumentation, and problems in data collection strategies and proposed methods. Other potential uses may be to answer a methodological question, or as part of the development of a research plan.

Definition
A small scale trial of the research method to ensure that the design is feasible

Example
Lopez, M.J. & Radford, N.H. (1985) District nurse training: a pilot survey of demand, provision and students. *Journal of advanced nursing* 10(4) 361-367   5 References

A pilot survey of district nurse training provision for the period April 1982 to March 1983 was undertaken to provide a profile of training institutions, their resources, courses and students. Information was obtained by postal questionnaire sent to 50 institutions. The survey showed the feasibility and value of collecting data in this way and it has provided the basis for a further study (Baseline Data Project) which will produce a package of survey material and software for analysis of subsequent data.

Annotations
2.23.1   Lackey, N.R. & Wingate, A.L. (1989) The pilot study: one key to research success. IN Brink, P.J. & Wood, M.J. A (eds) *Advanced design in nursing research.* Newbury Park: Sage   ISBN 0803927428   References   Chapter 13   285-292

Chapter defines a pilot study, its philosophies and purposes. Discusses conducting the study and evaluating the results (CR 2.36.3).

2.23.2   Ort, S.V. (1981) Research design: pilot study. IN Krampitz, S.D. & Pavlovich, N. (eds) *Readings for nursing research.* St Louis: Mosby   ISBN 0801627478   References   Chapter 6   49-53

Discusses the purposes and characteristics of a pilot study, its design and implementation. Ethical aspects are covered, reliability and validity of instruments, potential difficulties and guidelines are given for developing the study (CR 2.1.32).

2.23.3   Prescott, P.A. & Soeken, K.L. (1989) The potential uses of pilot work. *Nursing research* 38(1) 60-62   3 References

Following a review of published studies and research texts, the authors reported that pilot studies are under-discussed, under-used and under-reported. Article focuses on the separate components within a main study, and highlights the contribution of pilot work to each. Although increasing the time spent in preparation for a study it can enable defects to be corrected which cannot be removed or remedied after the study has commenced.

Suggested textbook readings

	Pages	Cross reference
Fox	43	2.1.25
Grady & Wallston	145-146	3.11.2
Lin	199-200	2.1.37
Locke, Spirduso & Silverman	66/68-69	2.99.6
Polgar & Thomas	33	2.1.55
Polit & Hungler (1987)	38-39	2.1.56
Treece & Treece	378-400	2.1.65

Nursing research abstracts
Kratz C.R.   R25 (Retrospective volume 1968-1976)

2.24   RELIABILITY

Reliability and validity are two major characteristics which need to be considered when undertaking both quantitative and qualitative research. The criteria for these need to be differentiated as the purpose, goals and intent of each type of research are different. Many students are taught to use quantitative reliability and validity criteria for qualitative studies. This is inappropriate and results in confusion (Leininger 1985). The item below outlines the essential difference in focus.

	Quantitative research	*Qualitative research*
Reliability	Focus is on measuring tool or its ability to assess the degree of consistency or accuracy with which it measures an attribute	Focus is on identifying and documenting features and phenomena in similar or different contexts

Definitions
Reliability − the degree of consistency or dependability with which an instrument measures the attribute it is designed to measure

Split-half reliability − a set of items is divided in half and the two halves are correlated

Test-retest reliability − an approach to reliability that compares two administrations of the same measuring instrument

Annotations
2.24.1 Carmines, E.G. & Zeller, R.A. (1979) *Reliability and validity assessment.* Beverly Hills: Sage   ISBN 0803913710   References

A clear basic text which introduces the issues in measurement theory. The concepts of reliability and validity are thoroughly discussed in light of current debate (CR 2.25).

2.24.2 **Hinds, P.S., Scandrett-Hibden, S. & McAulay, L.S.** (1990) Further assessment of a method to estimate reliability and validity of qualitative research findings. *Journal of advanced nursing* 15(4) 430-435 26 References

Discusses use of an evaluative strategy with qualitative data in order to assess the reliability and validity of findings. Four qualitative studies are briefly outlined to illustrate the technique and ways of interpreting evaluative results are explored (CR 2.25).

2.24.3 **Kirk, J. & Miller, M.L.** (1986) *Reliability and validity in qualitative research.* Beverly Hills: Sage ISBN 0803924704

Book concerns itself with the issues surrounding the scientific status of field data (CR 2.25).

2.24.4 **Knapp, T.R.** (1985) Validity, reliability and neither. *Nursing research* 34(3) 189-192 18 References

Explores misuse of the terms reliability and validity. Author believes that too liberal use is made of these technical terms (CR 2.25).

2.24.5 **Ryan, J.W., Phillips, C.Y. & Prescott, P.A.** (1988) Inter-rater reliability: the under-developed role of rater training. *Applied nursing research* 1(3) 148-150 (No references)

Discusses the process of establishing inter-rater reliability by developing a category scheme which has levels that are independent, mutually exclusive and exhaustive; training raters to use this scheme; evaluating raters and then assuming reliability in the setting for which the measure was designed.

2.24.6 **Yonge, O. & Stewin, L.** (1988) Reliability and validity: misnomers for qualitative research. *The Canadian journal of nursing research* (Nursing Papers) (20)2 61-67 21 References

Authors discuss their belief that the terms reliability and validity should not be applied to qualitative research methods. The essential differences, rigour in qualitative methods and the challenges are discussed (CR 2.25).

Suggested textbook readings

	Pages	*Cross reference*
Abdellah & Levine	151-152	2.1.1
Adams & Schvaneveldt	94-98	2.1.2
Brink P.J. IN Morse (1989)	151-168	2.36.8
Brink & Wood	162-166/172-181	2.1.7
Burns & Grove	291-294	2.1.12
Castles	103-105	2.1.15
Fox	255-260	2.1.25
Kidder & Judd	45-50	2.1.30

2.25 VALIDITY

The second major property required in any measuring instrument, in addition to reliability, is that of validity. The researcher should try to ensure that any existing tools used fulfil the required criteria and information on this should be sought prior to their use. The item below outlines the essential difference between the focus of validity in quantitative and qualitative research.

	Quantitative research	*Qualitative research*
Validity	Focus is on measurement	Focus is on gaining knowledge and understanding of the true nature of the phenomena under study

---

Definitions

Validity − the degree to which an instrument measures what it is intended to measure

  − in qualitative research validity refers to the extent to which the research findings represent reality

Construct validity − the degree to which a test measures the desired characteristic or construct of interest. It is estimated by validating the theory underlying the instrument

Content validity − the degree to which the desired domain (content) is adequately sampled and represented in the instrument. Also considered is the adequacy of the operational definition of the domain being sampled

Criterion related validity − the degree to which the instrument correlates with external variables or criteria believed to measure the concept under investigation. Concurrent and predictive validity are two types

External validity − the ability to generalise or frame a single study to other populations and conditions

Internal validity − the ability to believe in the conclusion drawn based on the design of the study. To assess this one asks if the treatment did indeed make a difference

Predictive validity − the degree to which an instrument can estimate the occurence of a criterion of interest in the future

---

Annotations

2.25.1 Imle, M.A. & Atwood, J.R. (1988) Retaining qualitative validity while gaining quantitative reliability and validity: development of the transition to parenthood concerns scale. *Advances in nursing science* 11(1) 61-75   26 References

Discusses the nature of validity in qualitative research and suggests ways of developing the reliability and validity associated with quantitative research. A set of procedures for testing qualitative scales is described and these provide a base for item and scale revisions and formal quantitative testing (CR 2.24).

2.25.2 McDaniel, C. (1988) Aspects of validity in clinical nursing research. *Applied nursing research* 1(2) 99-103   3 References

Discusses validity in field settings and the main interaction effects related to it.

2.25.3 Reason, P. & Rowan, J. (eds) (1981) Issues of validity in new paradigm research IN Authors *Human inquiry: a sourcebook of new paradigm research.* Chichester: Wiley   ISBN 0417279358   References   Chapter 21   239-250

Chapter gathers together material from a number of sources in order to create a coherent statement about the principles and practices which lead to a more valid inquiry within new paradigm research (CR 2.11.5).

2.25.4 Rew, L., Stuppy, D. & Becker, H. (1988) Construct validity in instrument development: a vital link between nursing practice, research and theory. *Advances in nursing science* 10(4) 10-22   24 References

Author examined 17 articles published in Advances in Nursing Science for evidence of construct validity which provides links between practice, research and theory. Fourteen provided such evidence, with factor analysis being the most commonly used method. Findings indicated the need to develop further links between the three areas.

2.25.5 Robinson, C.A. & Thorne, S.E. (1988) Dilemmas of ethics and validity in qualitative nursing research. *The Canadian journal of nursing research* (Nursing papers) 20(1) 65-76   30 References

Discusses the dilemmas of informed consent, influence of the researcher, immersion into the data and intervention during the research. The implications for nursing research are outlined (CR 2.17).

Suggested textbook readings

	Pages	*Cross reference*
Abdellah & Levine	148-151	2.1.1
Adams & Schvaneveldt	80-94	2.1.2
Brink P.J. IN Morse J.M. (1989)	151-168	2.36.8
Brink & Wood	166-181	2.1.7
Burns & Grove	232-241	2.1.12
Castles	105-107	2.1.15
Cook & Campbell	37-94	2.35.1
Fox	260-267	2.1.25
Kidder & Judd	50-59	2.1.30
Krathwohl	57-130	2.1.33
LoBiondo-Wood & Haber	247-264	2.1.38
Nieswiadomy	200-207	2.1.43
Notter & Hott	98-100	2.1.44
Phillips L.R.F. (critique)	212-216/218-221	2.98.11
Polgar & Thomas	37-58/99-100/ 117-119	2.1.55
Polit & Hungler (1987)	323-329	2.1.56
Seaman	317-329	2.1.62
Smith H.W.	61-79	2.98.14
Thomas	98-102	2.1.64
Williamson	160-167	2.1.67
Woods & Catanzaro	137-138	2.1.72

2.26 TRIANGULATION

The purpose of using triangulation is to provide a basis for convergence on truth. By using multiple methods and perspectives it is hoped that 'true' information can be sorted from 'error' information. In the final analysis this is not conceptually different from the process of estimating reliability and validity by quantitative researchers (Polit & Hungler 1987).

Definitions

Triangulation — the use of multiple methods or perspectives to collect and interpret data about some phenomena in order to converge on an accurate representation of reality

Data triangulation — use of multiple data sources in a study (e.g. interviewing multiple key informants about the same topic)

Investigator triangulation — use of many individuals to collect and analyse a single set of data

Methodological triangulation — use of multiple methods to address a research problem (e.g. observation, interviews, inspection of documents)

Theory triangulation − use of multiple perspectives to interpret a single set of data

---

Example
Hinds, P.S. & Young, K.J. (1987) A triangulation of methods and paradigms to study nurse-given wellness care. *Nursing research* 36(3) 195-198   12 References

Reports a longitudinal study of wellness in adults who participated in a community health nursing programme. Four methods of data collection were used in order to examine wellness as a multi-dimensional, dynamic phenomena.

Annotations
2.26.1 Campbell, D.T. & Fiske, D.W. (1959) Convergent and discriminant validation by the multitrait-multimethod matrix. *Psychological bulletin* 56(2) 81-105   References

A seminal paper advocating the use of cumulative evaluations rather than single methods of measurement.

2.26.2   Jick, T.D. (1983) Mixing qualitative and quantitative methods: triangulation in action. IN Van Maanen, J. (ed) *Qualitative methodology.* Newbury Park: Sage   References 135-148

Chapter defines triangulation, provides an illustration of how it works, discusses whether there is convergence in the data, and gives its advantages and disadvantages (CR 2.36.15).

2.26.3   Mitchell, E.S. (1986) Multiple triangulation: a methodology for nursing science. *Advances in nursing science* 8(3) 18-26   9 References

Discusses the process of triangulation which can assist in the study of complex human behaviour. Four basic types are described and issues relating to multiple triangulation are highlighted.

2.26.4   Morse, J.M. (1991) Approaches to qualitative/quantitative methodological triangulation. *Nursing research* 40(2) 120-123   16 References

Explores the principles underlying the use of methodological triangulation when combining qualitative and quantitative methods.

2.26.5   Sohier, R. (1988) Multiple triangulation and contemporary nursing research. *Western journal of nursing research* 10(6) 733-742   33 References

Author believes the utilisation of multiple methods in nursing research will enable the development of consistency between the theory, practice and research elements of research. It is not a substitute for poor design or sloppy research, but with clear questions and a sound theoretical base triangulation offers the means to increase reliability and validity, and reflect the holistic context of nursing.

Suggested textbook readings

	Pages	Cross reference
Burgess (1982)	143-165	2.1.9
Cohen & Manion	269-286	2.1.19
Denzin	471-475	2.1.23
Fielding & Fielding	23-35	2.89.3
Hakim	144-145	2.20.1
Hovland C.I. IN Denzin	476-494	2.1.23
Polit & Hungler (1987)	332	2.1.56
Silverman D. (1985)	105-106	2.36.14
Smith H.W.	271-292	2.98.14
Woods & Catanzaro	216-217	2.1.72
Vielich P.J. & Shapiro G. IN Denzin	512-522	2.1.23
Zelditch M. IN Denzin	495-511	2.1.23

Nursing research abstracts

Murphy S.A.	90/006

2.27   BIAS

A major consideration at many stages in any research project is the possibility of bias. If this factor is not taken into account then the results may be distorted.

Definition

Any influence that produces a distortion in the results of a study

---

Suggested textbook readings

	Pages	Cross reference
Brink & Wood	113-115	2.1.7
Bryman	37-38	2.9.1
Chenitz & Swanson	56-57	2.46.2
Christensen	100-117/141-142	2.1.17
Fox	184-186/282-283	2.1.25
Katzer, Cook & Crouch	50-58	2.98.8
Kidder & Judd	17-18	2.1.30

2.28   GENERALISABILITY

An important research goal is to try and understand what is taking place in a general way during a series of events. One isolated event may have considerable importance, particularly in qualitative research, but the ability to extrapolate beyond the specifics is a characteristic of the scientific method.

Definition
The extent to which the findings of research may be applied to other situations or settings

Suggested textbook readings

	Pages	*Cross reference*
Abdellah & Levine	216-217	2.1.1
Bryman	34-37	2.9.1
Christensen	315-328	2.1.17
Fox	268-269	2.1.25
Kidder & Judd	34-35/169-171	2.1.30
LoBiondo-Wood & Haber	353-355	2.1.38
Phillips L.R.F. (critique)	352	2.98.11
Polgar & Thomas	10/278	2.1.55
Polit & Hungler (1987)	16-17	2.1.56
Seaman	234	2.1.62
Thomas	84-98	2.1.64
Treece & Treece	454-459	2.1.65
Woods & Catanzaro	157	2.1.72

2.29 EXPERIMENTAL DESIGNS – GENERAL

Experimental research involves the active manipulation of variables under the control of the researcher. This approach attempts to study how subjects will react to the manipulated conditions through monitoring one or more outcome measures. If an experiment is well designed, the experimenter may, in principle, detect causal relationships between variables. However, there are many threats to the satisfactory detection of such relationships.

Experimental studies involve the following steps:

(a) definition of the problem
(b) selection of the sample - this should be representative of the population
(c) assignment procedures - participants allocated to groups who should be as similar as possible
(d) treatment – researcher administers the intervention(s) i.e. the independent variables in an unbiased way
(e) measurement of outcomes – this is measured via the dependent variable. It may be measured both before and after the treatment or only after

Definitions
Experiment – ... is characterised by randomisation, manipulation and control
Control group – the subjects who are not exposed to the experimental treatment
Random sample – a sample drawn from a population that assures that all possible sampling units have an equal probability of being selected

Annotations

2.29.1 Atwood, J.R. (1984) Advancing nursing science: quantitative approaches. *Western journal of nursing research* 6(3) 9-15   27 References

A keynote address indicating why, in the author's view, quantitative approaches to research are essential in health care.

2.29.2 Boruch, R.F., McSweeney, A.J. & Soderstrom, E.J. (1978) Randomised field experiments for programme planning, development and evaluation. *Evaluation quarterly* 2: 655-695

A bibliography listing 300 randomised field experiments in ten different categories. These are: criminal and civil justice, mental health, training re-education, mass communications, information collection and retrieval, research utilisation, commerce, industry and public utilities, social welfare, health services and medical treatment, fertility control. It is suggested that randomised tests are numerous and have been used in many settings, and the professional in one setting could learn from those conducted in another sphere.

2.29.3 Brown, G., Cherrington, D.H. & Cohen, L. (1975) *Experiments in the social sciences.* London: Harper & Row   SBN 063180146   References

Book is intended to show that experimental methods designed for research in the social sciences can be incorporated into academic courses. It contains 21 experiments applicable to the fields of psychology and sociology. Details are given at the end of the book for the teacher/organiser to show how each experiment should be conducted and analysed.

2.29.4 Campbell, D.T. & Stanley, J.C. (1963) *Experimental and quasi-experimental designs for research.* Chicago: Rand McNally College   ISBN 0528614002   References

Book examines 16 experimental/quasi-experimental designs with emphasis being given to factors affecting validity (CR 2.35).

2.29.5 Clark, E. (1988) *The experimental perspective.* Research Awareness, Module 9 London: Distance Learning Centre, South Bank Polytechnic   ISBN 0948250291   References

This is number 9 in a series of 13 modules, each of which deals with a different aspect of nursing research. It was developed to assist nurses, midwives and health visitors in understanding research in terms of their own professional practice. Modules can be used separately or as part of a programme. The reader is encouraged to work through a number of activities, self-assessment questions and answers, and progress summaries. Some articles/book extracts referred to in the text are reproduced in full.

This module is an introduction to experimental methods as used in nursing research. The topics discussed include variations in experimental design, statistics, the role of the practising nurse with particular reference to the protection of subjects, experimental research and evaluating an experimental research proposal (CR Appendix D).

2.29.6 Dumas, R. (1987) Clinical trials in nursing. *Recent advances in nursing* 17: 108-125   35 References

Outlines the need for clinical trials in nursing, their design and the value of conducting multi-centre trials. The use of meta-analysis is mentioned (CR 2.95).

2.29.7 Fairweather, G.W. & Tornatzky, L.G. (1977) *Experimental methods for social policy research.* Oxford: Pergamon   ISBN 0080212379   References

Aims to provide social scientists with an integrated series of research techniques that may be used to solve contemporary human problems. Experimental techniques for evaluating the processes of innovation and diffusion are presented.

2.29.8 Hicks, C.M. (1990) *Research and statistics: a practical introduction for nurses.* New York: Prentice Hall   ISBN 0138440778   References

Book concentrates on hypothesis testing and experimental design. Little statistical theory is included and worked examples are given for each test. Summaries of major points are given together with lists of key words and exercises. Text relates research principles directly to nursing issues. Advice is also given on preparing research for publication (CR 2.20, 2.102).

2.29.9 Louis, T.A. & Shapiro, S.H. (1983) Critical issues in the conduct and interpretation of clinical trials. *Annual review of public health* 4: 25-46   141 References

Some of the problems encountered with clinical trials are described and 18 key issues which need to be addressed prior to a trial are shown. Ethical issues involved are also discussed, together with planning a study and its management once underway (CR 2.17).

2.29.10 McLaughlin, F.E. & Marascuilo, L.A. (1990) *Advanced nursing and health care research: quantification approaches.* Philadelphia: Saunders   ISBN 0721630987   References

Written for advanced level students, graduates and experienced researchers this book covers initial and advanced research techniques and statistical procedures. An extensive research example is used throughout the text and others illustrate special issues in nursing research. New techniques are introduced and the range and variety of quantification techniques useful for hypothesis testing is included.

2.29.11 Meinert, C.L. (1986) *Clinical trials: design, conduct and analysis.* New York: Oxford University Press   ISBN 0195035682   References

A general text concerned with the design and conduct of clinical trials. The main focus is on trials involving uncrossed treatments and a clinical event as the outcome measure. Many designs and operating principles are also applicable to other types of research.

2.29.12 Open University (1983) Testing new drugs. IN *Statistics in society*. (MDST 242) Milton Keynes: Open University Press (MDST 242) ISBN 0035141366 Block C Data in context. Unit C1

Unit covers the processes involved in conducting clinical trials in the testing of new drugs.

2.29.13 Pocock, S.J. (1983) *Clinical trials: a practical approach*. Chichester: Wiley ISBN 0471901555 References

A comprehensive text on the principles and practice of clinical trials. Discusses their historical development, current status and future strategies.

2.29.14 Wilson-Barnett, J. (1991) The experiment: is it worthwhile? *International journal of nursing studies* 28(1) 77-87 30 References

Discusses how the experiment can be modified and interpreted to provide evidence for changes in nursing practice. A list of suggestions is given for improving the experimental approach with human subjects.

2.29.15 Wooldridge, P.J., Leonard, R.C. & Skipper, J.K. (1978) *Methods of clinical experimentation to improve patient care*. St Louis: Mosby ISBN 0801656222 References

Authors believe that controlled clinical trials are the way forward for nursing research. Emphasis in the book is on replication, theory building and inductively derived general principles from specific examples. Methodological issues are discussed throughout the text (CR 2.7, 2.13).

Suggested textbook readings

	Pages	Cross reference
Abdellah & Levine	164-170/176-200	2.1.1
Brink & Wood (1989)	27-56	2.36.3
Brophy E.B. IN Krampitz & Pavlovich	40-48	2.1.32
Burns & Grove	45-73	2.1.12
Castles	61-65	2.1.15
Cohen & Manion	193-216	2.1.19
Fox	176-193	2.1.25
Greene J. (DE 304) 3A	45-72	2.1.48
Grey M. IN LoBiondo-Wood & Haber	147-162	2.1.38
Kidder & Judd	69-101	2.1.30
Kovacs	55-65	2.1.31
Lawson L. IN Krampitz & Pavlovich	67-74	2.1.32
Leedy	217-232	2.1.35
Nieswiadomy	123-138	2.1.43
Notter & Hott	75-77	2.1.44

Note: The use of standard *notation* is helpful in understanding alternative experimental designs

R = Random assignment of subjects to experimental and control groups
O = Observation or measurement (O1 pre-test/O2 post-test)
X = Treatment or intervention

Four of the most commonly used designs are illustrated in the following sections (2.30−2.34) but it is also possible within any design to increase the number of treatments.

2.30 EXPERIMENTAL DESIGNS
Pre-test/Post-test Design

Measurements of the outcomes or dependent variables are taken both before and after the intervention. This allows the measurement of change in individual cases.

R	O1	X	O2	Experimental group
R	O3		O4	Control group

[Note: Key − please see 2.29]

The measurement process may itself produce change thereby introducing difficulties in attributing change to the intervention on its own.

Example
Dixon, J. (1984) Effects of nursing intervention on nutritional and performance status in cancer patients. *Nursing research* 33(6) 330-335   30 References

Cancer patients were assigned to a control group or one of four intervention groups receiving (a) nutritional supplementation, (b) relaxation training, (c) both (a) and (b) and (d) neither (a) nor (b). Findings suggested that the cachexia of cancer may be slowed or reversed through non-invasive interventions.

Suggested textbook readings

	Pages	Cross reference
Christensen	172-175	2.1.17
Fox	187	2.1.25
Polgar & Thomas	62	2.1.55
Williamson	133-135	2.1.67
Woods & Catanzaro	174-175	2.1.72

2.31 EXPERIMENTAL DESIGNS
Post-test Control Design

This design may be useful in situations where it is not possible to pre-test the participants or where they have been randomly assigned.

R	X	O	Experimental Group
R	O		Control Group

[Note: Key − please see 2.29]

Example

Dean, N.R. (1979) Effect of free time the day prior to mastery testing on student nurse scores. *Nursing research* 28 (1) 40-42   4 References

Study compared mastery test scores of students who had free time and those who were having clinical experience. Results showed that scores were not significantly different.

Suggested textbook readings

	Pages	Cross reference
Christensen	170-172	2.1.17
Fox	186-187	2.1.25
Polgar & Thomas	63	2.1.55
Williamson	135-136	2.1.67
Woods & Catanzaro	176	2.1.72

2.32 EXPERIMENTAL DESIGNS
Solomon Four Group design

A complex design useful in studies of developmental phenomena which permits the investigator to differentiate between many effects. Two experimental and two control groups are used.

R	O1	X	O2	Experimental Group 1
R	O3		O4	Control Group 1
R		X	O5	Experimental Group 2
R			O6	Control Group 2

[Note: Key — please see 2.29]

This design has potential for generating information about differential sources of effect of the dependent variable.

Example

Brock, A.M. (1978) Impact of a management-orientated course on knowledge and leadership skills exhibited by baccalaureate nursing students. *Nursing research* 27(4) 217-221   12 References

Study evaluated the impact on 80 baccalaureate students of a one month management course which was designed to aid development of management knowledge and skills. Results showed that students who had attended the course had gained knowledge and skills, demonstrated leadership behaviours and understanding of the concepts involved.

Suggested textbook readings

	Pages	Cross reference
Christensen	175-177	2.1.17
Williamson	136	2.1.67
Woods & Catanzaro	175-176	2.1.72

2.33   EXPERIMENTAL DESIGNS
Factorial designs

Factorial designs allow the researcher to analyse the effects of two or more factors simultaneously. They also provide information on whether factors interact to produce differences in the outcome that would not have occured if each factor was considered separately.

	Type of Surgery	
	Cholecystectomy	Herniorraphy
Treatment		
Specific booklet		
Non-specific booklet		
No pre-admission booklet		

Authors assessed whether the factors (type of surgery and type of instruction) had an interactive effect (Rice & Johnson 1984).

Example
Rice, V. & Johnson, J. (1984) Pre-admission self instruction booklets, post admission exercise performance and teaching time. *Nursing research* 33(3) 147-151 15 References

Aim of study was to determine if pre-admission clients would learn post-operative exercise activities from self instructional booklets sent to their homes, thus requiring less teaching time in hospital than a comparable group. Providing patients with such information can help to increase their sense of control over some aspects of the impending experience, which is an important factor in response to stressful situations. Subjects given booklets did perform more of the exercises and less teaching time was required.

Suggested textbook readings

	Pages	Cross reference
Christensen	180-187	2.1.17
Fox	187-188	2.1.25
Polgar & Thomas	63-64	2.1.55
Williamson	136-138	2.1.67
Woods & Catanzaro	176-177	2.1.72

2.34 EXPERIMENTAL DESIGNS
Single Case design

Single case research can be carried out in any setting where one individual can be studied intensively. One advantage of this method is that responses are not masked as they may be in grouped data. A number of terms are used to describe or name small sample research. These are single case design, intensive research, $N=1$ design, ideographic research, experimental analysis of behaviour, applied analysis of behaviour and case study designs (Holm & Llewellyn 1986, Woods & Catanzaro 1988).

Definition
An examination of a single subject in order to understand the specific causes of problems and the effectiveness of treatment applied to that individual

Example
Holm, K. (1983) Single subject research. *Nursing research* 32(4) 253-255 17 References

Discusses ways in which single subject research may be used in nursing research and clinical practice. Two brief examples are given and suggestions made for appropriate areas in clinical practice.

Annotations

2.34.1 Barlow, D.H. & Hersen, M. (1984) *Single case experimental designs: strategies for studying behaviour change.* 2nd edition New York: Pergamon ISBN 0080301363 References

Book provides a historical overview of the single case in basic and applied research and discusses general issues, procedures and assessment strategies. Different designs are covered in depth and many examples given. Methods of statistical analysis are included together with examples of direct, systematic and clinical replication (CR 2.13).

2.34.2 Kazdin, A.E. (1982) *Single case research designs: methods for clinical and applied settings.* New York: Oxford University Press ISBN 0195030214 References

Provides a concise description of single case experimental designs and places this methodology in the context of applied research in general. Examples are given from clinical psychology, psychiatry, education, counselling and other disciplines. The methodology covers assessment, design and data analysis.

2.34.3 Schroeder, H.E. & Wildman, B.G. (1988) Single case designs in clinical settings. *The hospice journal* 4(4) 3-24 8 References

Strengths and weaknesses of traditional experimental designs are explored, and the value of single case studies in clinical settings identified. The variety of designs are discussed together with approaches to interpreting results and threats to validity. Suggestions are made for overcoming some of the difficulties inherent in this type of research design.

Suggested textbook readings

	Pages	Cross reference
Berger & Patchner	125-143	2.1.6
Chinn	198-199	2.7.2
Christensen	235-271	2.1.17
Cohen & Manion	210-212	2.1.19
Holm & Llewellyn	92	2.1.26
Leedy	140-216	2.1.35
Polgar & Thomas	84-93	2.1.55
Polit & Hungler (1987)	169	2.1.56
Woods & Catanzaro	189-201	2.1.72

2.35 QUASI-EXPERIMENTAL DESIGNS

Quasi-experimental designs are a compromise between a true experiment with random assignment and a pre-experiment. They also represent a compromise between maximising internal and external validity.

Definition
Research design that has the features of manipulation and control, but in which participants are not randomly assigned to the treatment and control groups.

There are two major groups of quasi-experimental designs:

interrupted time series designs − effects of a treatment are inferred from comparing measures of performance taken at many time intervals

non-equivalent control group − those in which responses of a treatment group and a comparison group are measured before and after the treatment

Within each group there are several different designs and the interested reader is advised to consult the text listed below.

Example
Armitage, P., Champney-Smith, J. & Owen, K. (1989) Primary nursing in long-term psychiatric care. *Senior nurse* 9(9) 22-24   16 References

Reports a study which used a quasi-experimental approach to monitor the change from traditional care to primary nursing in a group of long-stay patients.

Annotation
2.35.1   Cook, T.D. & Campbell, D.T. (1979) *Quasi-experimentation: design and analysis issues for field settings.* Chicago: Rand McNally   (No ISBN number found) References

Book covers some quasi-experimental designs which can be used in many social research settings. The literature on causation is reviewed, aspects of validity are explored and the two major categories of quasi-experimental designs, non-equivalent group and interrupted time series are covered in detail. Further chapters on inferring cause from passive observation and the conduct of randomised experiments are included.

Suggested textbook readings

	Pages	Cross reference
Adams & Schvaneveldt	255-269	2.1.2
Brink & Wood (1989)	57-86	2.36.3
Castles	65-67	2.1.15
Christensen	197-232	2.1.17
Cook T.D. IN Morgan G.	74-94	2.8.6
Fox	174	2.1.25
Grey M. IN LoBiondo-Wood & Haber	154-158	2.1.38
Hakim	101-116	2.21.1
Kidder & Judd	102-126	2.1.30

	Pages	Cross reference
Lin	245-273	2.1.37
Polgar & Thomas	75-78	2.1.55
Polit & Hungler (1987)	130-140	2.1.56
Williamson	138-144	2.1.67
Wilson H.S. (1989)	167-169	2.1.69
Woods & Catanzaro	178-184	2.1.72

2.36 NON-EXPERIMENTAL DESIGNS/APPROACHES – GENERAL

Many studies which are undertaken to investigate aspects of the human condition are non-experimental in nature, and this is particularly true in nursing research. There are many characteristics in people's lives which cannot be manipulated and so it is not possible or indeed appropriate to perform experiments on them. Some examples might be height, age, social circumstances and personality. Much research undertaken in nursing aims to examine highly complex situations and many different designs have been utilised.

Sections 2.37−2.55 cover most non-experimental designs used in nursing research.

Definition

Research conducted in natural settings such as a ... public health agency, hospital or patient's home. This type of research is frequently retrospective

Annotations

2.36.1 Benoliel, J.Q. (1984) Advancing nursing science: qualitative approaches. *Western journal of nursing research* 6(3) 1-8   12 References

Keynote address which makes the case for the qualitative approach to scientific discovery. Covers a perspective on nursing knowledge, the qualitative paradigm, inquiry and nursing science.

2.36.2 Brewer, J. & Hunter, A. (1989) *Multi-method research: a synthesis of styles.* Newbury Park: Sage   ISBN 0803930771   References

Book discusses the value and use of multi-methods in social research. A strategy is suggested, its relationship to theory presented and each step of the research process is described.

2.36.3 Brink, P.J. & Wood, M.J. (eds.) (1989) *Advanced design in nursing research.* Newbury Park: Sage   ISBN 0803927428   References

An advanced text focusing on research designs for students and teachers who have a basic knowledge of the research process. Three major designs - exploratory/descriptive, survey and experiential are subdivided into further levels and fully discussed. Each one is contrasted with experimental design, and its strengths and weaknesses reviewed.

2.36.4 **Filstead, W.J.** (ed) (1970) *Qualitative methodology: first hand involvement with the social world.* Chicago: Markham   (No ISBN number)   References

Through a series of papers the many aspects of qualitative methodology are explored. Areas included are the direction of sociology, field work roles, data collection and analysis, problems of reliability and validity, ethical problems, qualitative methodology and theory.

2.36.5 **Lee, J.L.** (1988) Futures research IN Sarter, B. (ed) *Paths to knowledge: innovative research methods for nursing.* New York: National League for Nursing   ISBN 0887374158   References 61-75

Discusses futures research which is a means of forecasting change. Its history, vocabulary, philosophical basis, researcher characteristics, research process and representative techniques are included. These are scenario building, Delphi survey, nominal group technique, QUEST process (Quick Environmental Scanning Technique), trend impact analysis, cross impact analysis and INTERAX, a computer-based procedure. Validity, reliability and generalisation are discussed, the challenges of implementation and the potential for theory development (CR 2.1.61, 2.24, 2.25, 2.28, 2.68).

2.36.6 **Marshall, C. & Rossman, G.B.** (1989) *Designing qualitative research.* Newbury Park: Sage   ISBN 0803931573   References

Provides detailed guidance on developing acceptable qualitative research proposals. A series of vignettes provide illustrative material throughout the text (CR 2.99).

2.36.7 **Melia, K.M.** (1982) 'Tell it as it is' qualitative methodology and nursing research: understanding the student nurses world. *Journal of advanced nursing* 7(4) 327-335   8 References

Paper focuses on a study which describes student nurses accounts of being learners and demonstrates the value of qualitative methods for nursing research.

2.36.8 **Morse, J.M.** (ed) (1989) *Qualitative nursing research: a contemporary dialogue.* Rockville, Maryland: Aspen   ISBN 0834200112   References

Series of papers arising from a symposium in Chicago in 1987. Some of the more difficult issues relating to qualitative research are discussed and will add to the debate. Each chapter is preceded by a short dialogue where the problems are introduced, and ends with references. Areas covered include phenomenology, ethnography and epistemology, ethics and validity, use of self in ethnographic research, fieldwork, the evolving nature of qualitative methods, sampling, issues relating to reliability and validity, triangulation, funding, research proposals and teaching qualitative research (CR 2.6, 2.17, 2.24, 2.25, 2.26, 2.43, 2.52, 2.99, 3.12, 3.18).

2.36.9 **Parse, R.R., Coyne, A.B. & Smith, M.J.** (1985) *Nursing research: qualitative methods.* Bowie, Maryland: Brady Communications Co.   ISBN 0893037249   References

Intended for graduates and covers the basic elements of qualitative methods. These are demonstrated through one nursing perspective, the theory of man-living-health. Criteria are given for critical appraisal of qualitative studies.

2.36.10 Payne, G., Dingwall, R., Payne, J. & Carter, M. (1981) *Sociology and social research.* London: Routledge and Kegan Paul   ISBN 0710006268   References

Book examines the intellectual origins and recent growth in sociology in the UK. It describes the main styles of research − theories, ethnography, ethnomethodology and applied policy research. The final part concentrates on sociology as a research activity (CR 2.7, 2.43, 3.10).

2.36.11 Runcie, J.F. (1976) *Experiencing social research.* Homewood: Illinois The Dorsey Press   ISBN 0256018103   References

Author believes that students should be involved in doing research as well as reading about it. A series of research projects are suggested and methods of conducting the study and analysing the data are given in each chapter. The methods of data collection included are participant and non-participant observation, questionnaire, interview and ethnomethodological experimentation (CR 2.43, 2.70, 2.73, 2.76).

2.36.12 Sandelowski, M. (1986) The problem of rigour in qualitative research. *Advances in nursing science* 8(3) 27-37   40 References

Factors which complicate the debate about the scientific merits of qualitative research are discussed. A framework for understanding the similarities and differences in approach is given and a summary of strategies to achieve rigour in qualitative research.

2.36.13 Schwartz, H. & Jacobs, J. (1979) *Qualitative sociology: a method to the madness.* New York: The Free Press   ISBN 0029281709

Book provides a comprehensive and detailed examination of a broad range of qualitative methods. Its two parts cover reality construction and formal sociology. Various theories and methods are described, examples given and the strengths and weaknesses of each identified.

2.36.14 Silverman, D. (1985) *Qualitative methodology and sociology.* Aldershot: Gower   ISBN 0566008874   References

Book is mainly concerned with strategies rather than tactics. It discusses post-positivist methodologies and fundamental issues in social theory. Part 1 describes the problems which arise during the research process. Part 2 is concerned with the major conceptual polarities and Part 3 examines the practice of qualitative research. Three major research techniques are discussed, ethnography, interviews and conversational analysis and the analytical problems related to each (CR 2.43, 2.70, 2.80, 2.91).

2.36.15 Van Maanen, J. (ed) (1983) *Qualitative methodology.* Newbury Park: Sage ISBN 0803921179 References

Provides an updated reprint of the December 1979 issue of Administrative Science Quarterly. Papers cover ethnographic paradigms, multiple methods and a fresh outlook on some aspects of these complex methodologies.

2.36.16 Van Maanen, J., Dabbs, J.M. Jr & Faulkner, R.R. (1982) *Varieties of qualitative research.* Beverly Hills: Sage ISBN 0803918704 References

Monograph focuses on innovative ways of collecting and analysing qualitative data about organisations. In depth illustrations of three alternative strategies are given which highlight the opportunities and potential pitfalls of such approaches (CR 2.89).

2.36.17 Webb, E.J., Campbell, D.T., Schwartz, R.D. & Sechrestl, L. (1966) *Unobtrusive measures: non-reactive research in the social sciences.* Chicago: Rand McNally ISBN 0528686941 References

Monograph deals with methods of measurement appropriate to a wide range of social science studies. Authors stress the importance of using multiple data collection methods so that problems inherent in each may be minimised. Those examined are physical evidence, archival sources, simple and controlled observation, hidden hardware and control. No attempt is made to cover the ethical issues which arise (CR 2.26, 2.73, 2.77).

2.36.18 to 2.36.24 *Western journal of nursing research* (1988) 10(2) Edited by Knafl, K. A. Qualitative Research.

[NB The following entry differs in format as it documents a special issue of the journal *Western journal of nursing research*. These articles have not been annotated].

2.36.18 Artinian, B.A. Qualitative methods of inquiry. 138-149 13 References

2.36.19 Cowles, K.V. Issues in qualitative research on sensitive topics. 163-179 17 References

2.36.20 Faux, S.A., Walsh, M. & Deatrick, J.A. Intensive interviewing with children and adolescents. 180-194 39 References

2.36.21 Haase, J.E. & Myers, S.T. Reconciling paradigm assumptions of qualitative and quantitative research. 128-137 17 References

2.36.22 Knafl, K.A. Consider the possibilities of qualitative research. Editorial 125-127

2.36.23 Knafl, K.A. & Webster, D.C. Managing and analysing qualitative data. 195-209 26 References

2.36.24 Munhall, P.L. Ethical considerations in qualitative research. 150-162 10 References

Suggested textbook readings

	Pages	Cross reference
Abdellah & Levine	170-176/200-204/ 207-213	2.1.1
Adams & Schvaneveldt	101-118	2.1.2
Boyd C.O. IN LoBiondo-Wood & Haber	181-208	2.1.38
Brink & Wood (1988)	100-105	2.1.7
Burns & Grove	75-106	2.1.12
Castles	55-61	2.1.15
Field & Morse	19-31	2.1.24
Leininger	1-25	2.1.36
LoBiondo-Wood & Haber	165-179	2.1.38
Notter & Hott	72-75	2.1.44
Polgar & Thomas	94-102	2.1.55
Polit & Hungler (1987)	141-154	2.1.56
Roberts & Burke	164-183	2.1.59
Seaman	181-192	2.1.62
Smith H.W.	99-102	2.98.14
Thomas	83-84	2.1.64
Waltz & Bausell	125-157	2.21.4

Nursing research abstracts
Fowler, M.D.M   88/021

2.37 NON-EXPERIMENTAL DESIGNS
Action research

Action research is concerned with diagnosing a problem in a specific context and attempting to develop local solutions. As the results will only be applicable locally, generalisation will not be possible. Because researchers and practitioners work together and trust develops between them, implementation of findings is more likely to occur.

Definition
Develops new skills or approaches to solve problems with direct application to an applied setting

---

Example
Bradley, S. & Smith, G. (1984) The use of action research to evaluate schemes for the professional development of newly registered nurses. IN Workgroup of European Nurse-Researchers. *Nursing research: does it make a difference?* Proceedings of 2nd Open Conference, London − 10-13th April. London: Royal College of Nursing ISBN 0902606891 9 References 324-331

The use of action research in evaluating schemes for professional development is described. The characteristics of action research and its relevance to nursing are given, together with information on the scheme being evaluated and how the project was conducted (CR 3.26.4).

Annotations

2.37.1 Greenwood, J. (1984) Nursing research : a position paper. *Journal of advanced nursing* 9(1) 77-82   11 References

Research findings produced by conventional approaches are frequently perceived as irrelevant to practice. Because nursing is a practice discipline and a social phenonemon the author believes that action research is the most appropriate approach (CR 2.9).

2.37.2 McNiff, J. (1988) *Action research: principles and practice.* Basingstoke: Macmillan Education   ISBN 0333453182   References

Book is intended as a reference text for practising teachers who are urged to conduct their own research in order to open up educational debate about their work. The philosophies and practices of action research are explained and illustrated with case studies. Current trends are reviewed together with key concepts in its development (CR 2.39).

2.37.3 Nixon, J. (ed) (1981) *A teacher's guide to action research: evaluation, enquiry and development in the classroom.* London: Grant McIntyre   ISBN 0862160405   References

Describes several studies initiated and undertaken by teachers in their own classrooms, which illustrate the techniques of action research. Three groups of papers are included: classroom concerns, school concerns, and looking outside which identifies ways in which outside agencies can support action research. The editor believes that all teachers should develop the skills to study their own work throughout their professional lives.

2.37.4 Sanford, N. (1981) A model for action research. IN Reason, P. & Rowan, J. (eds) *Human inquiry: a sourcebook of new paradigm research.* Chichester: Wiley   ISBN 0471279358   References   Chapter 14   173-181

Discusses the position of action research today in terms of value, problems, funding and potential effects (CR 2.11.5).

2.37.5 Webb, C. (1989) Action research: philosophy, methods and personal experience. *Journal of advanced nursing* 14(5) 403-410 26   References

Author describes the processes involved in undertaking action research and discusses its underlying philosophy.

2.37.6 Winter, R. (1982) 'Dilemma analysis': a contribution to methodology for action research. *Cambridge journal of education* 12(3) 161-174   12 References

Discusses some of the problems experienced when trying to interpret data obtained in the action research/case study tradition, and focuses particularly on interview transcripts. Content analysis and thematic induction are examined. A new set of procedures was adopted, termed 'dilemma analysis'. The nature of this is explored and the author believes it has potential when dealing with complex data.

Suggested textbook readings

	Pages	*Cross reference*
Cohen & Manion	217-241	2.1.19
Fox	11-13	2.1.25
Payne, Dingwall, Payne, & Carter	163-180	2.36.10

2.38 NON-EXPERIMENTAL DESIGNS
Atheoretical research

Some purists may regard research which is not based on theoretical frameworks or conceptual orientations, as problem-solving rather than scientific research. However early studies in clinical nursing research tended to be problem-solving endeavours rather than scientific research. More recently, emphasis has been put on the use of theory as the appropriate grounding, but there is still room for work to be done in nursing while a theoretical base is being discovered (Phillips L.R.F. 1986).

Definition
Research that is formulated without a theory base which involves problem-solving in specific situations

Suggested textbook reading

	Pages	*Cross reference*
Phillips L.R.F.	364-365	2.98.11

2.39 NON-EXPERIMENTAL DESIGNS
Case study research

The term case study does not denote a single specific technique but rather a general strategy for research. Typically a case study involves one or several cases that are studied over time by multiple data gathering methods. Case studies have a contemporary, rather than historical focus. They are naturalistic and conducted in a setting which is not controlled by the researcher.

Definition
A research method that involves a thorough, in-depth analysis of an individual, group, institution or other social unit

Example
Baer, E.D. (1989) Nursing's divided loyalties: an historical case study. *Nursing research* 38(3) 166-171 50 References

Research explored nurses' conflicting loyalties at the turn of the century. One training school alumnae association was used to examine contributing factors.

Annotations
2.39.1 Adelman, C., Jenkins, D. & Kemmis, S. (1975) Re-thinking case study: notes from the second Cambridge Conference. *Cambridge journal of education* 6(3) 139-150 6 References

Article reports the deliberations of an international conference which explored the problems and potential of case study research. The value of the method in contributing to the body of knowledge is identified although its characteristics are poorly understood and its potential underdeveloped. The nature of case studies is explored, the practical difficulties involved, conduct of such research and the importance of triangulation is discussed. Possible consequences are highlighted because the data emerges from real life situations and six advantages are listed (CR 2.26).

2.39.2 Bromley, D.B. (1986) *The case study method in psychology and related disciplines.* Chichester: Wiley ISBN 0471908533 References

Book deals with the theory and practice of individual case studies. Details are given on how to conduct and evaluate them and use diagrams and decision analysis. Although the examples used are mainly psychological, the book would be of value to students and practitioners in the social and behavioural sciences.

2.39.3 Lane, H. (1977) *The wild boy of Aveyron.* London: Allen & Unwin ISBN 0041550072 References

The individual case study is sometimes viewed with scepticism but this book shows the value of an in-depth study in the teaching of deaf children. The techniques developed are now used throughout the world in the education of deaf, handicapped and young normal children.

2.39.4 Yin, R.K. (1983) *The case study method: an annotated bibliography 1983-1984 edition.* Washington DC: COSMOS Corporation ISBN 0942570022

Cites publications dealing with the case study as a research method. The six sections include general descriptions of the use of case studies; quality control issues; design and analysis; data collection; indirectly related topics and coverage by traditional social science textbooks.

2.39.5 Yin, R.K. (1984) *Case study research: design and methods.* Beverly Hills: Sage ISBN 080392058X References

Book is concerned with the design and conduct of single and multiple case studies for research purposes. It aims to answer some of the more difficult questions commonly neglected by existing research texts − for example how is the case under study defined, what sort of data should be collected and how can it be analysed?

Suggested textbook readings

	Pages	Cross reference
Boyd C.O. IN LoBiondo-Wood & Haber	199-201	2.1.38
Cohen & Manion	124-153	2.1.19
Hakim	61-75	2.21.1
Nieswiadomy	142-143	2.1.43
Phillips L.R.F. (critique)	370-372	2.98.11
Polit & Hungler (1987)	168-170	2.1.56
Seaman	151-152	2.1.62
Strauss A.L.	215-240	2.89.7
Wilson H.S. (1989)	142-145	2.1.69
Wiseman & Aron	73–82	2.66.1
Woods & Catanzaro	156-163	2.1.72

2.40 NON-EXPERIMENTAL DESIGNS
Correlational research

Correlational research examines the pattern of variation in two phenomena.

Definition
Investigations that explore the inter-relationships among variables of interest without any active intervention on the part of the researcher

---

Example
Fugleberg, B.B. (1986) Nursing research in the practice setting. *Nursing administration quarterly*: Fall 38-42   12 References

A descriptive correlational study undertaken to investigate the attitudes of nursing administrators and staff nurses towards nursing research. Factors associated with a favourable environment and perceived level of competence in the research process were also examined.

Suggested textbook readings

	Pages	Cross reference
Brink & Wood (1989)	104-118	2.36.3
Cohen & Manion	154-175	2.1.19
Fox	164	2.1.25
LoBiondo-Wood & Haber	168-170	2.1.38
Nieswiadomy	145-146	2.1.43
Polgar & Thomas	74-75	2.1.55
Polit & Hungler (1987)	142-143	2.1.56
Seaman	218-219	2.1.62
Waltz & Bausell	239-295	2.21.4
Woods & Catanzaro	150-152	2.1.72

2.41 NON-EXPERIMENTAL DESIGNS
Cross-cultural/Trans-cultural research

Cross-cultural research seeks to investigate variables which exist in one or more communities. These include age, sexual division of labour, habits of cleanliness, religious ceremonies, courtship patterns, kinship terminology, birth and death rites and the prevention and cure of disease. The major difficulties associated with it are cost, communication difficulties and the maintenance of cultural meanings in an instruments language (Treece & Treece 1986).

[Note: The terms cross-cultural and trans-cultural are sometimes used interchangeably in the literature.]

Definition
Nursing research within and across cultural contexts

Example
Whetstone, W.R. (1987) Perceptions of self-care in East Germany: a cross-cultural empirical investigation. *Journal of advanced nursing* 12(2) 167-176   33 References

This replication study aimed to compare self-care phenomena in a cross-cultural setting. Two self-reporting inventories were used to measure perceptual dimensions of self-care agency and self-concept. Samples comprised American students and adults living in East Germany. Limitations of the study are identified and cross-cultural implications of the findings are discussed (CR 2.13).

Annotations
2.41.1 Champion, V., Austin, J. & Tzeng, O.C.S (1987) Cross-cultural comparison of images of nurses and physicians. *International nursing review* 34(2) Issue 272 43-48   23 References

Study investigates attitudes related to the image of nurses and physicians across 30 cultures using six concepts. Differences were found with respect to the power held by physicians and nurses, and the authors suggest that nurses' influence in health care decisions can be reduced unless they address this deficit. Physicians were highly correlated with knowledge and independence and nurses were correlated with kindness.

2.41.2 Giger, J.N. & Davidhizar, R. (1990) Transcultural nursing assessment: a method for advancing nursing practice. *International nursing review* 37(1) 199-202   12 References

Discusses a systematic method for comprehensive nursing assessment necessary for practitioners and researchers under the following headings: communication, space, social organisation, time, environmental control and biological variations.

2.41.3 Leininger, M.M. (1984) *References sources for transcultural health and nursing.* Thorofare, New Jersey: Slack Inc. ISBN 0913590932 Part II D 33-38

Contains selected references on many aspects of trans-cultural nursing including theory and research methods.

2.41.4 Morse, J.M. (1986) Transcultural nursing research: process, problems and pitfalls. IN Stinson, S.M. & Kerr, J.C. (eds) *International issues in nursing research* London: Croom Helm ISBN 0709944373 References Chapter 4 61-75

Chapter explores the process, problems and pitfalls of clinical nursing research in different cultural settings. It aims to stimulate interest in this area and prepare those entering this field of research (CR 3.27.7).

2.41.5 Morse, J.M. (1987) Transcultural nursing : its substance and issues in research and knowledge. *Recent advances in nursing* 18: 129-141 34 References

Examines the progress of transcultural nursing and charts the contribution of research to the development of a knowledge base.

2.41.6 Morse, J.M. (ed) (1988) Issues in cross-cultural nursing. *Recent advances in nursing* 20: Edinburgh: Churchill Livingstone ISBN 0443039755 References

Articles cover various issues within cross-cultural nursing as described in research studies undertaken in several parts of the world. A brief history of this type of research is given.

2.41.7 Tripp-Reimer, T. & Dougherty, M.C. (1985) Cross-cultural nursing research. IN Werley, H.H. & Fitzpatrick, J.J. (eds) *Annual review of nursing research* Volume 3 New York: Springer ISBN 0826143520 References Chapter 4 77-104

A critical review of published literature on cross-cultural nursing research.

2.41.8 Warwick, D.P. & Osherson, S. (eds) (1973) *Comparative research methods.* Englewood Cliffs, New Jersey: Prentice Hall ISBN 013153940X References

Papers seek to show how the same problem may be studied in different societies and cultures using a combination of methods. The problems which may occur are included together with some successful outcomes. The five parts of the book cover an overview of comparative research methods; conceptual equivalence and cultural bias; equivalence of measurement and linguistics; translation and illustrative methods; survey research and participant observation (CR 2.55, 2.73).

Suggested textbook reading

	Pages	*Cross reference*
Treece & Treece	207-229	2.1.65

Nursing research abstracts

Jones, E.   87/218
Munet, V.F.   88/003

2.42   NON-EXPERIMENTAL DESIGNS
Epidemiological research

Epidemiological researchers have a special interest in data which may be retrospective in terms of diseases, epidemics or disasters, or prospective in trying to understand risk factors in the environment such as carcinogens or factors contributing to mental illness.

Definition
Study of the relationships of different factors that determine the frequency and distribution of health problems in people

Example
Buckle, P. (1987) Epidemiological aspects of back pain within the nursing profession. *International journal of nursing studies* 24(4) 319-324   19 References

Paper summarises some key epidemiological findings related to the extent of the back pain problem in nursing. The prevalence of back pain, its effects in terms of sickness/absence, nurses lost to the profession, comparison with other occupations, risks, factors associated with it and age effects are highlighted.

Annotations
2.42.1   Abramson, J.H. (1984) *Survey methods in community medicine: an introduction to epidemiological and evaluative studies.* 3rd edition Edinburgh: Churchill Livingstone   ISBN 0443030685   References

Book provides a systematic guide to conducting investigations concerned with health and disease. It covers all aspects of design, execution and analysis, and would assist those planning many types of study (CR 2.55).

2.42.2   Ahlbom, A. & Norell, S. (1984) *Introduction to modern epidemiology.* Chesnut Hill, Massachusetts: Epidemiology Resources Inc.   ISBN 091722700X References

An introductory text providing a concise description of the core ideas underlying epidemiological research. Exercises are included in each chapter to aid learning.

2.42.3   Breslow, N.E. & Day, N.E. (1980) *Statistical methods in cancer research.* Lyon: International Agency for Research on Cancer   ISBN 0197230326   References Volume 1

Outlines the nature of case control studies, their objectives, strengths, limitations, planning, implementation and interpretation. Chapters 2-7 cover measuring techniques and analysis of case control studies (CR 2.42.4).

2.42.4 Breslow, N.E. & Day, N.E. (1987) *Statistical methods in cancer research.* Lyon: International Agency for Research on Cancer   ISBN 9283211820   References Volume 2

Book is an introduction to the design and execution of cohort studies. Chapter 1 gives a general overview of cohort studies, their historical role, significance and strengths, limitations, implementation and interpretation. Problems relating to proportional mortality studies are outlined. Chapters 2-7 discuss the statistical techniques and development applicable in this type of study. Appendices give statistical data and details of design and conduct of studies cited in the text (CR 2.42.3).

2.42.5 Cook, R.L. (1981) Epidemiologic methodology for nurses. *Military medicine*: 146 July 469-472   21 References

Processes involved in epidemiological research are described and three types of studies outlined: retrospective, prospective and historical. The role of the nurse in such studies is discussed.

2.42.6 Copp, L.A. (1987) Implications of epidemiological research. *Recent advances in nursing* 17: 94-107   References

Areas which have been studied in particular populations are discussed, together with special methods which may be required and the implications this could have for nursing.

2.42.7 Grufferman, S., Delzell, E. & Delong, E.R. (1984) An approach to conducting epidemiologic research within co-operative clinical trial groups. *Journal of clinical oncology* 2(6) 670-675   12 References

Reports a case control study which examined the role of environmental factors in the aetiology of rhabdomyosarcoma in children. The methodology is described in detail and the advantages and disadvantages discussed. Practical problems encountered during the study are mentioned.

Suggested textbook reading

	Pages	Cross reference
Meininger J.C. IN Brink & Wood (1989)	201-222	2.36.3

Nursing research abstracts

Long, A.F.	85/378

2.43 NON-EXPERIMENTAL DESIGNS
Ethnomethods

The growth of a new cultural movement, based on the anthropological tradition, developed in the USA in the 1960s and it focused on discovering how people know and understand their world. The term ethnomethods is used to describe a group of techniques which seek to explain human care and health attributes which are part of the social structure, world views, language and different environmental contexts (Leininger 1987).

These qualitative approaches are defined below and literature included on some in this section.

Definitions

Ethnography — a systematic process of observing, detailing, describing, documenting and analysing the lifeways or particular patterns of a culture or sub-culture in order to understand people's behaviour in their own environment

Ethnology — a special application of ethnography in which the researcher develops theories of culture and society, rather than focusing on individuals in the setting

Ethnomethodology — an attempt to examine empirically the ways in which meanings are produced in social practice. It holds that all knowledge is a social creation

Ethnonursing — the study and analysis of the local or indigenous peoples' viewpoints, beliefs and practices about nursing care phenomena and processes of designated cultures

Ethnoscience — a formalised and systematic study of people from their viewpoint in order to obtain an accurate account of how the people know, classify and interpret their lifeways and the universe

Ethology — an observational technique, developed and adapted from research on animal behaviour, in which behaviours are recorded, coded, categorised and analysed

---

NB: Examples of each of the above have not been included but an overview of these approaches may be found in:

Field and Morse (1985)	19-31	(CR 2.1.24)
Leininger (1985)	33-71	(CR 2.1.36)
Leininger (1987)	12-36	(CR 2.43.13)

Grounded theory and phenomenology are also included in this group of techniques and may be found in sections 2.46 and 2.52 respectively.

Annotations
2.43.1 Aamodt, A.M. (1982) Examining ethnography for nurse researchers. *Western journal of nursing research* 4(2) 209-221 20 References

A critical examination is made of ethnography as a method for doing nursing research. Author contends that a growing body of knowledge in ethnographic techniques could be used to enhance the science of nursing. The methodology is briefly described together with some of the assumptions made about it, and various myths are explored.

2.43.2   Agar, M.H. (1980) *The professional stranger: an informal introduction to ethnography.* New York: Academic Press   ISBN 012043850X   References

Book explores the nature of ethnographic research and discusses the key issues involved. It is contrasted with hypothesis testing approaches and examples are given mainly from the author's own experience. Problems relating to ethnographic interviews and observation are discussed.

2.43.3   Benson, D. & Hughes, J.A. (1983) *The perspective of ethnomethodology.* London: Longman   ISBN 058229584X   References

Volume provides an introduction to ethnomethodology. Its intellectual background, in particular the work of Schutz, Garfinkel and Sacks, is examined and detailed discussions of research in the field is given.

2.43.4   Berreman, G.D. (1973) Behind many masks: ethnography and impression, management in a Himalayan village. IN Warwick, D.P. & Osherson, S. *Comparative research methods.* Englewood Cliffs, New Jersey: Prentice Hall   ISBN 013153940X   References   Chapter 13   268-312

Ethnographers rarely make explicit the ways in which their information is derived outside the conventional description of method. This chapter describes some features of the human experience in doing field research (CR 2.16, 2.41.8).

2.43.5   Dobson, S. (1986) Ethnography: a tool for learning. *Nurse education today* 6(2) 76-79   18 References

Author advocates the use of small-scale projects based on ethnographic research methods to enable nurse learners to develop cultural awareness and sensitivity.

2.43.6   Ellen, R.F. (ed) (1984) *Ethnographic research.* London: Academic Press   ISBN 0122371801   References

Volume is intended to provide an introduction to a series on ethnographic research by outlining practical matters and including a guide to existing literature. (1,130 entries are given in the reference list). Chapters cover theory, methodology, the research process, a history of field methods, approaches to ethnographic research, the fieldwork experience, ethical issues, producing data and writing reports.

2.43.7   Evaneshko, V. & Kay, M.A. (1982) The ethnoscience research technique. *Western journal of nursing research* 4(1) 49-64   19 References

Focuses on the process by which researchers obtain, analyse and interpret cultural data using the ethnoscience method which aims to identify the meaning of underlying group behaviour.

2.43.8   Garfinkel, H. (1967) *Studies in ethnomethodology.* Englewood Cliffs, New Jersey: Prentice Hall   (No ISBN number)   References

A series of studies undertaken over a period of 12 years which illustrate the properties and methodologies of ethnomethodological research.

2.43.9 Goetz, J. & LeCompte, M. (1981) Ethnographic research and the problem of data reduction. *Anthropology and education quarterly* 12: 51-70   88 References

Techniques are identified which enable ethnographic data to be reduced. The most commonly used are: analytic induction, typological analysis, the constant comparative, enumerative systems and standardised observational protocols. Each of these is defined and discussed.

2.43.10 Hammersley, M. & Atkinson, P. (1983) *Ethnography: principles in practice.* London: Tavistock   ISBN 0415045177   References   [Note: reprinted by Routledge]

Book provides an introduction to the principles and practice of ethnographic research, and is intended for students and experienced researchers. The principle of reflexivity* is thoroughly explored as the authors believe this is the key to development of both theory and methodology in social science generally, and in ethnographic work in particular. Ethnographic research is put in the context of other qualitative methods, and each step in the process is examined using a wide range of examples. An annotated bibliography of ethnographic texts is included − pages 238-245.

* Reflexivity is a recognition that we are part of the social world which we study.

2.43.11 Handel, W. (1982) *Ethnomethodology: how people make sense.* Englewood Cliffs, New Jersey: Prentice Hall   ISBN 0132917084   References

Book written for students which explores what ethnomethodologists study, their philosophical position, the approaches taken and the current state of knowledge.

2.43.12 Hilton, A. (1987) *The ethnographic perspective.* Research Awareness, Module 7 London: Distance Learning Centre, South Bank Polytechnic   ISBN 0948250283   References

This is number 7 in a series of 13 modules, each of which deals with a different aspect of nursing research. It was developed to assist nurses, midwives and health visitors in understanding research in terms of their own professional practice. Modules can be used separately or as part of a complete programme. The reader is encouraged to work through a number of activities, self-assessment questions and answers and progress summaries. Some articles/book extracts are reproduced in full.
   This module is one of three which deal with the practicalities of research (Module 8 covers the survey perspective and Module 9 the experimental). Ethnography is examined in detail and the following are included: definitions, action research, presentation of results, interpretation of findings, ethical issues and the psychological problems of the researcher (CR 2.16, 2.17, 2.37, 2.96, 2.97, Appendix D).

2.43.13 Leininger, M.M. (1987) Importance and uses of ethnomethods: ethnography and ethnonursing research. *Recent advances in nursing* 17: 12-36   48 References

Article provides a review of the nature, purposes, characteristics and uses of ethno-methods in nursing. Definitions of terms are included. Brief accounts are given of ethnoscience, grounded theory and phenomenological research methods. Each stage of an ethnographic and ethnonursing research study are described. (CR 2.46, 2.52).

2.43.14 Livingston, E. (1987) *Making sense of ethnomethodology.* London: Routledge & Kegan Paul   ISBN 0710212623   (no references)

A general introduction to methodological studies. Some of the problems involved are illustrated together with an introduction to conversational analysis. An extended ethnomethodological investigation is discussed (CR 2.89).

2.43.15 Robertson, M.H.B. & Boyle, J.S. (1984) Ethnography : contributions to nursing research. *Journal of advanced nursing* 9(1) 43-49   24 References

Describes the processes involved in conducting ethnographic research and suggests how it may be used to extend the knowledge base of nursing.

2.43.16 Rosenthal, T.T. (1989) Using ethnography to study nursing education. *Western journal of nursing research* 11(1) 115-127   38 References

Provides an overview of the procedures involved in ethnographic research.

2.43.17 Sharrock, W. & Anderson, B. (1986) *The ethnomethodologists.* Chichester: Ellis Horwood and London Tavistock   ISBN 0853129495   References

Provides a clear and authoritative introduction to the main thinkers in ethnomethodology. Following a critical reception as a technique, this book gives a base on which a more balanced assessment can be made.

2.43.18 Turner, R. (ed) (1974) *Ethnomethodology.* Harmondsworth: Middlesex Penguin Education   ISBN 0140809627   References

A collection of readings focusing on examples of research conducted in an ethnomethodological vein. There is some disagreement about its true nature because of its diversity, but working papers illustrate what is, and might be done by ethnomethodologists. Major sections are on the name and its uses; theorising as practical reasoning; practical reasoning in organisational settings and methodological bases of interaction.

Suggested textbook readings

	Pages	*Cross reference*
Aamodt A.M. IN Munhall & Oiler	163-172	2.1.42
Atkinson P. (DE 304) 3B	41-81	2.1.49
Boyd C.O. IN LoBiondo-Wood & Haber	187-190	2.1.38
Evaneshko V. IN Leininger (1985)	133-147	2.1.36
Field P.A. IN Morse (1989)	79-91	2.36.8
Germain C. IN Munhall & Oiler	147-162	2.1.42
Hammersley M. (DE 304) 4	89-177	2.1.50

	Pages	Cross reference
Hammersley M. (DE 304) 6	9-40	2.1.52
Honigmann J.J. IN Burgess (1982)	236-252	2.1.9
Leininger (1985)	33-71/237-249	2.1.36
Lipson J.G. IN Morse (1989)	61-75	2.36.8
Omery A. IN Sarter	17-31	2.1.61
Payne, Dingwall, Payne & Carter	87-141	2.36.10
Silverman D. (1985)	95-117/140-145	2.36.14
Wilson M.J. (DE 304) 1	79-90	2.1.45
Wiseman & Aron	237-252	2.66.1
Woods & Catanzaro	133-149	2.1.72

Nursing research abstracts

Cressler D.L. & Tomlinson P.S.	89/085

2.44 NON-EXPERIMENTAL DESIGNS
Evaluation research

'The practice of evaluation involves the systematic collection of information about the activities, characteristics and outcomes of programmes, personnel and products in order for judgements to be made about specific aspects of what these are doing or affecting' (Patton 1981).

Definition
Research that investigates how well a programme, practice or policy is working

---

Example
Lathlean, J., Smith, G. & Bradley, C. (1986) *Post-registration development schemes evaluation.* London: Nursing Education Research Unit, Kings College, University of London   (No ISBN number)   NERU Report No.4

Report of a study which evaluated three schemes for the professional development of newly registered nurses. Findings are discussed under the following headings: development needs, opportunities for development and support, developments occuring in newly registered nurses, processes of development, developments and changes in a wider context, constraints and resource requirements.

Annotations
2.44.1 Crow, R. (1984) Criteria for evaluation research. IN *Nursing research - does it make a difference?* Proceedings of the 7th Workgroup Meeting/ 2nd Open Conference of European Nurse Researchers 10-13th April London: Royal College of Nursing   ISBN 0902606891   149-157   17 References

Evaluation research is defined and discussed with particular reference to the difficulties arising when trying to evaluate the quality of nursing care (CR 3.26.4).

2.44.2 Levine, R.A., Solomon, M.A., Hellstern, G.M. & Wollman, H. (eds) (1981) *Evaluation research and practice: comparative and international perspectives.* Beverly Hills: Sage ISBN 0803915616 References

Collection of papers generated from an American/German workshop on evaluation research held in Berlin in June 1979. These discuss the spread of evaluation research, evaluation in the administrative machinery, improving evaluation research strategies, translating research into policy and future needs and prospects.

2.44.3 Luker, K. (1981) An overview of evaluation research in nursing. *Journal of advanced nursing* 6(2) 87-93 29 References

Explores some of the general issues relating to evaluation research in nursing. The evaluation and nursing processes are contrasted and the author urges nurses to emphasise more this phase of the nursing process. The methods used in evaluative research are described.

2.44.4 Parlett, M.R. & Dearden, G.J. (eds) (1981a) *Introduction to illuminative evaluation: studies in higher education.* Cardiff-by-the-Sea, California: Pacific Soundings Press (No ISBN number) References

(Re-issued in 1981 by the Society for Research into Higher Education: University of Surrey, Guildford)

A compilation of excerpts from published and unpublished papers on illuminative evaluation. This procedure aims to assist teachers evaluate their programmes. The four parts cover the rationale and design of illuminative evaluation; the approach in action; study of a college and illuminating educational practice.

2.44.5 Parlett, M.R. & Hamilton, D. (1981b) Evaluation as illumination. IN Parlett, M.R. & Dearden, G.J. (eds) *Introduction to illuminative evaluation: studies in higher education.* Cardiff-by-the-Sea, California: Pacific Soundings Press (No ISBN number) References 2, 9-29

Paper discusses illuminative evaluation which is a reappraisal of previous techniques used for programme evaluation. Innovation is examined in the school context and the methodological strategies described. Practical aspects discussed are problems and potential; applicability; validity and generalisability; the skills and obligations of the researcher; the development of theory and its value to decision makers (CR 2.44.4).

2.44.6 Patton, M.Q. (1990) *Qualitative evaluation and research methods.* 2nd edition Beverly Hills: Sage ISBN 0803937792 References

Book aims to encourage expansion of the evaluation skills of social scientists. It recognises that quantitative research is not 'better' than qualitative research but different methods are appropriate for different situations. The emphasis is on developing strategies for using qualitative evaluation methods (CR 2.9).

2.44.7 Rossi, P.H., Freeman, H.E. & Wright, S.R. (1979a) *Evaluation: a systematic approach*. Beverly Hills: Sage ISBN 0803911793 References

A comprehensive text designed for practitioners in many disciplines which covers the role of evaluation research in the planning, design and implementation of programmes and projects. Examples of each stage are given throughout the text.

2.44.8 Rossi, P.H. & Wright, S.R. (1979b) Evaluation research: an assessment of theory, practice and politics. IN Pollitt, C., Lewis, L., Negro, J. & Patten, J. (eds) *Public policy in theory and practice*. Sevenoaks: Hodder & Stoughton in association with the Open University Press ISBN 0340247797 References Chapter 11 197-221

[A reader for the Policies, people and administration course of the Open University No D 336. This course has now been discontinued]

Discusses the problems when undertaking evaluation research in two chief areas: political and methodological. The techniques available are described, as are their main features and inherent problems (CR 3.10).

2.44.9 Struening, E.L. & Guttentag, M. (eds) (1975) *Handbook of evaluation research*. Beverly Hills: Sage ISBN Volume 1 0803904282 ISBN Volume 2 0803904290 References

Handbook provides expert views on evaluation research and alternative strategies which may be considered. Volume 1 emphasises strategies and methods of evaluation under the following headings: policy and strategy in evaluation research, conceptualisation and design of studies, development of measures, data collection through interview and records, evaluation through social ecology, data analytic methods and communication of results. Volume 2 focuses on evaluation in context, politics and values in evaluation research, cost-benefit approach to evaluation, evaluation of mental health programmes and selected content areas.

Suggested textbook readings

	Pages	Cross refereces
Adams & Schvaneveldt	315-329	2.1.2
Christensen	272-292	2.1.17
Fox	162	2.1.25
Kidder & Judd	404-426	2.1.30
LoBiondo-Wood & Haber	218-223	2.1.38
Polit & Hungler (1987)	158-163	2.1.56
Seaman	222-223	2.1.62
Smith H.W.	293-311	2.98.14
Wood M.J. IN Brink & Wood (1989)	223-237	2.36.3

2.45 NON-EXPERIMENTAL DESIGNS
Ex-post facto research

In this type of research attempts are made to explain or describe events which have already occured, and this has value when research problems cannot be studied by experimentation. Studies investigate cases where variables have been manipulated by life events, for example environmental pollution, the effects of thalidomide, and those which have taken place in natural settings rather than in a laboratory.

Definition
Examines the relationships among variables after the variations have occurred

---

Example
Lynn, M.R. (1985) Reliability estimates: use and disuse. *Nursing research* 34(4) 254-256   8 References

Article examines the extent of the reliability estimates in published nursing research. Two major nursing research publications were studied from 1978-1982 using two questions: to what extent are reliability estimates included in research reports, and did such reporting increase significantly over the research period (CR 2.24).

Suggested textbook readings

	Pages	Cross reference
Castles	65-67	2.1.15
Cohen & Manion	176-192	2.1.19
LoBiondo-Wood & Haber	170-171	2.1.38
Polit & Hungler (1987)	141-151	2.1.56
Seaman	217-218	2.1.62
Thomas	73-76	2.1.64
Wilson H.S. (1989)	169-170	2.1.69

2.46 NON-EXPERIMENTAL DESIGNS
Grounded theory research

Grounded theory is a highly systematic research approach for the collection and analysis of qualitative data. Its purpose is to generate explanatory theory that furthers the understanding of social and psychological phenomena.It represents an advance in the technology for handling qualitative data gathered in the natural, everyday world. It has its roots in the social sciences, specifically in the symbolic interaction tradition* of social psychology and sociology.

* a theory about human behaviour and an approach to the study of human conduct and group life.

Definition
An approach to collecting and analysing qualitative data with the aim of developing theories and theoretical propositions grounded in real-world observations

Example
Hinds, P.S. (1984) Inducing a definition of 'hope' through the use of grounded theory methodology. *Journal of advanced nursing* 9(4) 357-362   19 References

Describes how grounded theory methodology guided conceptualisation processes to induce a construct definition of hope. Twenty-five adolescents participated in the study to define hope. Four categories emerged which seemed to form a contiuum of degree and are the basis for the 'hopefulness' scale for adolescents.

Original text
Glaser, B.G. & Strauss, A.L. (1967) *The discovery of grounded theory: strategies for qualitative research.* Chicago: Aldine   ISBN 297763180 (CR 2.46.3).

Annotations
2.46.1 Atwood, J.R. & Hinds, P.S. (1986) Heuristic heresy: application of reliability and validity criteria to products of grounded theory. *Western journal of nursing research* 8(2) 135-154   30 References

Using data from a study which examined 'well' and 'impaired' adolescents, authors discuss reliability and validity considerations in grounded theory methodology. Commentaries and authors responses are also included (CR 2.24, 2.25).

2.46.2   Chenitz, W.C. & Swanson, J.M. (eds) (1986) *From practice to grounded theory: qualitative research in nursing.* Menlo Park, California: Addison-Wesley   ISBN 0201129604   References

Book is designed for nurses undertaking qualitative research using grounded theory. It discusses the entire research process in grounded theory and six studies are included to illustrate the method. A final chapter shows how this type of research can be used to improve nursing care.

2.46.3   Glaser, B.G. & Strauss, A.L. (1967) *The discovery of grounded theory: strategies for qualitative research.* Chicago: Aldine   ISBN 297763180   References

A seminal work in the field of qualitative research which guides those planning such an approach.

2.46.4   Stern, P.N. (1980) Grounded theory methodology: its use and processes. *Image: the journal of nursing scholarship* 7(1) 20-23   14 References

Appropriate uses of grounded theory are described and the method is explained in jargon free language.

2.46.5 Stern, P.N., Allen, L.M. & Moxley, P.A. (1982) The nurse as grounded theorist: history, process and uses. *Review journal of philosophy and social science* 17: 200-215   36 References

Describes the grounded theory approach to research, its history and the method. Examples are given of ways in which it has been used. A short description of symbolic interactionism and the computer methodology of factor analysis are also included.

Suggested textbook readings

	Pages	*Cross reference*
Boyd C.O. IN LoBiondo-Wood & Haber	190-193	2.1.38
Bowers B.J. IN Sarter	33-59	2.1.61
Hutchimon S. IN Munhall & Oiler	109-130	2.1.42
Phillips L.R.F. (critique)	128-130	2.98.11
Polit & Hungler (1987)	351-352/361-362	2.1.56
Stern P.N. IN Leininger (1985)	149-160	2.1.36
Strauss A.L.	22-39	2.89.7
Wilson H.S. IN Munhall & Oiler	131-144	2.1.42
Woods & Catanzaro	133-149	2.1.72

2.47   NON-EXPERIMENTAL DESIGNS
Historical research (a) documentary

The historical approach involves using literature, records, diaries, verbatim reports, letters, artefacts and other sources of data from the past to arrive at conclusions. It can provide some predictive insights of value to the profession.

Definition
The critical investigation of events, developments and experiences of the past, the careful weighing of evidence of validity of sources of information about the past, and the interpretation of the weighed evidence

Example
Davies, C. (1988) The health visitor as mother's friend: a woman's place in public health, 1900 – 1914. *Social history of medicine* 1(1) 39-59   54 Notes and References

Paper explores aspects of the debate about health visiting at the turn of the century and asks whether it was an appropriate form of work for women. The struggle of the sexes in terms of employment is identified and discussed.

Annotations
2.47.1 Carr, E.H. (1973) *What is history?* Harmondsworth, Middlesex: Penguin ISBN 0140206523

A classic text which explores historical theory, the origins of history, its relationship to science and morality, causation in history, its progress and how it expands the horizon of learning.

2.47.2 Christy, T.E. (1975) The methodology of historical research: a brief introduction. *Nursing research* 24(3) 189-192   7 References

Provides guidance on three essential steps in historical research: the gathering of data, criticism of the data and the presentation of findings.

2.47.3 Christy, T.E. (1981) Can we learn from history? IN McCloskey, J.C. & Grace, H.K. (eds) *Current issues in nursing.* Oxford: Blackwell Scientific   ISBN 086542005X   References   Part 2   Chapter 13   122-129

Author discusses the reasons for including the history of nursing in the curriculum and the value of undertaking historical research in preventing 'the rediscovery of the wheel'.

2.47.4 Church, O.M. (1985) New knowledge from old truths: problems and promises of historical enquiry in nursing. IN McCloskey, J.C. & Grace, H.K. (eds) *Current issues in nursing.* 2nd edition Boston: Blackwell Scientific   ISBN 086542019   References   Part 2   Chapter 15   182-189

Value of nursing history is discussed as a link between the past and future. This sense of history enables us to examine current ideas and take them forward in the development of the profession.

2.47.5 Church, O.M. (1987) Historiography in nursing research. *Western journal of nursing research* 9(2) 275-279   12 References

First article relating to history published in this journal. The importance of history in relation to the development of nursing is discussed.

2.47.6 Floud, R. (1979) *An introduction to quantitative methods for historians.* 2nd edition London: Methuen   ISBN 0416716601   References

A number of quantitative techniques are discussed in relation to their application to historical problems and historical evidence.

2.47.7 Kerr, J.C. (1986) Historical nursing research. IN Stinson, S.M. & Kerr, J.C. (eds) *International issues in nursing research.* Beckenham: Croom Helm   ISBN 0709944373   References   Part 1   Chapter 2   28-40

Chapter discusses the relevance of historical research in professional disciplines; issues in historical research methods and the state of the art in nursing. Nurses are urged to learn the necessary skills in order to widen our understanding of the past and present to underpin progress in the future (CR 3.27.7).

2.47.8 Maggs, C.J. (1989) *Exploring history: an introduction to nursing's past.* London: Continuing Nurse Education Programme, Barnet College ISBN 0948910119 References Section 2 11-22

Part of a workbook which covers various aspects of nursing history. Book contains exercises, sources of primary and secondary information, and how to find and use them.

2.47.9 Sarnecky, M.T. (1990) Historiography: a legitimate research methodology for nursing. *Advances in nursing science* 12(4) 1-10 36 References

Examines the historical approach, discusses its relevance to nursing and contrasts it with other epistemologies and ontologies.

2.47.10 Sorenson, E.S. (1988) Archives as sources of treasure in historical research. *Western journal of nursing research* 10(5) 666-670 11 References

Discusses the use of historical archives and gives some of the sources available for the study of nursing history.

Suggested textbook readings

	Pages	Cross reference
Abdellah & Levine	204-207	2.1.1
Cohen & Manion	47-69	2.1.19
Fitzpatrick M.L. IN Munhall & Oiler	195-225	2.1.42
Fox	143-158	2.1.25
Glass L.K. IN Brink & Wood (1989)	183-200	2.36.3
Kerr IN Stinson & Kerr	28-40	3.27.7
Kovacs	140-142	2.1.31
Kruman M.W. IN Leininger	109-118	2.1.36
Lee J.L. IN Sarter	5-16	2.1.61
Lin	213-217	2.1.37
LoBiondo-Wood & Haber	212-217	2.1.38
Matejski IN Munhall & Oiler	175-193	2.1.42
Nieswiadomy	140-142	2.1.43
Polit & Hungler (1987)	164-168	2.1.56
Seaman	185-188	2.1.62
Treece & Treece	203-207	2.1.65
Woods & Catanzaro	348-352	2.1.72

2.48 NON-EXPERIMENTAL DESIGNS
Historical research (b) oral

The validity of oral history as a field of study has been questioned by some historians because of the difficulties of trying to reconstruct the past on minimal and perhaps biased evidence. Agreement can never be reached about what the past was really like, but oral history can assist in filling in some of the gaps about the more recent past.

Definitions

History − a branch of knowledge that records and explains past events as steps in the sequence of human activities

Historiography − the principles, theory and history of historical writing

Oral historiography − information transmitted orally, in a personal exchange, of a kind likely to be of historical or long-term value

Example

Nolan, P.W. (1989) *Psychiatric nursing past and present: the nurses' viewpoint.* PhD Thesis (unpublished) University of Bath

Thesis examines the state of psychiatric nursing by focusing on four periods, the second half of the 19th century, the 1920s, 1940s and 1980s. The historical background to the development of psychiatric practice is examined and three cohorts of nurses were questioned about their work. The 1982 syllabus of training for mental nurses is reviewed to assess its contribution to changes in practice. Many problems still exist which require radical changes in organisation and attitude.

Annotations

2.48.1 Allemang, M.M. (1987) Oral historiography. *Recent advances in nursing* 17: 2-11   30 References

Author presents an assessment of the requirements for the creation, evaluation and interpretation of oral materials which will add to historical understanding.

2.48.2 Allen, B. (1984) Re-creating the past: the narrator's perspective in oral history. *Oral history review* 12: 1-12   19 References

Article discusses the different perspectives of the narrator and interviewer and identifies the points of view from which each approaches the oral history interview. The differing emphases and the researchers interest in reconstructing the past along chronological lines are outlined, whereas that of the client is one of association. Both angles are needed in order to create a composite picture.

2.48.3 Becker, H.S. (1970) The relevance of life histories. IN Denzin, N.K. *Sociological methods: a sourcebook.* London: Butterworths   ISBN 0408701250 References

Discusses the value of life histories in developing understanding of the complex mosaic of the social world. Such studies may help to fill in some of the gaps or challenge assumptions which researchers can make. It is never possible to study all aspects of a problem in detail as selection always takes place to a greater or lesser extent (CR 2.1.23).

2.48.4 Davis, C., Back, K. & Maclean, K. (1977) *Oral history: from tape to type.* Chicago: American Library Association   ISBN 0838902308   References

140

An instructional and operating manual designed to guide those beginning an oral history programme and a textbook for instructors. Illustrations and exercises are included to enable the novice to practice certain skills. Sample forms show how to do the paperwork which accompanies oral history interviewing and processing. A glossary is included and a list of additional sources.

2.48.5 Humphries, S. (1984) *The handbook of oral history: recording life stories.* London: Inter-Action Inprint ISBN 0904571467 References

Book shows how a more accurate and authentic picture of the past may be created by talking to the people who were actually there. It includes sections on organising a project, working with different groups and all aspects of presentation and publication.

2.48.6 Mandelbaum, D.G. (1982) The study of life history. IN Burgess, R.G. (ed) *Field research: a sourcebook and field manual.* London: Allen & Unwin ISBN 0043120148 References Chapter 20 146-151

Examines the value of life history in obtaining the views of individuals on how they cope in the society in which they live (CR 2.1.9).

2.48.7 Perks, R. (ed) (1990) *Oral history.* London: British Library ISBN 071230505X

An annotated bibliography giving a wide range of health topics in over 2100 entries. Sources of information on the processes involved in oral history are also included.

2.48.8 Samuel, R. (1982) Local history and oral history. IN Burgess, R.G. (ed) *Field research: a sourcebook and field manual.* London: Allen & Unwin ISBN 0043120148 References Chapter 19 136-145

Identifies sources of available material and highlights the value of oral evidence (CR 2.1.9).

2.48.9 Seldon, A. & Pappworth, J. (1983) *By word of mouth: 'elite oral history'.* London: Methuen ISBN 0416367402 References

A practical guide to the oral history of elite figures, i.e. from or about people eminent in their field. Book analyses the advantages of using oral history, offers advice on aspects of interviewing and gives information on the establishment and maintenance of an oral archive. A series of case studies showing the use of oral evidence by contemporary authors are included.

2.48.10 Thompson, P. (1987) *The voice of the past: oral history.* Oxford: Oxford University Press ISBN 0192158333 References

The accepted myths of the nature of historical scholarship are challenged. Author traces oral history through its past and into the future showing how the method could be developed. This new material can be evaluated alongside traditional sources to construct a more democratic record (CR 2.70).

Suggested textbook readings

	Pages	*Cross reference*
Adams & Schvaneveldt	291-314	2.1.2
Leedy	125-139	2.1.35
Leininger	119-132	2.1.36
Krampitz IN Krampitz & Pavlovich	54-58	2.1.32

2.49   NON-EXPERIMENTAL DESIGNS
Longitudinal/developmental research

This research strategy is useful for detecting change in individuals or groups over time, for example examining health maintenance or illness recovery.

[Note: The above terms are often used interchangeably]

Definition

Collection of data from the same subjects at different points in time

---

Example

Bradshaw, P., Brown, H., Couchman, W. & Moore, D. (1988) The same or different. *Senior nurse* 8(11) 15-17   10 References

Describes a longitudinal study which aimed to investigate attitude and value changes in students undertaking a conversion course from Enrolled Nurse (General) to Registered General Nurse.

Annotations

2.49.1   Barnard, K.E., Magyary, D.L., Booth, C.L. & Eyres, S.J. (1987) Longitudinal designs: considerations and applications to nursing research. *Recent advances in nursing* 17: 37-64   34 References

Discusses the value of longitudinal studies as nurses are interested in changes in peoples' health over time. Studies based on large samples are described together with use of the case study approach incorporated within this type of design.

2.49.2   Goldstein, H. (1979) *The design and analysis of longitudinal studies: their role in the measurement of change.* London: Academic Press   ISBN 0122895800 References

Provides comprehensive coverage of the theoretical background to this type of design together with a practical approach to the problems encountered in human field studies. Statistical aspects of longitudinal studies are thoroughly explored.

Suggested textbook readings

2.50 NON-EXPERIMENTAL DESIGNS
Methodological/instrumentation research

The development of new measurement techniques is a complex task requiring expertise in the clinical area, research and statistics. Once a tool has been developed its use should be replicated with large samples so that it demonstrates precision, stability, accuracy and sensitivity.

Definition
Development or evaluation of measurement devices

Example
Brooking, J.I. (1989) A scale to measure use of the nursing process. *Nursing times* 85(15) April 12 44-48   12 References

Describes a methodological study in which a scale was developed to measure use of the nursing process. The tool was tested in eight general wards with follow-up studies at two and eighteen months.

Annotations
2.50.1 to 2.50.11 *Nursing research* (1981) 30(5) Instrumentation for nursing research.

[NB: The following entry differs in format as it documents a special issue of the journal *Nursing research*. These articles have not been annotated]

2.50.1 Brandt, P.A. & Weinart, C. The PRQ − a social support system. 277-280   20 References

2.50.2 Cranley, M.S. Development of a tool for the measurement of maternal attachment during pregnancy. 281-284   12 References

2.50.3 Doerr, B.T. & Hutchins, E.B. Health risk appraisal: process, problems and prospects for nursing practice and research. 299-306   35 References

2.50.4 Fleming, J. An evaluation of the Denver Developmental Screening Test. 290-293   13 References

2.50.5 Goetz, A.A. & McTyre, R.B. Health risk appraisal: some methodologic considerations. 307-313   35 References

2.50.6 Goodwin, L.D., Prescott, P.A., Jacox, A. & Collar, M.R. The Nurse Practitioner Rating Form Part 2: methodological development. 270-276   (No references)

2.50.7 Lowery, B.J. Misconceptions and limitations of locus of control and the I-E Scale 294-298   41 References

2.50.8 Miller, T.W. Life events scaling: clinical methodological issues. 316-321   40 References

2.50.9 Mishel, M.H. The measurement of uncertainty in illness. 258-263   19 References

2.50.10 Norbeck, J.S., Lindsey, A.M. & Carrieri, V.L. The development of an instrument to measure social support. 264-269   27 References

2.50.11 Palisin, H. The neonatal perception inventory: a review. 285-298   29 References

Suggested textbook readings

	Pages	*Cross reference*
LoBiondo-Wood IN LoBiondo-Wood & Haber	217-218	2.1.38
Mishel M.H. IN Brink & Wood (1989)	238-284	2.36.3
Nieswiadomy	147-148	2.1.43
Phillips L.R.F. (critique)	146-148	2.98.11
Polit & Hungler (1987)	178-179	2.1.56
Seaman	223-224/226-227	2.1.62
Waltz & Bausell	83-99	2.21.4
Wilson H.S. (1989)	255-256	2.1.69

2.51 NON-EXPERIMENTAL DESIGNS
Panel research

Panel studies typically yield more information than trend studies because the investigator can usually reveal patterns of change and reasons for the changes (Polit & Hungler 1987).

Definition
A type of longitudinal study in which the same subjects are used to provide data at two or more points in time

---

Example
Mercer, R. (1985) The process of maternal role attainment over the first year. *Nursing research* 34(4) 198-204   29 References

Describes the development of role attainment behaviours of mothers of three different age groups towards their babies.

Annotation
2.51.1   Wiseman, J.P. & Aron, M.S. (1970) *Field projects for sociology students.* Cambridge, Massachusetts: Schenkman   (No ISBN number)   References   Assignment 12 Panel analysis 150-164

Chapter describes the nature, advantages and disadvantages of panel studies, gives details of a project assignment and concludes with references (CR 2.66).

Suggested textbook readings

	Pages	*Cross reference*
Polit & Hungler (1987)	200	2.1.56
Treece & Treece	181	2.1.65
Woods & Catanzaro	142-145/181-184	2.1.72

2.52   NON-EXPERIMENTAL DESIGNS
Phenomenological research/approaches

'Phenomenology is that kind of thinking which guides one back from theoretical abstraction to the reality of lived experience ... it is not just a research method but also a philosophy and an approach' (Field & Morse 1985, Psathas 1978).

Definition
A method of study that attempts to understand human experience through analysis of the participants description of an experience

---

Example
Field, P.A. (1981) A phenomenological look at giving an injection. *Journal of advanced nursing* 6(4) 291-296   8 References

Author attempts to answer the question, 'what is it like to give an injection?' Nurses and patients were asked to describe their experiences in order to discover its deeper meaning. The phenomenologist never reaches a conclusion but further understanding of both groups' views is gained.

Annotations
2.52.1   Cohen, M.Z. (1987) A historical overview of the phenomenological movement. *Image: the journal of nursing scholarship* 19(1) 31-34   21 References

A brief historical overview of phenomenology is given. Key figures and important concepts are highlighted to clarify some of its more complex aspects.

2.52.2   Drew, N. (1989) The interviewers experience as data in phenomenological research. *Western journal of nursing research* 11(4) 431-439   References

Discusses the use of a diary as data, the new categories which emerged and the significance of the researchers experience (CR 2.16, 2.69).

2.52.3   Knaak, P. (1984) Phenomenological research. *Western journal of nursing research* 6(1) 107-114   9 References

Article examines the philosophy, historical perspective, characteristics and roles of the subject and researcher in phenomenological research. Its methodology is described, together with its application to nursing (CR 3.16).

2.52.4   Oiler, C. (1982) The phenomenological approach in nursing research. *Nursing research* 31(3) 178-181   18 References

Phenomenology is a philosophy, an approach and a method. Article introduces the major themes and method of phenomenology and suggests ways in which nurses may use this approach to develop nursing knowledge.

2.52.5   Omery, A. (1983) Phenomenology: a method for nursing research. *Advances in nursing science* 5(2) 49-63   33 References

Describes the phenomenological method, its origins and implementation and discusses how it differs from other research methods. Its value to nursing research is explored.

2.52.6   Swanson-Kauffman, K.M. (1986) A combined qualitative methodology for nursing research. *Advances in nursing science* 8(3) 58-69   16 References

Describes the experience of miscarriage using a combination of ethnography, grounded theory and phenomenological techniques. The step by step process used by the researcher is outlined and the value of this combined approach to examine human responses is highlighted (CR 2.43, 2.46).

Suggested textbook readings

	Pages	Cross reference
Anderson J.M. IN Morse (1989)	15-26	2.36.8
Bergum V. IN Morse (1989)	43-57	2.36.8
Boyd C.O. IN LoBiondo-Wood & Haber	194-199	2.1.38
Chenitz & Swanson	3-7	2.46.2
Denzin N.K. IN Morgan G.	129-146	2.8.6
Leininger IN Cahoon	25-26	2.1.14
Lynch-Sauer J. IN Leininger	93-107	2.1.36
Oiler IN Munhall & Oiler	69-84	2.1.42

	Pages	Cross reference
Polit & Hungler (1987)	21	2.1.56
Ray M.A. IN Leininger	81-92	2.1.36
Riemen D.J. IN Munhall & Oiler	85-108	2.1.42
Swanson-Kaufmann K &		
Schonwald E. IN Sarter	97-105	2.1.61
Wilson H.S. (1989)	490-493	2.1.69
Woods & Catanzaro	133-149	2.1.72

2.53 NON-EXPERIMENTAL DESIGNS
Prescriptive theory research

Empirical validation of prescriptive theory has lagged behind other methodologies, as multiple studies over a long period of time are essential for this process.

Definition
Theory whose aims include controlling, promoting and changing nursing phenomena. Its elements include the aim or goal, prescriptions to produce the goal, and a survey list

---

Example
Kogan, H. & Betrus, P. (1984) Self-management: a nursing mode of therapeutic influence. *Advances in nursing science* 6(4) 55-73   12 References

Study aimed to assess the reduction in stress following self-management training sessions. Results showed that it was successful in reducing symptoms.

Suggested textbook reading

	Pages	Cross reference
Woods & Catanzaro	202-212	2.1.72

2.54 NON-EXPERIMENTAL DESIGNS
Simulation and gaming

Role-playing has been used as a technique in educational research and in the social sciences for assessing personality, in business training, and in psychotherapy. Its value is in the possibility of using it for assessment, teaching, and as a therapeutic procedure.

Definitions
Role-playing − a function performed in a particular situation, process or operation
Simulation − to imitate, represent or feign

Example
Maerker, M., Lisper, H-O. & Rickberg, S-E. (1990) Role-playing as a method in nursing research. *Journal of advanced nursing* 15(2) 180-186   14 References

Describes a study which investigated the way in which patients were informed about their illness. Advantages are listed of commissioning research on certain problems and by role playing studies with healthy people.

Annotations
2.54.1 Cohen, L. & Manion, L. (1989) Role-playing IN Authors *Research methods in education*. 3rd edition London: Routledge ISBN 0415036488 References Chapter 12   287-306

Chapter provides a brief introduction to role-playing; discussion of the argument about the technique and deception; its role and uses in educational settings; its strengths and weaknesses, organising and evaluating a session (CR 2.1.19).

2.54.2 Megarry, J. (ed) (1977) *Aspects of simulation and gaming: an anthology of SAGSET Journal Volumes 1-4.* London: Kogan Page ISBN 0850380588 References

Book comprises a series of articles which first appeared in the journal of the Society for Academic Gaming and Simulation. It does not include information about this research technique, but provides background materials for those unfamiliar with it.

2.54.3 Phillips, B.S. (1976) Simulation and computer simulation. IN Author *Social research: strategies and tactics*. 3rd edition New York: Macmillan ISBN 0023952601 References Chapter 8   179-203

Chapter discusses the role of simulation and computer simulation in research. Simulation can give increased insight into the situation under study and may reveal assumptions not considered initially. Its strengths and weaknesses are identified.

2.54.4 Smith, H.W. (1975) Simulation and gaming. IN Author *Strategies of social research: the methodological imagination.* London: Prentice Hall ISBN 0138511217 References Chapter 11   254-270

Discusses the use of simulation as a research technique with its dimensions and properties outlined. Man, machine and man-machine simulation are discussed (CR 2.98.14).

2.54.5 Stevens, F. (1987) The use of simulations for purposes of research. IN Crookall, D., Greenblat, C.S., Coote, A., Klabbers, J.H.G. & Watson, D.R. (eds) *Simulation-gaming in the late 1980's.* Oxford: Pergamon Press ISBN 0080341586 References 187-192

Reports a workshop which aimed to show participants how simulations could be used in research.

2.55 NON-EXPERIMENTAL DESIGNS
Survey research

Surveys are a commonly used research design where information is sought from a group of people, usually by means of interviews or questionnaires. It is a flexible method and broad in its scope. There are several types and forms of survey depending on semantics. Writers and researchers may interchange the names of similar types of studies which can lead to confusion.

Definitions

Survey − type of research plan undertaken to study a large population by systematically selecting samples from the group to discover the incidence, distribution, inter-relationships and behaviour of variables

Comparative survey − results from two groups or techniques are compared

Cross-cultural survey − study of more than one culture

Cross-sectional survey − several groups in various stages of development are studied simultaneously

Evaluation survey − researcher looks back at previous activities with a critical eye and evaluates results

Field survey − study conducted in the real world as opposed to in a laboratory

Long term/longitudinal survey − a sequence of events is observed over more than five years but there is no control over the outcome

[NB Long term/longitudinal surveys are given different names in the following disciplines:

psychology and education − longitudinal
anthropology and sociology − historical
economics − time-series]

Short term − sequence of events observed over less than five years

---

Example
Bircumshaw, D. (1989) A survey of attitudes of senior nurses towards graduate nurses. *Journal of advanced nursing* 14(1) 68-72   6 References

Describes a small survey, within a larger study, which examined the role and functions of a graduate nursing course as seen by senior nurse managers.

Annotations
2.55.1 Casley, D.J. & Lury, D.A. (1981) *Data collection in developing countries.* Oxford: Clarendon Press   ISBN 019877124X   References

Book covers the range of enquiring techniques from case study to the census, but gives major emphasis to data collection by sample survey. The practical aspects of conducting surveys in developing countries are discussed. It aims to combine theory and practice in a simple, practical way.

2.55.2 Cartwright, A. (1983) *Health surveys in practice and potential: a critical review of their scope and methods.* London: King Edward's Hospital Fund for London   ISBN 0197246230   References

Outlines some of the ways that surveys have contributed to the understanding of health and health care. A range of subject areas is covered which used different methodological approaches and the value and limitations of these are discussed.

2.55.3 Crosby, F.E., Ventura, M.A. & Feldman, M.J. (1989) Examination of a survey methodology: Dillman's total design method. *Nursing research* 38(1) 56-58   13 References

Total design method is a specific set of techniques which are associated with high response rates. Article discusses its background and implementation.

2.55.4 Deming, W.E. (1970) On errors in surveys. IN Denzin, N.K. *Sociological methods: a sourcebook.* London: Butterworths   ISBN 0408701250   References

Discusses thirteen factors which affect the value of surveys and must be taken into consideration when planning this type of research approach (CR 2.1.23).

2.55.5 Fink, A. & Kosecoff, J. (1985) *How to conduct surveys: a step by step guide.* Beverly Hills: Sage   ISBN 0803924569   References

This practical text outlines the basic essentials required to organise a rigorous survey or evaluate the credibility of others.

2.55.6 Fowler, F.J. (1984) *Survey research methods.* Beverly Hills: Sage   ISBN 0803923481   References

Book discusses the standards and practical procedures required for surveys designed to provide statistical descriptions of people by asking questions, usually of a sample. Surveys combine sampling, question design and interviewing techniques and each of these is explored to show how precision, accuracy and credibility are achieved.

2.55.7 Frey, J.H. (1983) *Survey research by telephone.* Beverly Hills: Sage   ISBN 0803919964   References

The history of telephone surveying is outlined, and comparisons made with mail, and face to face methods. Sampling procedures and question wording are discussed and procedures suggested for administering and implementing this method of data collection. Ethical issues are discussed together with the future of telephone surveys (CR 2.17, 2.22, 2.72).

2.55.8 Hoinville, G., Jowell, R. & Associates (1978) *Survey research practice.*
Aldershot: Gower   ISBN 0566051567   References

Book covers many of the organisational problems involved in conducting surveys.
All stages are covered in a practical way, to give students and commissioners of
research, insight into how good surveys are conducted.

2.55.9 Marsh, C. (1982) *The survey method: the contribution of surveys to
sociological explanation.* London: Allen & Unwin   ISBN 0043100155   References

Examines some of the criticisms made about surveys and shows the potential they
have for addressing major questions in the social sciences. A history of surveys is
given and some political applications discussed. An annotated bibliography of major
survey literature is included.

2.55.10 Moser, C.A. & Kalton, G. (1971) *Survey methods in social investigation.*
2nd edition London: Heinemann Educational   ISBN 0435826034   References

A classic text covering all aspects of social surveys.

2.55.11 Open University (1983) Surveys. IN *Statistics in society.* (MDST 242)
Milton Keynes: Open University Press   ISBN 0335141293   Block A, Exploring
the data: Unit A 4

Part of unit covers surveys and sampling techniques (CR 2.22).

2.55.12 Rogers, J. (1988) *The survey perspective.* Research Awareness, Module
8 London: Distance Learning Centre, South Bank Polytechnic   ISBN 0948250372
References

This is number 8 in a series of 13 modules, each of which deals with a different
aspect of nursing research. It was developed to assist nurses, midwives and health
visitors in understanding research in terms of their own professional practice. Modules
can be used separately or as part of a programme.

The reader is encouraged to work through a number of activities, self-assessment
questions and answers and progress summaries. Some articles/ book extracts referred
to in the text are reproduced in full.

This module is an introduction to the understanding of survey research. Types
of survey and sampling are described, the ways in which information is collected
and the advantages and disadvantages if these methods. The construction of
questionnaires, interview schedules, check lists and attitude scales is examined.
Advice is given about issues which need to be considered by nurses when approached
by researchers wishing to question patients or colleagues (CR Appendix D).

Suggested textbook readings

	Pages	Cross reference
Brink & Wood (1989)	89-103	2.36.3
Cohen & Manion	97-123	2.1.19

	Pages	*Cross reference*
Fox	159-175	2.1.25
Kidder & Judd	127-142	2.1.30
Kovacs	52	2.1.31
Lin	220-244	2.1.37
LoBiondo-Wood & Haber	167-168	2.1.38
Marsh C. IN Bulmer	82-102	2.1.8
Marriner A. IN Krampitz & Pavlovich	59-66	2.1.32
Nieswiadomy	144-147	2.1.43
Polgar & Thomas	71-83/94-102	2.1.55
Polit & Hungler (1987)	155-158	2.1.56
Oppenheim R.N. (DE 304) 4	33-87	2.1.50
Seaman	214-216	2.1.62
Smith H.W.	169-199	2.98.14
Swift B. (DE 304) 3A	73-110	2.1.48
Treece & Treece	175-182	2.1.65
Wilson H.S. (1989)	145-154	2.1.69
Wilson M.J. (DE 304) 1	15-19	2.1.45
Wiseman & Aron	37-48	2.66.1
Woods & Catanzaro	152-155	2.1.72

Nursing research abstracts

Amramson, J.H.	80/376, 85/006
Belson, W.A.	86/001
French, K.	81/402
Hockey, L. et al	84/137
Long, A.F.	85/378

MEASUREMENT

2.56 MEASUREMENT – GENERAL

The process of measurement involves the delineation of what needs to be measured in terms of the research problem, the development of an instrument to measure it and then analysis of the resulting data. Measurement in the natural sciences has been established over many decades but in the behavioural sciences it has a much shorter history. Movement has been slow and progress limited because many aspects of human functioning are difficult to measure. Nurses are now beginning to come to grips with these problems and are adding to the body of nursing knowledge.

Definitions
The assignment of some numerical value to objects or events to represent the kind or amount of some characteristic of those objects or events. Measurement as used in this context, includes qualitative data, in which objects are assigned to categories that represent the kind of characteristics they possess and that are mutually exclusive and exhaustive

There are several different approaches to measurement i.e. norm-referenced, criterion referenced and other sources of information such as physiological functions, thoughts and feelings. The individual and others can be information sources as well as written records.

Criterion referenced measures – techniques appropriate for determining whether or not an individual has acquired a set of behaviour or mastered a specific task

Norm referenced measures – techniques appropriate for evaluating the performance of an individual relative to some other individuals in a group

Annotations
2.56.1 **Berry, W.D. & Lewis-Beck, M.S.** (eds) (1986) *New tools for social scientists: advances and applications in research methods.* Beverly Hills: Sage   ISBN 0803926251   References

Volume is in three parts, each of which deals with a major methodological problem confronting sociological research. These are measurement strategies, techniques for non-interval level data and how to make inferences about the determinants of a dynamic process. Each paper includes both method and application which makes the book unusual. Book is intended to be accessible to readers with a limited knowledge of quantitative methods but the level of sophistication does vary within the chapters.

2.56.2 Llewellyn-Thomas, H. & Sutherland, H. (1987) Procedures for value assessment. *Recent advances in nursing* 17: 169-185 46 References

Provides an overview of strategies available for determining the 'weight' or 'value' given to the constituent dimensions within a measurement scale. The Quality of Life Index is used for illustration.

2.56.3 Miller, D.C. (1977) *Handbook of research design and social measurement.* 3rd edition New York: David McKay ISBN 067930312X References

A reference guide to research design, sampling, collection of data, statistical analysis, selection of sociometric scales or indexes, research funding, costing and reporting. Contains extensive references to resource materials and includes examples of psychometric, social psychological, demographic and sociometric scales (CR 2.21, 2.22, 2.57, 2.66, 2.90, 3.12).

2.56.4 Tierney, A., Closs, J., Atkinson, J., Murphy-Black, T. & Macmillan, M. (1988) On measurement and nursing research. *Nursing times* 84(12) March 23 55-58 25 References Occasional Paper

A background picture is provided of the importance and relevance of measurement in nursing today, e.g., measuring quality and standards of care and allocation of resources. It is suggested that researchers can help by developing measurement tools. Topics included are the definition of measurement, levels of measurement, measurement instruments and their accuracy. The purpose of measurement and whether it is always necessary in nursing research is discussed. Examples are given which emanate from the work of the Nursing Research Unit in Edinburgh (CR 3.13.19, 3.13.20).

2.56.5 Waltz, C.F., Strickland, O.L. & Lenz, E.R. (1984) *Measurement in nursing research.* Philadelphia: Davis ISBN 0803690460 References

A comprehensive text for students and experienced researchers who are consumers or developers of nursing measures. The theories and principles of sound measurement practices are discussed together with the processes involved in designing, selecting and testing instruments. The appendix contains information on compilations of existing tools, a selection of nursing theories and their measurement implications and guidance on resources useful for locating suitable tools (CR 2.57).

Suggested textbook readings

	Pages	Cross reference
Abdellah & Levine	125-163	2.1.1
Adams & Schvaneveldt	149-172	2.1.2
Bello A. IN LoBiondo-Wood & Haber	291-308	2.1.38
Brink & Wood	86-92	2.1.7
Burns & Grove	281-333	2.1.12
Bynner, et al (DE 304) 5	85-133	2.1.51

	Pages	*Cross reference*
Castles	101-109	2.1.15
Fox	232-254	2.1.25
Grady & Wallston	84-100	3.11.2
Holm & Llewellyn	127-141	2.1.26
Jaeger	85-110	2.83.8
Kidder & Judd	39-45/191-218	2.1.30
Kovacs	149-152	2.1.31
Lin	166-194	2.1.37
Nieswiadomy	190-194	2.1.43
Nuttall D.L. (DE 304) 5	39-83	2.1.51
Polgar & Thomas	114-128	2.1.55
Polit & Hungler (1987)	336-346	2.1.56
Seaman	303-316	2.1.62
Smith H.W.	132-165	2.98.14
Waltz & Bausell	39-82	2.21.4
Williamson	145-167	2.1.67
Wilson H.S. (1989)	503-509	2.1.69
Woods & Catanzaro	221-245	2.1.72

Nursing research abstracts
Gift A.	90/005
McLaughlin F.E. & Marascuilo L.A.	90/108

2.57 SELECTING AND USING EXISTING INSTRUMENTS

An issue that frequently faces nurses undertaking research is whether to use instruments developed by others or to develop new ones. It is generally less costly and time-consuming to use existing ones and this is beneficial from the knowledge building perspective. Use of existing tools provides an increasing data base for evaluating the properties of the instruments themselves. However in many instances existing instruments may not be adequate and high priority should be given to developing new ones appropriate for nursing measurement.

Definition
An instrument/tool is the device or technique that a researcher uses to collect data e.g., questionnaires, tests, observation schedules

Annotations
2.57.1 Ventura, M.R., Hinshaw, A.S. & Atwood, J.R. (1981) Instrumentation: the next step. *Nursing research* 30(5) 257 Guest Editorial

ledge, assess current practice and develop nursing interventions to positively influence health care and client behaviour.

2.57.2   Ward, M.J. (1986) Nursing research instruments: some considerations and recommendations. IN Stinson, S.M. & Kerr, J.C. (eds) *International issues in nursing research*. Beckenham: Croom Helm   ISBN 0709944373   References   Part 1   Chapter 3   41-60

Chapter lists the various approaches to data collection and then examines the properties of a research instrument. A series of questions which should be asked about an existing instrument to determine its appropriateness for the particular purpose is included together with suggested steps for developing one's own instruments. The Nursing Research Instruments Compilations Projects are outlined and nurses in other countries are urged to set up similar libraries of instruments (CR 3.27.7).

Suggested textbook readings

	Pages	Cross reference
Grady & Wallston	105-107	3.11.2
Jacobson S.F. IN Frank-Stromberg	3-19	2.63.3
Miller D.C.	211-459	2.56.3
Phillips L.R.F. (critique)	365-370	2.98.11
Sweeney & Olivieri	173-201	2.1.63
Waltz & Bausell	311-317	2.21.4
Williamson	208-212	2.1.67
Wilson H.S. (1989)	333-364	2.1.69

Nursing research abstracts
Moores, B.	81/4

Note: Sections 2.58 to 2.65 include compendia that list or describe instruments of possible relevance to nursing. They are grouped under the following headings:

2.58   Attitudinal
2.59   Behavioural
2.60   Health Related'
2.61   Medical
2.62   Mental Measures
2.63   Nursing
2.64   Physiological
2.65   Sociological/Occupational

The list is not exhaustive and there is some overlap between compilations, but it illustrates the wide variety of tools already available.

Before developing new tools existing ones should be carefully examined to see if their validity for nursing practice can be further strengthened by repeated use.

2.58 SOURCES OF INSTRUMENTS
Attitudinal

Annotations

2.58.1 Henerson, M.E., Morris, L.L. & Fitz-Gibbon, C.T. (1978) *How to measure attitudes*. Beverly Hills: Sage   ISBN 0803910703   References   Number 5

Book is part of the Program Evaluation Kit which comprises 8 books, each covering a topic commonly confronted by evaluators of educational programmes. It should enable the development of basic skills in designing and using instruments for the assessment of attitudes. Included are essential preliminary questions, selecting from alternative approaches, finding measures, developing measures, validity and reliability of attitudinal instruments, analysing the data and its presentation.

2.58.2 Robinson, J.P. & Shaver, P.R. (1973) *Measures of social psychological attitudes*. Ann Arbor, Michigan: Institute for Social Research, University of Michigan   ISBN 0879440694

A compilation of 126 instruments measuring attitudes organised under the general headings of self-esteem and related constructs, locus of control, alienation, authoritarianism, socio-political attitudes, values, attitudes towards people, religious attitudes and social desirability scales. Bibliographical information is included for 30 additional self-concept measures. For each tool the following are described, variables, format, samples to whom it has been given, reliability and validity, bibliographical sources in which it was described or used and the method of administration. An evaluation is also made.

2.58.3 Shaw, M.E. & Wright, J.M. (1967) *Scales for the measurement of attitudes*. New York: McGraw-Hill   (No ISBN number)

A compilation of 176 attitude scales which fall into the general categories of social practices, social issues and problems, international issues, abstract concepts, political and religious attitudes, ethnic and national groups, significant others and social institutions. Each tool is described together with subjects used for testing, measurement properties of the response mode, scoring, reliability and validity data together with an evaluation.

2.59 SOURCES OF INSTRUMENTS
Behavioural

Annotations

2.59.1 Andrulis, R.S. (1977) *A source book of tests and measures of human behaviour*. Springfield, Illinois: Charles Thomas   ISBN 0398036039   References

Volume contains descriptions of 155 commercially available tests to assess adult behaviour. Tests are categorised under intelligence and aptitude; achievement; cognitive style; general measures of personality; personality adjustment; vocational and interest inventories; attitude devices; personality performance; managerial and creativity tests. Each description includes variables measured, type of measure, where to obtain it, psychometric properties, its purpose, scoring and groups used for testing. Some reliability and validity data are available for about 90% of the tools.

2.59.2 Ciminero, A.R., Calhoun, K.S. & Adams, H.E. (eds) (1977) *Handbook of behavioural measurement*. New York: Wiley   ISBN 047115797X

A comprehensive review of general and specific issues in behavioural measurement. The book is divided into three parts − a general overview; basic issues in behavioural assessment; and a system to classify psychological responses that could be used as a framework for research. Part 2 covers general approaches to behavioural assessment and chapters on interviews, self-report tools, direct observation and psycho-physiologic techniques. Part 3 describes how these measurement approches may be used. A number of sources are included and some instruments are described (CR 2.70, 2.73, 2.79).

2.59.3 Lake, D.G., Miles, M.B. & Earle, R.B. Jr. (1973) *Measuring human behaviour: tools for the assessment of social functioning*. New York: Teachers College Press   ISBN 0807716480

84 behavioural instruments are described and critiqued and they include personal, inter-personal, group or organisational variables. Each tool is described, variables tested and its scoring, administration, development, critique and evaluation are discussed. Most have been tested for reliability and validity.

2.59.4 Pfeiffer, W.J., Heslen, R. & Jones, J.E. (1976) *Instrumentation in human relations training*. 2nd edition La Jolk: California University Associates Inc.   ISBN 0883901161

Part 1 of this book deals with instrumentation issues such as administration, validity, reliability, instrument development and problems of instrumentation. Part 2 contains a guide to 92 instruments appropriate for use in the behavioural sciences. These are categorised as personal, inter-personal and organisational in focus. A variable amount of information is included for each instrument, although for each the test length and time to complete, descriptions of scales and sub-scales and purchase information are provided.

2.60   SOURCES OF INSTRUMENTS
Health Related

Annotations
2.60.1   Karoly, P. (ed) (1985) *Measurement strategies in health psychology*. New York: Wiley   ISBN 0471893951   References

Book describes the current state of health psychology assessment and potential new directions. Many tests used have their applications discussed and references are given. In most instances the tests themselves are not included but research using them is reported. Assessments given include quality of life, life-styles, risk factors, medical compliance, pain, illness cognition, and life stress events. Methodological considerations are discussed.

2.60.2 McDowell, I. & Newell, C. (1987) *Measuring health: a guide to rating scales and questionnaires.* New York: Open University Press   ISBN 0195041011
References

Book brings together scattered information on several types of health measurement techniques and aims to provide data necessary to choose, apply and score the chosen method. 50 measures are reviewed and chapter topics include physical disability, psychological well-being, social health, pain and quality of life and general health. Descriptions cover the purpose of each test, its conceptual basis, reliability and validity and a copy of each is included. Alternative forms, a discussion of the method and the test developer's address are also given.

2.60.3 Reeder, L.G., Ramacher, L. & Gorelnik, S. (1976) *Handbook of scales and indices of health behaviour.* Pacific Palisades, California: Goodyear   ISBN 0876203799

78 studies are included and grouped under preventive health behaviour, health status, health orientation, illness behaviour and use of health services. Information is presented under the steps of the research process. Approximately 85% of studies used the survey method of data collection and for about 25% the tools or sections from them are included.

2.61   SOURCES OF INSTRUMENTS
Medical

Annotation
2.61.1   Weed, L.L. (1971) *Medical records, medical education and patient care.* Chicago: Year Book Medical Publishers   ISBN X1125838

A systematic approach to the organisation of patient data — the Problem Orientated Medical Record is described. The procedure has four phases — the establishment of a data base, identification of patient problems, development of initial plans to deal with each problem together with written progress notes. This procedure facilitates dealing with the complexities of patient care. It is particularly useful for formulating nursing care plans as a framework to evaluate the quality of patient care. Information on its uses, reliability and validity, and references are also included.

2.62   SOURCES OF INSTRUMENTS
Mental Measures

Annotations
2.62.1   British Psychological Society (1990) *Psychological testing: a guide.* Leicester: British Psychological Society (No ISBN number)   References

Booklet, developed by the Steering Committee of the Society, aims to give guidance mainly to non-psychologists and other prospective users on test standards. It includes an introduction to testing, different applications, various quality control issues, details of what to look for in a test and further information.

2.62.2 Buros, O.K. (ed) (1974) *Tests in print II*. Highland Park, New Jersey: Gryphon Press ISBN 0910674140

A guide to the tests of mental measurement in print up to 1974 and a cumulative index to the first seven Mental Measurements Yearbooks. Volume contains 2467 entries. It includes bibliographical sources, a cumulative index of all tests with references, publishers, author index, title index of tests in and out of print, and an index stating populations for whom each test is intended. Editor recommends using the 8th Mental Measurements Yearbook for a complete index to all tests (CR 2.62.3).

2.62.3 Buros, O.K. (ed) (1978) *The eighth mental measurements yearbook.* Highland Park, New Jersey: Gryphon Press ISBN 0910674248

Compilation is divided into 3 sections – firstly a list of 1184 tests, 898 of which are critically reviewed. The remainder have reviews excerpted from journals. Part 2 lists 576 books on testing with reviews of 229 books. Part 3 comprises six indices, author, title of test, book title, publishers, periodical and scanning index.

Tests are organised into 14 categories: achievement tests, English, fine arts, foreign language, intelligence, mathematics, miscellaneous, reading, science, sensory and motor, social studies, speech and hearing and vocations. Entries include title, population, variables, available forms and copyright information. This volume and Tests in Print II (2.62.2) provide a complete index to all tests of mental measurements.

Tests of personality, intelligence, reading and vocational skills have been separated into individual volumes (please see 2.62.4–2.62.9).

2.62.4 Buros, O.K. (ed) (1968) Volume 1 *Reading Tests and Reviews* ISBN 0910674094

2.62.5 Buros, O.K. (ed) (1975a) Volume 2 *Reading Tests and Reviews* ISBN 0910674205

2.62.6 Buros, O.K (ed) (1975b) *Intelligence Tests and Reviews* ISBN 0910674175

2.62.7 Buros, O.K (ed) (1970) Volume 1 *Personality Tests and Reviews* ISBN 0910674108

2.62.8 Buros, O.K. (ed) (1975c) Volume 2 *Personality Tests and Reviews* ISBN 0910674191

2.62.9 Buros, O.K. (ed) (1975d) *Vocational Tests and Reviews* ISBN 091067423X

(all the above are published by Gryphon Press)

2.62.10 Chun, K.T., Cobb, S. & French, J.R.P. Jr. (1975) *Measures for psychological assessment: a guide to 3000 original sources and their applications.* Michigan: University of Michigan, Institute for Social Research ISBN 0879441682 References

A compilation of annotated references to the measures of mental health and related variables and their uses. A bibliography of all quantitative research which used these measures between 1960 and 1970 is included. Volume consists of two major sections, primary references, applications and two indexes. The section on primary sources lists approximately 3000 references to articles or other publications in which the measures were first described. The section on application provides over 6000 instances in which the measures are described. Details relating to each test are not included.

2.62.11 Comrey, A.L., Backer, T.E. & Glaser, E.M. (1973) *A sourcebook for mental health measures.* Los Angeles: Human Interaction Research Institute (ISBN number not found).

Contains abstracts of approximately 1100 psychological and mental health-related tools with major well known tools excluded. Topics of interest to nurses are alcoholism, drugs, family interaction, geriatrics, mental handicap and evaluation of professional service delivery. Abstracts include title, source, authors name and address, purpose of the tool, a description, major applications and how it may be obtained. It also indicates for most tools where information on reliability and validity may be obtained.

2.62.12 Goldman, B.A. & Saunders, J.L. (1974) Volume 1 & (1978) Volume 2 *Directory of unpublished experimental measures.* New York: Behavioural Publications ISBN (Volume 1 not found), Volume 2 0877051305

Two volumes cover 1034 mental measures which were identified by reviewing psychology, sociology and educational journals from 1970 to 1972. Measures are organised under 23 headings. Authors excluded tests commercially available. Information for each test includes its name, purpose, description, reliability, validity, bibliographical information and related research references.

2.62.13 Lyerly, S. (1973) *Handbook of psychiatric rating scales.* 2nd edition Rockville, Maryland: National Institute of Mental Health (ISBN number not found)

Describes 61 rating scales which have been used in psychiatric settings. 38 of these include detailed descriptions and a table gives information on the population, type of rater, source of data, reliability and validity.

2.62.14 Mittler, P.J. (ed) (1970) *The psychological assessment of mental and physical handicaps.* London: Methuen SBN 416045707 References

Text is designed to assist those who are concerned with systematic assessment of the handicapped. It does not cover the psychometric aspects of testing which may be found in other standard texts but covers comprehensively the diagnostic and assessment aspects. Individual tests are commented upon and extensive references given. Principles of psychological assessment, assessment of children and adults and experimental advances are included.

2.62.15 *NFER-Nelson 1991 Catalogue* (Clinical catalogue) (obtainable from NFER-Nelson, Darville House, 2 Oxford Road East, Windsor, Berkshire SL4 1DF)

Lists many assessment tools in the following major categories: developmental assessment, child care and health, mental ability, neuropsychological assessment, functional assessment, assessment of older people, mental health, personality assessment, counselling, interpersonal relations, learning difficulties, communication – child and adult. Tests in preparation are also listed. Information on each test includes: its purpose, who is likely to use it, results which may be obtained, its advantages, contents and costs.

2.63 SOURCES OF INSTRUMENTS
Nursing

Annotations

2.63.1 Ball, J.A., Goldstone, L.A. & Collier, M.M. (1984) *Criteria for care: the manual of the north west nurse staffing levels project.* Newcastle upon Tyne: Newcastle upon Tyne Polytechnic Products   ISBN 0906471249

Describes an interactive means of assessing the current workload on medical and surgical wards together with a means of analysing the demands made on staff by that workload. Manual outlines the development of this system, entitled MONITOR, and gives detailed information on the methods, analysis and uses of it (CR 2.63.6, 2.63.7).

2.63.2 Baxter, B., Cox, N., Freeman, D., Harrison, S., Heaton, M., Mazza, J. & Shaw, H. (1987) *Quality Assurance Tool.* 2nd edition Harrogate: National Association of Theatre Nurses in conjunction with BUPA Hospitals

This tool sets standards and measureable criteria for the preparation of personnel, pre-operative care, care in the operating room, recovery room and the departmental organisation of the theatre complex. Standards are set for the environment, equipment, positioning and movement of patients, nursing care and management of each specialist area. It can be used in various ways to highlight good care as well as demonstrating areas where improvements can be made.

[Note: the above annotation has kindly been provided by Maureen Bonner, Secretary of the National Association of Theatre Nurses.
This tool is available from: BUPA Printing Division, Unit 3, Nugent Park Industrial Estate, Cray Avenue, St Mary Cray, Kent BR5 2LF]

2.63.3 Craig, D. (1987) Audit design. *Recent advances in nursing* 17: 65-93   45 References

Describes the development of a retrospective nursing audit tool for use in public health nursing. The quality of care was evaluated by examining the nursing process records for discharged patients and a set of criteria developed for a new audit tool.

2.63.4 Frank-Stromberg, M. (ed) (1988) *Instruments for clinical nursing research.* Norwalk, Connecticut: Appleton & Lange   ISBN 0838542964   References

Book developed from a project undertaken by the Oncology Nursing Society which aimed to describe available instruments. It reviews the tools currently obtainable to measure a selected phenomenon; describes the psychometric properties; details the sample or studies which have utilised the tool; identifies their strengths and weaknesses and discusses their use in all areas of nursing. Part 1 relates to evaluating research instruments: Part 2 contains those to assess health and function: Part 3 discusses commonly occuring clinical problems. Most chapters are summarised and have extensive reference lists.

2.63.5 Goodinson, S.M. & Singleton, J. (1989) Quality of life: a critical review of current concepts, measures and their clinical implications. *International journal of nursing studies* 26(4) 327-341   47 References

Discusses quality of life measures which are used to justify or refute various forms of medical treatment, to identify the results of disease or treatment and provide a basis for the allocation of resources. The rationale for using such measures, approaches to management, examples and patients' coping strategies are all explored.

2.63.6 Haussmann, R.K.D., Hegyvary, S.T. & Newman, J.F. (1976) *Monitoring quality of nursing care. Part II: Assessment and study of correlates.* Washington DC: United States Government Printing Office, Department of Health and Welfare Publication No HRA 76-7   (No ISBN number found)

The Rush-Medicus Quality Monitoring Instrument used to evaluate the quality of nursing care is described. It comprises 6 major objectives: a plan of care is formulated, the physical and non-physical needs of the patient are addressed, achievement of nursing care objectives is evaluated, unit procedures are followed for the protection of all patients and the delivery of care is facilitated by administrative and managerial services. Sub-objectives are defined for each of the above.

Information is given on its development, format, application, administration, scoring, interpretation, reliability, validity, uses and references illustrating its use (CR 2.63.7).

[Note: MONITOR is an adaptation for the UK of the Rush Medicus Quality Monitoring Instrument]

2.63.7 Illsley, V.A. & Goldstone, L.A. (1985) *A guide to MONITOR for nursing staff.* Newcastle upon Tyne: Newcastle upon Tyne Polytechnic Products Ltd   ISBN 0906471338

Provides a brief introduction to MONITOR and answers basic questions about it. A list of further reading is included (CR 2.63.6).

2.63.8 Jacox, A.K., Prescott, P.A., Collar, M.K. & Goodwin, L.D. (1981) *The nurse practitioner rating form: a primary care process measure.* Wakefield, Massachusetts: Nursing Resources (No ISBN number found)

Instrument aims to assess dimensions of the direct patient care role of the nurse practitioner in ambulatory settings. The measure covers particular activity areas, the content of teaching and global scales to rate the communication style of the nurse and client participation. Information on its development format, application, administration, scoring, interpretation, reliability, validity and its uses is included.

2.63.9 Kemp, N. & Richardson, E.W. (1990) *Quality assurance in nursing practice.* Oxford: Butterworth-Heinemann ISBN 0433016086 References Chapter 5 66-79

Chapter contains brief descriptions of QUALPACS (2.63.19), the Phaneuf Nursing Audit (2.63.12), Rush Medicus (2.63.6), MONITOR (2.63.7), National Association of Theatre Nurses Quality Assurance Tool (CR 2.63.2), and PA Nursing Quality Measurement Scale.

2.63.10 Meyer, D. (1978) *Grasp: a patient information and workload management system.* Volume 1 Morganston: North Carolina ISBN 0932150004

AND

2.63.11 Meyer, D. (1981) *Grasp Too: application and adaptations of the Grasp Workload Nursing management System.* Volume 2 Morganston: North Carolina ISBN 0932150012

[Note: this volume is an update of Volume 1]

Volume 1 contains information on the original development of a Nursing Workload System called Grasp*. The system measures patient care based on patient need/requirements and centres around the instrument which is called the PCH chart. All care given over a 24 hour period is recorded and is divided into the following categories: nutrition, elimination, hygiene, observations, mobility, respiratory, medication/fluids and other. Indirect care is also included.

* Grasp is a registered trademark

Volume 2 discusses applications of this system. Nursing process activities, teaching and emotional support were identified separately from other basic measurements. The data collected was patient specific and resulted in hours of care per day. All data for the entire ward/unit is totalled and used to determine the number of staff needed. Examples of workload instruments are given together with details of their use.

[Note: This annotation has been adapted from information kindly given by Ruth Brenner, FCG–UK Regional Co-ordinator].

2.63.12 Phaneuf, M.C. (1976) *The nursing audit: self regulation of nursing practice.* New York: Appleton-Century-Crofts ISBN 0838570054

A 50 item instrument designed to assess the quality of nursing care received by a patient in any setting as reflected in the patient care record once the cycle of care has been completed. Seven functions of professional practice are examined: application and execution of physician's legal order, observations of signs, symptoms and reactions, supervision of the patient and those participating in care, reporting and recording, application and execution of nursing procedures and techniques and promotion of physical and emotional health by direction and teaching. Some references are included illustrating its use. Information on its development, application, administration, scoring, reliability, validity and its uses are included.

2.63.13 Rinke, L.T. (ed) (1987a) *Outcome measures in home care.* New York: National League for Nursing   ISBN 088737378X   References   Volume 1 Research Publication No. 21-2194

Anthology provides a single reference to the classic and current literature addressing outcomes in home care. Part 1 includes: basic issues in evaluating the quality of health care; the relationship of nursing process to nursing outcomes; criterion measures of nursing care quality and status of quality assurance in public health nursing. Parts 2,3,4 & 5 include two studies on maternal and child health; using records as a data source; a community based demonstration project and instrument development (CR 2.63.14).

2.63.14 Rinke, L.T. & Wilson. A.A. (eds) (1987b) *Outcome measures in home care.* New York: National League for Nursing   ISBN 0887373798   References Volume 2 Service Publication No. 21-2195

Volume covers a sample of both published and unpublished measurement outcome indicators for community based nursing services. The six parts give a historical overview; examples of promulgated outcome standards; programmatic approaches; medical diagnosis approach; discipline specific indicators and a functional approach (CR 2.63.13).

2.63.15 Senior, E. (1988) Manpower planning objectives and information systems. *Recent advances in nursing* 19: 34-63   38 References

Briefly outlines several systems for measuring nurses workload, calculating demand and identifying supply sources. Amongst those included are MONITOR (pages 37-38) and GRASP (pages 39-40) (CR 2.63.1, 2.63.7, 2.63.10, 2.63.11).

[Note: GRASP is an American time-based workload measurement and information system. For further information contact: MIS, PO Box 1774, Morganton, North Carolina 28655 USA]

2.63.16 Strickland, O.L. & Waltz, C.F. (eds) (1988a) *Measurement of nursing outcomes.* New York: Springer   ISBN 0826152724   Volume 2, Measuring nursing performance, practice education and research

A collection of tools focusing on provider-centred outcomes. Some of the major topic areas include measuring professionalism, clinical performance, educational outcomes, research and measurement and future directions. Measurement protocol for each tool includes:

(a) critical review and analysis of the literature
(b) review and analysis of existing tools and procedures for measuring the variable
(c) conceptual basis of the measure
(d) purpose and/or objective of the measure
(e) procedures for construction, revision or future development of the tool
(f) procedures for administration and scoring
(g) methodology for testing the reliability and validity of the measure, including approach to data collection, protection of human subjects and statistical analysis procedures (CR 2.63.18).

2.63.17 Walker, L.O., Sandor, M.K. & Sands, D. (1989) Designing and testing self-help interventions. *Applied nursing research* 2(2) 96-102   9 References

Article discusses a three phase process for developing and testing nursing interventions using a paper and pencil medium. An illustration is given of a workbook developed to promote confidence in adolescents in coping with problems in the everyday world.

2.63.18 Waltz, C.F. & Strickland, O.L. (eds) (1988b) *Measurement of nursing outcomes*. New York: Springer   ISBN 0826152716   Volume 1, Measuring client outcomes

Aim of publication, and its companion volume (CR 2.63.16) is to disseminate information about the measurement of clinical and educational nursing outcomes. They include measurement tools, protocols for these tools, results including reliability and validity, results and conclusions. Tools were the result of the Measurement of Clinical and Educational Outcomes Project. Volume contains tools applicable to clinical settings grouped under the following sections; illness-orientated measures, assessing the whole person − measuring wellness, factors in community based care, quality of care and future directions (CR 2.63.16).

2.63.19 Wandelt, M.A. & Ager, J. (1975a) *Quality patient care scale (QUALPACS)*. New York: Appleton-Century-Crofts   (ISBN number not found)

QUALPACS is a 68 item observation scale which assesses the quality of nursing care received by patients in any care setting. It is subdivided into 6 categories: psychosocial, group and individual, physical, general, communications and professional implications. Each category is defined and there is a 20 page cue sheet giving examples of activities. QUALPACS draws heavily from the Slater Nursing Competencies Rating Scale but the focus of measurement is the care received by a patient rather than the competencies displayed by a nurse.

Information is given about its development, format, application, administration, scoring, interpretation, reliability, validity, uses and some illustrations of its use (CR 2.63.20).

2.63.20 Wandelt, M.A. & Stewart, D.S. (1975b) *Slater nursing competencies rating scale*. New York: Appleton-Century-Crofts   (ISBN number not found)

An 84 item observation scale intended for use by an observer-rater to assess the competencies displayed by a nurse while caring for a patient. The scale is divided into 6 categories – psychosocial, individual and group, physical, general, communication and professional implications. Tool is accompanied by a 20 page cue sheet listing examples of activities or behaviours illustrative of each item. Information is given about its development, application administration, scoring, reliability, validity and its uses. Some references illustrating its use are also included (CR 2.63.19).

2.63.21 Ward, M.J. & Fetler, M.E. (1979a) *Instruments for use in nursing education research.* Boulder, Colorado: Western Interstate Commission for Higher Education   (No ISBN number found)

A major barrier to conducting research is the lack of appropriate data collecting instruments so this compilation aims to provide a collection relating specifically to nursing education research. It contains descriptions, critiques and reproductions of 78 instruments; brief descriptions and references to another 40; an annotated bibliography of other published compilations; a glossary and appendices. Each tool is described with key concepts, title, author variables measured, nature and content of the instrument, its administration and scoring, rationale for its development and sources of the items. Data on reliability and validity are included together with studies where it has been used, selected comments, references, name and address of the person to contact for further information and the name of the copyright owner.

2.63.22 Ward, M.J. & Lindeman, C.A. (1979b) *Instruments for measuring nursing practice and other health care variables.* Hyattsville, Maryland: Department of Health and Welfare Publication Nos. Volume 1, HRA 78-53 & Volume 2, HRA 78-54   (No ISBN number found)

Volumes contain descriptions, critiques, and reproductions of 138 psychosocial research instruments; descriptions of 19 instruments which measure physiological parameters; an annotated bibliography of other selected compilations and a glossary of physiological instrument terms.

2.63.23 Werley, H.H. & Lang, N.M. (eds) (1988) *Identification of the nursing minimum data set.* New York: Springer   ISBN 0826153402   References

Book describes the development of the nursing minimum data set. This is information unique to nursing practice and represents nursing's essential data.It enables nurses to use computers to assemble comparable nursing data across clinical populations, geographical areas and time through the use of consensually derived data categories, variables and uniform definitions. It contains conceptual considerations, existing information about the data set, perspectives on data requirements across settings, multiple perspectives, effectiveness of nursing care, control of practice standards, quality assessment, health policy, work of the Task Force which generated the data set and future directions.

[Note: Acknowledgement is made to Waltz, Strickland and Lenz (CR 2.56.5) as the source for many of the instruments cited in this section]

2.64 SOURCES OF INSTRUMENTS
Physiological

Physiological functioning can often be measured very precisely by scientific instruments which yield numerical values and so allow a wide range of statistical procedures to be employed in their analysis.

Both nurses and doctors obtain physiological data but because of rapid changes in technology, sources of instruments and procedures quickly become outdated. For this reason it is most important that steps are taken to ensure that the latest editions of the annotated compilations are consulted. Later editions of some books listed here have not been found.

Annotations

2.64.1 Bauer, J.D., Ackerman, P.G. & Toro, G. (1974) *Clinical laboratory methods.* 8th edition St Louis: Mosby   (No ISBN number found)

Laboratory methods in urinalysis, haematology, clinical chemistry, enzymology, stool analysis, parasitology, toxicology and tissue examination are described. Information included is general principles, equipment, methodology, physiological variation, calculations, normal values and interpretation.

2.64.2 Cromwell, L., Weibell, F.J. & Pfeiffer, E.A. (1980) *Biomedical instrumentation and measurements.* 2nd edition Englewood Cliffs, New Jersey: Prentice Hall   (No ISBN number found)

General overview of instrumentation with specific classes of instruments being described in some depth. For each major body system basic physiology is presented, variables are identified and principles of instrumentation discussed. Chapters on intensive care monitoring and biomedical computer applications are included.

2.64.3 Lindsey, A.M. (1982) Phenomena and physiological variables of relevance to nursing: review of a decade of work. Part 1 *Western journal of nursing research* 4(4) 343-364   73 References

AND

2.64.4 Lindsey, A.M. (1983) Phenomena and physiological variables of relevance to nursing: review of a decade of work. Part 2 *Western journal of nursing research* 5(1) 41-63   79 References

This two part article reports a study which examined the nature and scope of clinical nursing research in selected journals between 1970 and 1980, where physiological phenomena and variables were examined by investigators. The aim of this was to establish the knowledge base underlying nursing practice. The author concluded there was no evidence to confirm or refute findings about these phenomena so the contribution to knowledge is fragmentary and it is not possible to generalise or apply findings from single studies.

Studies reviewed came under the broad headings of the individual, the individual's environment, and nursing therapeutics. Information is presented in table form and summarised in narrative. Variables and methodological issues are briefly discussed together with the limitations of this review.

2.64.5 Shaver, J.F. & Heitkemper, M.M. (1988) Using biological measures. IN Woods, N.F. & Catanzaro, M. *Nursing research: theory and practice.* St. Louis: Mosby   ISBN 0801657032   References   Unit 3, 16 260-277

Chapter reviews ideas about human physiological functions and how these may be measured (CR 2.1.72).

2.64.6 Weiss, M. (1973) *Biomedical instrumentation.* Philadelphia: Chilton Book Company   (No ISBN number found)

Information enabling an understanding of biomedical instrumentation is presented. Descriptions of some monitoring devices are included e.g. sensors, ECGs, bedside monitors and telemetry. Equipment used to assess cardiovascular and pulmonary function is described. The use of computer systems is discussed.

Suggested textbook readings

	Pages	*Cross reference*
Grady & Wallston	126-133	3.11.2
Holm & Llewellyn	124-125	2.1.26
LoBiondo-Wood & Haber	156-160	2.1.38
Polit & Hungler (1987)	289-299	2.1.56
Waltz & Bausell	241-248	2.21.4

2.65 SOURCES OF INSTRUMENTS
Sociological/Occupational

Annotations

2.65.1 Beere, C.A. (1979) *Women and women's issues: a handbook of tests and measurements.* San Francisco: Jossey-Bass   (No ISBN number found)   References

Volume contains 235 instruments obtained from literature published in 1977. They are divided into 11 categories: sex roles, sex stereotypes, sex role prescriptions, childrens' sex roles, gender knowledge, marital and parental roles, employee roles, multiple roles, attitudes towards womens' issues, somatic and sexual issues and some unclassified.

Each category constitutes a chapter and included for many of the instruments is the title, author, date, variables, type of instrument, item content, length, group for whom it is intended, sample items, scoring method, theoretical basis, reliability, validity, possible modifications, source and bibliographical information.

2.65.2 Bonjean, C.M., Hill, R.J. & McLemore, S.D. (1967) *Sociological measurement: an inventory of scales and indices.* San Francisco: Chandler (No ISBN number found)

Contains bibliographical information for 2080 sociologic scales and indices. 78 conceptual categories were used to classify the instruments and some of these were authoritarianism, family cohesion and attitudes towards medicine and health. Extent of the discussion varies but generally includes information on its development, use, administration, scoring and the sample used.

2.65.3 Miller, D.C. (1977) *Handbook of research design and social measurement.* 3rd edition New York: David McKay ISBN 067930312X

Book is concerned with all phases of research design. 48 sociological scales and indices are included and come under the general headings of social status, group structure and dynamics, social indicators, measures of organisational structure, evaluation research and organisational effectiveness, community, social participation, leadership in the work organisation, morale and job satisfaction and scales of attitudes, norms and values. Descriptive information is given for most scales.

Reliability and validity information is difficult to evaluate because of minimum description of the methodologies used. An inventory of all instruments used in the American Sociological Review between 1965 and 1974 is also included.

2.65.4 Murray, A., Strauss, M.A. & Brown, B.W. (1978) *Family measurement techniques: abstracts of published instruments 1935-1974.* Revised edition Minneapolis: University of Minnesota Press ISBN 0816607990

Includes abstracts of 813 instruments to measure the properties of the family or the behaviour of people in family roles. Four broad categories are husband−wife relationships, parent−child and sibling to sibling relationships, husband−wife and parent−child variables and sex and pre-marital relationships.

Abstract includes author, test name, variables, test description, sample item, length, availability and references. Psychometric properties of the instruments are not included.

2.65.5 Price, J.L. (1972) *Handbook of organisational measurement.* Lexington: Massachusetts DC Heath ISBN 0669752002

Book is structured under 22 organisational concepts some of which are absenteeism, autonomy, centralisation communication, effectiveness, satisfaction and span of control. Each chapter contains a general discussion and definition of the concept, issues pertaining to its measurement and descriptions of 1-3 relevant instruments.

Descriptive information includes; a definition, data collecting information, computation methods, reliability and validity of some instruments, evaluative comments and bibliographical source.

2.65.6 Raynes, N.V. (1988) *Annotated directory of measures of environmental quality for use in residential services for people with a mental handicap.* Manchester: Department of Social Policy and Social Work, University of Manchester (No ISBN number found).

Contains summaries of 62 instruments which can be used to evaluate aspects of the environment provided for mentally handicapped people although some may be of relevance to other client groups. Each instrument is described using a standard format which includes title, authors, date of most recent edition, purpose content, administration, scientific credibility − focusing on standardisation, reliability and validity and references. An appendix gives names and addresses of people to contact for further information.

2.65.7 Robinson, J.P., Athanasiou, R. & Head, K.B. (1969) *Measures of occupational attitudes and occupational characteristics.* Ann Arbor, Michigan: Institute for Social Research, University of Michigan (No ISBN number found)

77 scales used to measure occupational-related variables are cited. Ten general headings are used: job attitudes for particular occupations, satisfaction with specific job features, concepts related to job satisfaction, occupational values, leadership styles, other work-related attitudes, vocational interests and occupational status.

Information provided for most tests includes variable, description, sample, reliability, validity, source, results and comments. There is a wide variation in details of reliability and validity. Several chapters discuss topics such as status inconsistency, occupational similarity and social mobility. An overview of research and survey of literature related to job attitudes and performance is also included.

Suggested textbook reading

	Pages	*Cross reference*
Thomas	110-126	2.1.64

DATA COLLECTION

2.66 DATA COLLECTION – GENERAL

Data collection refers to ways in which information can be obtained from the real world, recorded in a systematic way and quantified. There are many data collection techniques and sections 2.67 to 2.80 will guide the reader towards appropriate sources.

High quality data collection methods will increase the value of the research. Choices therefore need to be made in terms of the degree of structure which is possible or desirable, whether or how the data can be quantified, the obtrusiveness of the researcher which may lead to ethical problems and how objective or subjective the data are or need to be.

There is sometimes confusion between the following terms: research methodology, research design and methods of data collection.

Research methodology is an umbrella term embracing the whole process

Research design includes all the plans which must be made prior to the actual collection of data

Methods of data collection are the actual tools or instruments used to collect the information.

Definitions
Data – pieces of information obtained in the course of a study
Data collection – the gathering of data relevant to the problem under investigation

Annotation
2.66.1 Wiseman, J.P. & Aron, M.S. (1970) *Field projects for sociology students.* Cambridge, Massachusetts: Schenkman (No ISBN number found) References

Book contains a series of project assignments designed to give students experience in collecting data in the real world. Different types of research approaches are included within broad sociological categories. Definitions, advantages and disadvantages, applications, assignments which include steps to be taken, action in the field and presenting the results, and selected bibliographies are given for each approach.

Suggested textbook readings

	Pages	Cross reference
Abdellah & Levine	232-244	2.1.1
Burns & Grove	433-456	2.1.12

2.67   METHODS OF DATA COLLECTION
Critical incident technique

The critical incident technique employs a set of principles for collecting data on observable human activities. It provides a flexible way of examining interpersonal communication skills and has been used in many nursing studies, especially in the USA. Incidents are of particular value because it is reality which is being described rather than hypothetical situations.

Definition

A set of procedures for collecting direct observations of human behaviour which have special significance and meet systematically defined criteria. An incident is an observable type of human activity which is sufficiently complete in itself to permit inferences and predictions to be made about the person performing the act. To be critical it must be performed in a situation where the purpose or intent of the act seems fairly clear to the observer, and its consequences are sufficiently definite so there is little doubt concerning its effects (Flanagan 1947, 1954).

Original articles
Flanagan, J.C. (1947) *The aviation psychology programme in the army air forces.* AAF psychology programme research report No 1 Washington DC: Government Printing Office

Flanagan, J.C. (1954) The critical incident technique. *Psychological bulletin* 51(4) 327-358   74 References (CR 2.67.5)

Example
Clamp, C.G.L. (1984) *Learning through incidents: studies in the development and use of critical incidents in the teaching of attitudes in nursing.* M.Phil Thesis (unpublished) University of London, Institute of Education

Study aimed to develop a teaching method which could increase attitude awareness and develop interpersonal communication skills in nursing education. Critical incidents were used as triggers for in-depth discussions on the behaviour, attitudes and feelings reported by nurses. Many aspects of learning and areas of personal growth were highlighted.

Annotations
2.67.1   Bermosk, L.S. & Corsini, R.J. (1973) *Critical incidents in nursing.* Philadelphia: Saunders   ISBN 0721616968

Book concentrates on 38 current controversial issues documented in the form of critical incidents under the headings of: nurse and the patient, her peers, doctors, the family, supervision and the system. The background to each incident is given, the incident itself described and this is followed by opinions, reactions and some suggestions for resolution from experienced nurses who examined each one from various viewpoints. The complex world in which nurses work is portrayed.

2.67.2   Cormack, D.F.S. (ed) (1984) Flanagan's critical incident technique. IN Author *The research process in nursing.* Oxford: Blackwell Scientific   ISBN 0632010134   References   Chapter 12   118-125

Describes the origins and uses of critical incidents in nursing (CR 2.1.20).

2.67.3   Cortazzi, D. & Roote, S. (1975) *Illuminative incident analysis.* London: McGraw Hill   ISBN 0070844526

Using critical incidents as the focal point, authors describe the process of learning through illuminative incident analysis. The aim of the book is to encourage constructive team development by drawing the incident, rather than discussing it. This method has been shown to develop understanding of attitudes, role perceptions and motivation. Solutions emerge which can become a 'health care plan' for the team.

2.67.4   Dunn, W.R. & Hamilton, D.D. (1986) The critical incident technique: a brief guide. *Medical teacher* 8(3) 207-215   26 References

Authors maintain that the technique has stood the test of time as a means of identifying those activities essential to good practice in a profession, and as a tool to delineate the competencies needed by those members. Article reviews the technique and addresses the questions, what is the technique and when can it be applied in medical education?

2.67.5 Flanagan, J.C. (1954) The critical incident technique. *Psychological bulletin* 51(4) 327-358   74 References

Article describes the development of critical incident methodology, its fundamental principles and status. Studies using this technique are reviewed and possible future uses identified.

2.67.6 Hayes, D.M., Fleury, R.A. & Jackson, T.B. (1979) Curriculum content from critical incidents. *Medical education* 13(3) 175-182   6 References

Describes a study designed to create a medical school curriculum which would meet the needs of students, teachers and the community. Data was collected using the critical incident technique and ten major areas of behaviour were identified. These areas of clinical activity were then subdivided and subsequently formed the basis for the curriculum.

2.67.7 Rimon, D. (1979) Nurses' perception of their psychological role in treating rehabilitation patients: a study employing the critical incident technique. *Journal of advanced nursing* 4(4) 403-413   14 References

Study reports on the psychological role of nurses whose perceptions were explored using the critical incident technique. From these the aims and objectives of psychological care were generated and were found to support the limited available literature.

Suggested textbook readings

	Pages	*Cross reference*
Polit & Hungler (1987)	230	2.1.56
Treece & Treece	354-356	2.1.65
Waltz, Strickland & Lenz	382	2.56.5

2.68   METHODS OF DATA COLLECTION
Delphi technique

The Delphi concept may be seen as a spin off from defence research. 'Project Delphi' was the name given to an Air Force sponsored, Rand Corporation study in the early 1950s concerning the use of expert opinion. The aim of this study was to select an optimal US industrial target system, and to estimate the number of atom bombs required to reduce the munitions output by a prescribed amount. The study set out to obtain the most reliable concensus of opinion of a group of experts . . . by a series of intensive questionnaires interspersed with controlled opinion feedback (Linstone & Turoff 1975).

[Apollo became master of Delphi upon slaying the dragon Pythos and he was renowned not only for his youth and perfect beauty but even more for his ability to see the future.]

Definition
Technique employed to quantify the judgements of experts, to assess priorities or to make long range forecasts

---

Example
Hitch, P.J. & Murgatroyd, J.D. (1983) Professional communications in cancer care: a Delphi survey of hospital nurses. *Journal of advanced nursing* 8(5) 413-422   27 References

Examined some nurses perceptions of communication difficulties with cancer patients. A Delphi survey among nurses in northern England highlighted the following major areas: dealing with patients questions and fears; pain control and relationships with other professional groups inside and outside the hospital. Suggestions were made for improving communications.

Major text
Linstone, H.A. & Turoff, M. (eds) (1975) *The Delphi method: techniques and applications.* Reading, Massachusetts: Addison-Wesley ISBN 0201042940 References (CR 2.68.6)

Annotations
2.68.1   Bond, S. & Bond, J. (1982) A Delphi survey of clinical nursing research priorities. *Journal of advanced nursing* 7(6) 565-575   19 References

A full description is given of a Delphi survey carried out in the north of England. Its purpose was to establish the clinical nursing research priorities as seen by 271 nurses of various grades and specialities throughout the region.

2.68.2   Couper, M.R. (1984) The Delphi technique: characteristics and sequence model. *Advances in nursing science* 7(1) 72-77   5 References

An attempt is made to design a sequential model in order to clarify the processes in this technique.

2.68.3   Farrell, P. & Scherer, K. (1983) The Delphi technique as a method for selecting criteria to evaluate nursing care. *Nursing papers* 15(1) 51-60   27 References

An example of a study using this technique is shown. Its purpose was to help in the development of nursing standards as part of the Manitoba Nursing Standards Project.

2.68.4 Goodman, C.M. (1987) The Delphi technique: a critique. *Journal of advanced nursing* 12(6) 729-734   15 References

The development of the technique is described together with examples of its use. Its key characteristics are examined and its value as an aid to policy making discussed (CR 3.10).

2.68.5 Lindeman, C.A. (1975) Delphi survey of priorities in clinical nursing research. *Nursing research* 24(6) 434-441   17 References

The Delphi technique is described and the results of four survey rounds is reported. Three questions were studied − is clinical nursing research an area in which nursing should assume primary research responsibility; how important is research on this topic for the nursing profession, and what is the likelihood of change in patient welfare because of research on this topic?

2.68.6 Linstone, H.A. & Turoff, M. (eds) (1975) *The Delphi method: techniques and applications.* Reading, Massachusetts: Addison-Wesley   ISBN 0201042940 References

A major text covering the technique and applications of the Delphi technique. Its principal area of application has been technological forecasting but it has also been used in many other contexts.These include normative forecasts, the ascertainment of values and preferences, estimates concerning the quality of life, simulated and real decision making and planning. Despite many applications Delphi lacks a completely sound theoretical basis. Book includes philosophy, general applications, evaluation, cross-impact analysis, specialised techniques, computers and the future of Delphi, a checklist of pitfalls and an extensive bibliography.

2.68.7 Prophit, P. (1983) Delphi study: clinical nursing research priorities. IN University of Edinburgh Nursing Research Unit, *Seventh Report: January 1983-February 1984* Edinburgh: University of Edinburgh, Nursing Research Unit

A description of the Delphi technique and its application by the Nursing Research Unit to determine priorities in clinical nursing research.

Suggested textbook readings

	Pages	*Cross reference*
Polit & Hungler (1987)	303-305	2.1.56
Treece & Treece	367-368	2.1.65
Waltz, Strickland & Lenz	281-285	2.56.5
Woods & Catanzaro	109/326/328	2.1.72

2.69 METHODS OF DATA COLLECTION
Diaries

Diaries can provide information which it is not possible to obtain in any other way. However skilful the questionnaire or interview schedule, inevitably the researcher imposes the structure. A diary may also be structured to a certain extent in that people can be asked to record particular things, but additional insights may be gained.

Definition
A ... source of data which can provide an intimate descriptive comment on everyday life for an individual

Example
Boyle, J.S. (1985) Use of the family health calendar and interview schedules to study health and illness. IN Leininger, M.M. (ed) *Qualitative research methods in nursing.* Orlando: Grune & Stratton   ISBN 0808916769   References 14   217-235

Describes a study carried out in Guatemala which aimed to explore the experiences of health-illness situations. Two research tools were used to collect the data: the health beliefs interview schedule and a family health calendar recording. The latter took the form of a health diary which showed how each family member or household unit had developed specific characteristics in maintaining health, preventing illness, experiencing morbidity and treating illness (CR 2.1.36).

Annotations
2.69.1 Burgess, R.G. (1981) Keeping a research diary. *Cambridge journal of education* 11(1) 75-83   16 References

Describes purposes for which diaries are used in social and educational settings, and how they may be kept by both the subject and the researcher.

2.69.2 Malinowski, B. (1982) The diary of an anthropologist. IN Burgess, R.G. (ed) *Field research: a sourcebook and field manual.* London: Allen & Unwin   ISBN 0043120148   References   Chapter 27   200-205

An actual diary extract is reproduced (2.1.9).

2.69.3 Roghmann, K.J. & Haggerty, R.J. (1972) The diary as a research instrument in the study of health and illness behaviour. *Medical care* 10(2) 143-163   30 References and footnotes

A health calendar was completed over a 28 day period by a random sample of 512 families in a New York community. Over 71,316 personday descriptions yielded information inaccessible by retrospective interview. These included everyday complaints, well-being, taking of medicines and things that went wrong. Study yielded data on family mechanisms and the quantity of data gave greater potential for complex analysis.

2.69.4 Ruffing-Rahal, M.A. (1986) Personal documents and nursing theory develpoment. *Advances in nursing science* 8(3) 50-57   36 References

Discusses the use of personal documents as a means of providing insights into the nature of health and experiences of illness. Triangulated research strategies are advocated in order to incorporate these experiences into nursing research (CR 2.26).

2.69.5 Verbrugge, L. (1980) Health diaries. *Medical care* 18(1) 73-95   52 References

A review and methodological discussion of studies which used health diaries. Evidence is given on the following aspects: levels of reporting compared to retrospective interview, recall error, validity of health reports, value of diary data for a broad view of symptoms and health behaviour for individual-level analysis and studies of health dynamics, respondent co-operation, conditioning effects, quality of diary data, survey costs, complexity of data collection, processing and analysis (CR 2.25, 2.70).

2.69.6 Woods, N.F. (1981) The health diary as an instrument for nursing research: problems and promise. *Western journal of nursing research* 3(1) 76-92   16 References

Discusses use of a health diary as a means of obtaining valid data about symptoms. Its advantages and disadvantages are discussed together with reliability and validity, and its purpose. Paper is illustrated by a study where 96 women completed a diary for three weeks. Results were weakly correlated with the Cornell Medical Index Health Questionnaire, but the author believes the method should be further explored in nursing research.

2.69.7 Wykle, M.L. & Morris, D.L. (1988) The health diary. *Applied nursing research* 1(1) 47-48   3 References

Outlines the advantages and disadvantages of this technique and illustrates it with a study which aimed to identify the self-care practices of community dwelling elders.

2.69.8 Zimmerman, D.H. & Wieder, D.L. (1977) The diary-interview method. *Urban life* 5(4) 479-499   42 References

Describes a study of the counter-culture i.e. freedom from a conventional schedule of activities, where participants were asked to record all their activities over one week in diary form and were subsequently interviewed in depth. The value of keeping diaries is discussed but authors believe that they need to be used in conjunction with interviews based around their content. They believe this method is an adjunct to or approximation of the process of direct observation which is central to the ethnographic research tradition (CR 2.43).

Suggested textbook readings

	Pages	*Cross reference*
Burgess (1982)	128-142	2.1.9
Field & Morse	85-86	2.1.24

2.70 METHODS OF DATA COLLECTION
Interview

Interviews are used for a variety of purposes in nursing research but most frequently to obtain factual information about the respondent, events, situations or other people. It is one of the most common methods of data collection and requires considerable skill on the part of the researcher.

Definition
A data collection method employing a verbal questioning technique

---

Example
Luker, K.A. & Chalmers, K.J. (1989) The referral process in health visiting. *International journal of nursing studies* 26(2) 173-185   20 References

Discusses the process of referral used by health visitors. A grounded theory approach was used to discover more of this little described area of practice (CR 2.46).

Annotations
2.70.1 Bernstein, L. & Bernstein, R.S. (1985) *Interviewing: a guide for health professionals.* 4th edition Norwalk, Connecticut: Appleton-Century-Crofts   ISBN 0838543170   References

Although primarily written for health professionals who wish to develop their skills in clinical interviews, many of the principles outlined are also applicable in research interviews.

2.70.2 McCracken, G. (1988) *The long interview.* Newbury Park: Sage   ISBN 0803933533   References

Provides a systematic guide to the theory and method of the long qualitative interview. Key theoretical and methodological issues are identified, research strategies, and a simple four step model of enquiry is described. Its value as a tool in scientific studies is outlined and nine key issues discussed.

2.70.3 McCrossan, L. (1984) *A handbook for interviewers: a manual of social survey practice and procedures on structured interviewing.* London: HMSO   ISBN 0116910011   Number M 134

Guide produced by the Social Survey Division of the Office of Population Censuses and Surveys which is based on many years experience of interviewing the public.

It contains chapters on the work of this government department, sampling, approaching the public, questionnaires and types of questions, asking the questions, recording the answers, classification of definitions, general points and procedures, supervision and training of interviewers and the analysis of a survey (CR 2.22, 2.55, 2.76).

2.70.4 McHaffie, H. (1988) The artistry of interviewing. *Senior nurse* 8(1) 34   3 References

Author suggests that an interview can be a beneficial experience for both respondent and researcher. Some of the advantages are described and advice given on how to facilitate this outcome.

2.70.5 Mishler, E.G. (1986) *Research interviewing: context and narrative.* Cambridge: Massachusetts Harvard University Press ISBN 0674764609 References

Examines current views and practices of interviewing and concludes that they reflect a restricted conception of the interview process. Author makes the proposition that an interview is a form of discourse which is shaped and organised by asking and answering questions. He advocates using a family of methods as a framework for developing an alternative.

2.70.6 Spradley, J.P. (1979) *The ethnographic interview.* New York: Holt, Rinehart & Winston ISBN 0030444969 References

This book, together with its companion volume 'Participant Observation' (CR 2.73.8), aims to provide a systematic handbook for doing ethnography and develops techniques initially used largely by anthropologists. Part 1 sets ethnographic research in context and Part 2 identifies a series of steps designed to develop skills in this type of interviewing The text is illustrated by many examples from the authors own and others research (CR 2.43).

2.70.7 Stone, S. (1984) CRUS Guide 6. *Interviews.* Sheffield: University of Sheffield, Centre for Research on User Studies ISBN 0906088178 References

An introductory booklet whose purpose is to enable researchers to assess the feasability of using interviews as the main data collection device. Use of interviews for exploratory purposes or to follow up issues raised by studies using other data collection devices is considered.

2.70.8 Whyte, W.F. (1982) Interviewing in field research. IN Burgess, R.G. (ed) *Field research: a sourcebook and field manual.* London: Allen & Unwin ISBN 0043120148 References Chapter 16 111-122

Chapter concentrates on the method in which the interviewer does not follow a standard order or wording of questions (CR 2.1.9).

2.70.9   Williams, J.A. (1973) Interviewer-respondent interaction: a study of bias in information interviews. IN Cochrane, R. (ed) *Advances in social research: a reader.* London: Constable   ISBN 0094581908   References   Chapter 13   229-248

Chapter reports on research undertaken to examine the extent to which characteristics of interviewers and respondents influence the information elicited (CR 2.27).

2.70.10   Wragg, E.C. (undated) *Conducting and analysing interviews.* Maidenhead: TRC Rediguides Ltd No. 11   References (Series edited by Youngman, M.B. Nottingham University School of Education)   (No ISBN number)

A short, practical text which discusses the processes in conducting and analysing interviews.

Suggested textbook readings

	Pages	Cross reference
Adams & Schvaneveldt	213-229	2.1.1
Brink & Wood	146-159	2.1.7
Burgess (1982)	101-122	2.1.9
Carr P. IN Cormack	81-89	2.1.20
Castles	92-95	2.1.15
Chenitz & Swanson	66-90	2.46.2
Chisnall	131-144	2.1.16
Cohen & Manion	291-314	2.1.19
Fox	223-224	2.1.25
Grey M. IN Lobiondo-Wood & Haber	235-238	2.1.38
Kidder & Judd	265-278	2.1.30
Nieswiadomy	231-246	2.1.43
Phillips L.R.F. (critique)	229-230	2.98.11
Polgar & Thomas	105-113	2.1.55
Polit & Hungler (1987)	227-248	2.1.56
Seaman	288-294	2.1.62
Smith H.W.	171-199	2.98.14
Treece & Treece	298-317	2.1.65
Walker	45-91	2.1.66
Waltz, Strickland & Lenz	263-274	2.56.5
Williamson	197-200	2.1.67
Wilson H.S. (1989)	148-149/436-442	2.1.69
Wiseman & Aron	27-36	2.66.1
Woods & Catanzaro	300-333	2.1.72

Nursing research abstracts
Belson W.A.	86/001

2.71 METHODS OF DATA COLLECTION
Interview – group (focus group)

Interviewing subjects as a group is much less frequently used as a data collection method than talking to individuals, but in some circumstances may be of particular value.

Definition
The process of asking a group of subjects verbally in order to obtain data

Example
Nyamathi, A. & Shuler, P. (1990) Focus groups interview: a research technique for informed nursing practice. *Journal of advanced nursing* 15(11) 1281-1288   31 References

Paper describes the use of focus group interviews to promote development of a programme, which aimed to reduce risk behaviour of minority populations in order to prevent AIDS. Historical, methodological and philosophical perspectives are given, issues of reliability and validity discussed, together with its advantages and disadvantages.

Annotations
2.71.1 Goldman, A.E. & McDonald, S.S. (1987) *The group depth interview: principles and practice.* Englewood Cliffs, New Jersey: Prentice Hall ISBN 013365396X   References

Covers both the theory and practice of group interview methodologies particularly in marketing research. The practical aspects are covered in depth including designing and conducting a study, data analysis and writing the report. Verbatim quotations are used throughout the book to demonstrate 'probing skills'.

2.71.2 Krueger, R.A. (1988) *Focus groups: a practical guide for applied research.* Newbury Park: Sage ISBN 0803931875   References

Book provides a comprehensive and detailed analysis of focus group interviewing techniques. Part 1 presents an overview of focus groups and identifies the differences between this and other similar methodological procedures. Part 2 describes the processes used in conducting focus group interviews and Part 3 outlines the involvement of non-researchers, variations of focus groups and ways for contracting focus group assistance.

2.71.3 Morgan, D.L. (1988) *Focus groups as qualitative research.* Newbury Park: Sage ISBN 0803932081   References

Describes uses for focus groups, gives a historical perspective and discusses it as a qualitative method. Its strengths and weaknesses are outlined and advice is given on planning, conducting the study and analysing the data.

2.71.4 Morgan, D.L. & Spanish, M.T. (1984) Focus groups: a new tool for qualitative research. *Qualitative sociology* 7: 253-270   17 References

Authors describe ways in which focus groups may differ and illustrate this from their own research. This method of data collection is contrasted with individual interviews and observation and applications are discussed. The value of such groups in triangulating data is discussed (CR 2.26).

Suggested textbook readings

	Pages	Cross reference
Chisnall	148-150	2.1.16
Stone	21-23	2.70.7
Walker	71-91	2.1.66

2.72 METHODS OF DATA COLLECTION
Interview – telephone

Telephone interviews are one of the tools used particularly in market research to ascertain people's views on a wide range of topics, for example customer services provided by a particular company, or aspects of health care. New developments in this field include the use of computer-assisted telephone interviewing and direct computer interviewing.

Definition
Questioning by telephone

Example
Hill, A. & Mayon-White, R.T. (1987) A telephone survey to evaluate an AIDS leaflet campaign. *Health education journal* 46(3) 127-129   5 References

Discusses the methods and uses of telephone surveys in the evaluation of health education campaigns.

Annotations
2.72.1 Howard, B.J., Meade, P.A., Booth, D. & Whall, A. (1988) The telephone interview. *Applied nursing research* 1(1) 45-46   5 References

Discusses the advantages and disadvantages of telephone interviewing and how such a survey may be successfully conducted. A survey is briefly described which aimed to obtain data regarding care of people with Alzheimer's disease (CR 2.55).

2.72.2 Lavrakas, P.J. (1987) *Telephone survey methods: sampling, selection and supervision.* Beverly Hills: Sage   ISBN 0803926340   References

Three major elements of telephone survey techniques are explored in depth: generating and processing telephone survey sampling pools, selecting a respondent and securing co-operation and structuring the work of interviewers and supervisors. Areas not covered in the text are clearly listed.

Contains a glossary of terms relevant to this method (CR 2.55.7).

Suggested textbook readings

	Pages	Cross reference
Adams & Schvaneveldt	219-220	2.1.2
Chisnall	123-130/180	2.1.16
Kidder & Judd	226-229	2.1.30
Nieswiadomy	239	2.1.43
Seaman	293-294	2.1.62
Stone	19-21	2.70.7

2.73   METHODS OF DATA COLLECTION
Observation

Observation is one of the major methods by which data are gathered and is particularly appropriate for complex research situations. These may be viewed as complete entities and would be difficult to measure either as a whole or separately (Fox 1982).

Definitions

Observation − a method of collecting data in which the researcher scientifically watches and records pertinent information

Non-participant observation − observer watches and records but does not participate as a member of the group of study subjects being observed

Participant observation − observer watches, collects and records data while interacting with the group of study subjects as a member of the group

---

Example

Wolf, Z.R. (1988) Nursing rituals. *The Canadian journal of nursing research* 20(3) 59-69   16 References

Reports an ethnographic study which aimed to explore the beliefs, values and patterns of nursing rituals. Participant observation was used as a major data collection method together with event analysis and semi-structured interviews. Rituals focused upon were post-mortem care, admission to and discharge from hospital, medication administration, bed baths, handling excreta and the products of infection and the change of shift report. Author believes that rituals enable nurses to carry out caring activities for patients (CR 2.43).

Annotations

2.73.1   Becker, H.S. & Geer, B. (1982) Participant observation: the analysis of qualitative field data. IN Burgess, R.G. (ed) *Field research: a sourcebook and field manual.* London: Allen & Unwin   ISBN 0043120148   References   Chapter 32   239-250

Discusses the role of participant observation as a data collection method and describes three stages of analysis using a study of medical students for illustration (CR 2.1.9).

2.73.2   Buckingham, R., Kack, S.A., Mount, B.M., Maclean, L.D. & Collins, J.T. (1976) Living with the dying: use of the technique of participant observation. *Canadian Medical Association journal* 115: December 18 1211-1215   19 References

Describes the experience of an anthropologist who assumed the role of a terminally ill patient when admitted firstly to a surgical ward and then to a palliative care unit. Both units are compared and contrasted with particular reference to treatment, attitudes and interactions of staff, terminally ill patients and their families. Of particular note was the effect of this hospitalisation on the researcher (CR 2.16).

2.73.3   Friedrichs, J. & Ludtke, H. (1975) *Participant observation: theory and practice.* Farnborough, Hants: Saxon House/Lexington Books   ISBN 0347010490   References

Book contributes to laying methodological foundations for participant observation and aims to bring it closer to the status of a rigorous scientific method. Part 1 covers the theory and methodology of participant observation; Part 2 discusses practical field problems and Part 3 gives guidance on the instruction and preparation of observers.

2.73.4   Leininger, M.M. (1985) Audio-visual methods in nursing research. IN Author (ed) *Qualitative research methods in nursing.* Orlando: Grune & Stratton   ISBN 0808916769   References   Part 20 331-341

Chapter discusses the purpose of audio-visual methods in research, gives guidelines for their use, together with the advantages and limitations (CR 2.1.36).

2.73.5   Luker, K.A. & Box, D.F. (1985) Clinical nursing research in context. *Nursing practice* 1(2) 109-113   7 References

Study examines the attitudes and role of nurses involved in the teaching and management of patients undergoing Continuous Ambulatory Peritoneal Dialysis, and is an example of a clinical nursing study using participant observation. The strengths and weaknesses of the technique are described and the difficulty of applying it to the real world of nursing. Mention is also made of other practical difficulties encountered (CR 2.16).

2.73.6   McCall, G.J. & Simmons, J.L. (eds) (1969) *Issues in participant observation: a text and reader.* Reading, Massachusetts: Addison-Wesley   ISBN 0201070278   References

Discusses the range of problems and issues together with statements and solutions available in the literature at the time. Contents include the nature and uses of participant observation; methodological and ethical issues; data collection; recording and retrieval; quality of data; generating and evaluating hypotheses and publication of results. It is also compared with other methods of data collection (CR 2.17, 2.66).

2.73.7   Robertson, C.M. (1982) A description of participant observation of clinical teaching. *Journal of advanced nursing* 7(6) 549-554   14 References

A description is given of participant observation undertaken by the author. The purpose of it, and its differing forms and disadvantages are described and discussed. Examples are given both from this study and the literature.

2.73.8   Spradley, J.P. (1980) *Participant observation.* New York: Holt, Rinehart & Winston   ISBN 003044501   References

Book describes the techniques of participant observation when carrying out ethnographic research. Part 1 defines ethnography, identifies assumptions which underly it and distinguishes it from other approaches. Part 2 discusses the 'Developmental Research Sequence' which is a series of 12 tasks designed to guide the reader through each stage of observations in ethnographic research (CR 2.43).

[Companion volume – The Ethnographic Interview 2.70.6]

2.73.9   Stubbs, M. & Delamont, S. (eds) (1976) *Explorations in classroom observation.* Chichester: Wiley   ISBN 0471995932   References

Papers explore different methods of directly observing, recording and describing the complex behaviour of teachers and pupils inside classrooms. Authors maintain that this area is under-researched because of its complexity. Different theoretical backgrounds are used to explore the field.

Suggested textbook readings

	Pages	Cross reference
Adams & Schvaneveldt	231-254	2.1.2
Brink & Wood	139-146	2.1.7
Burgess (1984)	78-100	2.1.10
Castles	89-92	2.1.15
Chenitz & Swanson	48-65	2.46.2
Crow R. IN Cormack	90-104	2.1.20
Fox	196-211	2.1.25
Gans H.J. IN Burgess (1982)	53-61	2.1.9
Grady & Wallston	117-125	3.11.2
Grey M. IN LoBiondo-Wood & Haber	232-235	2.1.38
Holm & Llewellyn	115-118	2.1.26
Kidder & Judd	168-188/279-299	2.1.30
Lin	205-213	2.1.37
Nieswiadomy	247-252	2.1.43

	Pages	Cross reference
Phillips L.R.F. (critique)	230-231	2.98.11
Polit & Hungler (1987)	266-288	2.1.56
Seaman	251-273	2.1.62
Smith H.W.	200-253	2.98.14
Thomas	120-121	2.1.64
Treece & Treece	332-347	2.1.65
Walker	92-100/167-171	2.1.66
Waltz, Strickland & Lenz	248-255	2.56.5
Wiseman & Aron	15-26/49-59	2.66.1
Wilson H.S. (1989)	433-436	2.1.69
Woods & Catanzaro	278-299	2.1.72

Nursing research abstracts

James, N.   85/116

Note: In the literature on qualitative research methods many writers use the terms field work/research interchangeably with participant observation. This usage should be distinguished from that of more structured methods e.g. a social survey based on a questionnaire where the term field work has been used to denote the practical problems involved in data gathering.

2.74 METHODS OF DATA COLLECTION
Projective Techniques

Projective techniques encompass many different measurement tools, devices, and strategies which may be used to examine fundamental aspects of psychological functioning (Waltz, Strickland & Lenz 1984).

Definition

A method for collecting data in which the subjects are asked to respond to non-structured or ambiguous stimuli − an ambiguity that the investigator has made no attempt to conceal

---

Example

Wood, S.P. (1983) School aged children's perceptions of the causes of illness. *Pediatric nursing* 9: March/April 101-104   12 References

Study examined the perceptions of causes of illness in a group of 65 children. Pictures were used with brief sentences attached to explore their ideas. Two major theories emerged as causes, illness as punishment and the germ theory.

Suggested textbook readings

	Pages	Cross reference
Adams & Schvaneveldt	271-289	2.1.2
Kidder & Judd	260-262	2.1.30
Oppenheim	160-196	2.76.5
Polit & Hungler (1987)	305-307	2.1.56
Walker	6-7/101-121	2.1.66
Waltz, Strickland & Lenz	285-297	2.56.5
Wiseman & Aron	126-137	2.66.1

2.75 METHODS OF DATA COLLECTION
Q Sort

This is a technique used extensively in nursing to assess the similarity of perceptions about the quality of nursing care, behaviours of patients and attitudes of nurses towards roles and illness (Woods & Catanzaro 1988)

Definition
A research method comprised of rank ordering objects by sorting, and then assigning numbers to the subsets for statistical purposes

Example
Irwin, B.L. & Meier, J.S. (1973) Supportive measures for relatives of the fatally ill. *Communicating nursing research: collaboration and competition* 6: 119-128   19 References

The Q sort technique was used to generate a group of descriptive statements about supportive care. Three categories were derived: religious-philosophical, non-verbal-action, and verbal non-religious. Staff,and relatives of people with fatal diagnoses were given these items, and asked to sort them according to their feelings of agreement or disagreement.

Original text/articles
Stephenson, W. (1953) *The study of behaviour: Q technique and its methodology.* Chicago: University of Chicago Press   (No ISBN number found)

Stephenson, W. (1935a) Technique of factor analysis. *Nature* 136: August 24 297

Stephenson, W. (1935b) Correlating persons instead of tests. *Character and personality* 4: September 17-24

Annotations

2.75.1 Brown, S.R. (1986) Q Technique and method: principles and procedures. IN Berry, W.D. & Lewis-Beck, M.S. (eds) *New tools for social scientists: advances and applications in research methods.* Beverly Hills: Sage ISBN 083926251 References Chapter 3 57-76

Although an old technique, having been introduced in the 1930's, author feels it is a neglected tool which has considerable value. Much of the chapter is devoted to discussion of two studies where the technique was used, and it closes with some methodological pointers (CR 2.56.1).

2.75.2 Dennis, K.E. (1986) Q methodology: relevance and application to nursing research. *Advances in nursing science* 8(3) 6-17 16 References

Explores the value of Q methodology, which is much more than the Q sort data collection method, for the expansion of nursing knowledge. An overview of the technique is given and suggestions made as to how it may be used.

2.75.3 McKeown, B. & Thomas, D. (1988) *Q methodology.* Newbury Park: Sage ISBN 0803927533 References

Covers the principles, techniques and procedures of the Q method.

2.75.4 Nyatanga, L. (1989) The Q sort: theory and technique. *Nurse education today* 9(5) 347-350 12 References

Paper focuses on the theoretical assumptions of the Q sort technique, summarises the self-theory of Carl Rogers, describes the procedure, and highlights its strengths and limitations.

2.75.5 Tetting, D.W. (1988) Q-sort update. *Western journal of nursing research* 10(6) 757-765 16 References

Article gives a brief review of the literature; discusses processes used to develop and sort the cards in a study related to job activity; offers suggestions for analysis and shares examples for displaying results.

Suggested textbook readings

	Pages	Cross reference
Kovacs	83-87	2.1.31
Phillips L.R.F. (critique)	233	2.98.11
Polit & Hungler (1987)	301-303	2.1.56
Strickland & Waltz	409-419	2.63.16
Treece & Treece	352-353	2.1.65
Waltz, Strickland & Lenz	297-305	2.56.5
Woods & Catanzaro	326-328	2.1.72

2.76 METHODS OF DATA COLLECTION
Questionnaire

The questionnaire is a relatively direct method of obtaining information which may be factual, attitudinal, beliefs, opinions, intentions, standards and levels of knowledge. Since no verbal exchange is involved a questionnaire can be handed or mailed to the respondent.

Definition
A data collection technique consisting of a set of written items requesting a response from subjects

Example
Blackmore, S. (1989) A survey of general medical knowledge among university students: its implications for informed consent and health education. *Senior nurse* 9(10) 17-21   18 References

Study aimed to elicit student's knowledge about health in terms of basic anatomy, physiology and pathology of selected organs and also their attitudes to health. Questionnaires were used together with a short interview. Concerns are expresssed about the findings which show the need for more health education.

Annotations
2.76.1 Atkinson, I. (1987) Are we asking the right questions? *Senior nurse* 7(1) 55   1 Reference

Stresses the importance of the questions used in the compilation of questionnaires and interview schedules.

2.76.2 Belson, W.A. (1981) *The design and understanding of survey questions.* Aldershot: Gower   ISBN 0566004208   References

Reports the findings of an exploratory study which aimed to investigate respondent misunderstanding of survey questions and to provide insights into the processes involved. 265 people were interviewed about 29 experimental questions spread within four carrier questionnaires. Recommendations were that regular use of standard question testing technique should be made to detect misunderstanding of survey questions. The 15 sets of hypotheses which emerged should be further examined to obtain more understanding of these difficulties. Study has implications which go beyond the boundaries of survey research as the efficiency of mass communication is also in question.

2.76.3 Bennet, A.E. & Ritchie, K. (1975) *Questionnaires in medicine.* Oxford: Oxford University Press for the Nuffield Provincial Hospitals Trust, Oxford   ISBN 019721390

Author draws heavily on Oppenheim's publication but applies the principles to the field of health care. Examples are included which are relevant to many nursing projects (CR 2.76.5).

2.76.4 Champion, P.J. & Sear, A.M. (1973) Questionnaire response rates: a methodological analysis. IN Cochrane, R. (ed) *Advances in social research: a reader.* London: Constable ISBN 0094581908 References Chapter 15 263-271

Report of a study which aimed to investigate the differential effects of three important variables on response rates of a mailed questionnaire. The variables examined were length of the questionnaire; type of postage used and the incentives given to respondents.

2.76.5 Oppenheim, A.N. (1966) *Questionnaire design and attitude measurement.* London: Heinemann ISBN 043582676X References

A classic text on questionnaire design which provides step by step guidance on question writing, both factual and attitudinal, attitude scaling and projective techniques. (CR 2.74).

2.76.6 Robin, S.S. (1973) A procedure for securing returns to mail questionnaires. IN Cochrane, R. (ed) *Advances in social research: a reader.* London: Constable ISBN 0094581908 References Chapter 16 272-284

Describes a technique which has resulted in high returns of questionnaires in ten independent samples.

2.76.7 Robinson, D.K. (1989) Response rates in questionnaires. *Senior nurse* 9(10) 25-26 29 References

Outlines findings from mainly older literature on response rates to questionnaires. No conclusions are drawn.

2.76.8 Simpson, M.A. (1984) How to design and use a questionnaire in evaluation and educational research. *Medical teacher* 16(4) 122-127 24 References

Article discusses the points which contribute to a well designed questionnaire and takes the reader step by step through the process.

2.76.9 Youngman, M.B. (1978) *Designing and analysing questionnaires.* Nottingham: University of Nottingham, School of Education ISBN 094606900X References Rediguide 12: Guides in Educational Research

A small, practical booklet which discusses the design and analysis of questionnaires.

Suggested textbook readings

	Pages	*Cross reference*
Adams & Schvaneveldt	202-213	2.1.2
Brink & Wood	146-159	2.1.7
Castles	92-95	2.1.15
Chisnall	104-130	2.1.16
Fox	212-231	2.1.25
Grey M. IN LoBiondo-Wood & Haber	235-239	2.1.38
Henerson, Morris & Fitz-Gibbon	57-83	2.58.1
Holm & Llewellyn	106-114/118-120	2.1.26
Kidder & Judd	219-265	2.1.30
Kovacs	70-75	2.1.31
Nieswiadomy	209-229	2.1.43
Phillips L.R.F. (critique)	231	2.98.11
Polgar & Thomas	105-113	2.1.55
Polit & Hungler (1987)	227-248	2.1.56
Seaman	276-287	2.1.62
Sheehan J. IN Cormack	110-117	2.1.20
Smith H.W.	171-199	2.98.14
Treece & Treece	277-297	2.1.65
Waltz, Strickland & Lenz	275-281	2.56.5
Williamson	195-197/217-229	2.1.67
Woods & Catanzaro	300-333	2.1.72

Nursing research abstracts
Atkinson, I.   88/101

2.77 METHODS OF DATA COLLECTION
Records/archival data

Records are a readily available and valuable source of research data and may be found everywhere. Sources include government records, those kept by institutions and individuals.

Definition
Compilations of writing, photographs and figures that individuals have collected

---

Example
Harris, R.B. & Hyman, R.B. (1984) Clean versus sterile tracheostomy care and level of pulmonary infection. *Nursing research* 33(2) 80-85   39 References

Patients' charts were examined before and after tracheostomy for clinical and laboratory data related to infection. Hospital infection survey reports were also studied in order to make comparisons and a tool developed to examine these records.

Annotations

2.77.1 Burgess, R.G. (ed) (1982a) Keeping field notes. IN Author, *Field research: a sourcebook and field manual.* London: Allen & Unwin ISBN 0043120148 References 25: 191-194

Covers aspects of keeping field notes and outlines the three types which may be kept; substantive, methodological and analytic (CR 2.1.9).

2.77.2 Burgess, R.G. (ed) (1982b) Personal documents, oral sources and life histories. IN Author, *Field research: a sourcebook and field manual.* London: Allen & Unwin ISBN 0043120148 References 18: 131-135

Discusses the value of different sources of data in field research (CR 2.1.9).

2.77.3 Webb, B. (1982) The art of note taking. IN Burgess, R.G. (ed) *Field research: a sourcebook and field manual.* London: Allen & Unwin ISBN 0043120148 References 26: 195-199

Chapter discusses the processes involved in note-taking which are essential for the creation of accurate records (CR 2.1.9).

2.77.4 While, A.E. (1987) Records as a data source: the case for health visitor records. *Journal of advanced nursing* 12(6) 757-763 26 References

It is suggested that health records are a useful source of research data, and a case study approach was used to evaluate health visitor records. Consideration must however also be given to their limitations.

Suggested textbook readings

	Pages	*Cross reference*
Burgess (1982)	123-128/166-176	2.1.9
Fox	155	2.1.25
Grady & Wallston	91-100	3.11.2
Grey M. IN LoBiondo-Wood & Haber	238-239	2.1.38
Hakim	36-46	2.94.2
Kidder & Judd	299-311	2.1.30
Polit & Hungler (1987)	299-301	2.1.56
Treece & Treece	318-331	2.1.65
Woods & Catanzaro	334-352	2.1.72

2.78 METHODS OF DATA COLLECTION
Repertory Grid Technique

Personal construct theory, which forms the basis of the repertory grid technique, stresses the importance of eliciting the individuals own constructs rather than those supplied by a researcher. A construct is a way of viewing elements as alike or different where these objects of study are provided by the researcher. These elements are then developed into a grid, the constructs examined and scores generated.

Definitions
Personal construct — a cover term for each of the ways in which a person attempts to perceive, understand, predict and control the world

Repertory grid — a series of judgements made by a person, using his constructs, on some aspect of the world

Example
Heyman, R., Shaw, M.P. & Harding, J. (1983) A personal construct theory approach to the socialisation of nursing trainees in two British general hospitals. *Journal of advanced nursing* 8(1) 59-67 8 References

A longitudinal study with British student and pupil nurses which aimed to examine changes in their perceptions of nursing using a personal construct theory framework and a repertory grid technique. Trainees were found to be more identified with, and attracted to, a medical role and less with lower status non-medical roles. Some other measures derived from the grids included wastage and satisfaction with the hospital.

Original texts
Kelly, G.E. (1955) *The psychology of personal constructs.* New York: Norton Volumes 1 and 2 (No ISBN numbers)

Kelly, G.E. (1963) *A theory of personality.* New York: Norton & Coy ISBN 0393001520

Major reference
Fransella, F. & Bannister, D. (1977) *A manual for repertory grid technique.* London: Academic Press ISBN 0122654560 References [contains annotated bibliography 149-169] (CR 2.78.6)

Annotations
2.78.1 Bannister, D. (1970) Concepts of personality: Kelly and Osgood. IN Mittler, P.J. (ed) *The psychological assessment of mental and physical handicaps.* London: Methuen SBN 416045707 References Chapter 26 761-779 (CR 2.62)

Outlines two techniques for exploring interpretive man; the repertory grid and the semantic differential.*

*a technique used to measure attitudes that asks the respondents to rate a concept of interest on a series of seven-point bipolar scales

2.78.2 Bannister, D. (1981) Personal construct theory and research method. IN Reason, P. & Rowan, J. (eds) *Human inquiry: a sourcebook of new paradigm research.* Chichester: Wiley ISBN 0471279358 References Chapter 16 191-199

Outlines the personal construct theory developed by Kelly in the 1950's and discusses use of the repertory grid technique as a tool in various psychological fields (CR 2.11.5).

2.78.3 Bannister, D. & Fransella, F. (1986) *Inquiring man: the theory of personal constructs.* 3rd edition London: Croom Helm   ISBN 0709939516   References

Book summarises personal construct theory and reviews the research it has generated. It examines its value for psychologists and psychotherapists and challenges orthodox thinking.

2.78.4 Beail, N. (ed) (1985) *Repertory grid technique and personal constructs: applications in clinical settings.* London: Croom Helm   ISBN 0709932642   References

A collection of readings which explore various applications of repertory grid technique. Included are a brief introduction to the technique and seven sections covering − construct systems; constructs and disability; evaluation of change; exploring relationships through grids; practical applications in education; constructs of handicap and a caveat on some aspects of validity.

2.78.5 Cohen, L. & Manion, L. (1989) *Research methods in education.* 3rd edition London: Routledge   ISBN 0415036488   References   Chapter 14   336-358

Outlines the personal construct theory of George Kelly and discusses the structure and development of repertory grids. Its strengths and weaknesses are identified and some examples of its use in education are given (CR 2.1.19).

2.78.6 Fransella, F. & Bannister, D. (1977) *A manual for repertory grid technique.* London: Academic Press   ISBN 0122654560   References

Manual describes a technique developed from George Kelly's personal construct theory which aimed to 'look beyond words'. A variety of commonly used grid formats are discussed and the many difficulties which may be encountered are outlined. The reader is given guidance to enable him to design his own grid while also becoming aware of its limitations. Appendix 1 contains an example of the use of grids and Appendix 2 contains the first published annotated bibliography on grid usage.

2.78.7 Pollock, L.C. (1986) An introduction to the use of repertory grid technique as a research method and clinical tool for psychiatric nurses. *Journal of advanced nursing* 11(4) 439-445   24 References

Provides summary of the repertory grid technique as a research method.

Nursing research abstracts
Andrew C.   86/469
Heyman R., Shaw M.P. & Harding J.   83/389

2.79 METHODS OF DATA COLLECTION
Self and other reports

Self-reporting techniques are used in nursing research because they offer straightforwardness and flexibility, and may yield information which could not otherwise be obtained. Their major weaknesses are lack of validity and accuracy.

Definition
An indirect method for assessing health status

Example
Maruyama, M. (1981) Endogenous research*: the prison project. IN Reason, P. & Rowan, J. (eds) *Human inquiry: a sourcebook of new paradigm research.* Chichester: Wiley ISBN 0471279358 References Chapter 23 267-281

Chapter describes a project undertaken to investigate prison violence where the researchers were largely the inmates themselves. The abilities of the endogenous researchers to conceptualise, record, code and analyse data are discussed. A list of criteria for selecting such researchers is given (CR 2.11.5).

*Endogenous research is where a culture is studied by its insiders

Annotations
2.79.1 Grady, K.E. & Wallston, B.S. (1988) *Research in health care settings.* Newbury Park: Sage ISBN 0803928742 References Chapter 7 101-116

Chapter explores areas where self-report may be appropriate, gives examples and discusses possible biases (CR 3.11.2).

2.79.2 Hersen, M. (1973) Self-assessment of fear. *Behaviour therapy* 4(2) 241-257 47 References

Self-assessment measures are reviewed in terms of their reliability, validity, factorial structure, sex and population differences and correlations with other personality scales.

2.79.3 Lipson, J.G. (1989) The use of self in ethnographic research. IN Morse, J.M. (ed) *Qualitative nursing research: a contemporary dialogue.* Rockville, Maryland: Aspen ISBN 0834200112 References Chapter 5 61-75

Discusses the contributions researchers can make when conducting research. The background and assumptions inherent in this are discussed, together with influences on the use of self and advice given on how this technique may be improved (CR 2.36.8).

Suggested textbook readings

	Pages	Cross reference
Barlow & Hersen	132-135	2.34.1
Polit & Hungler (1987)	228-248	2.1.56

2.80 METHODS OF DATA COLLECTION
Talk/conversation

Talk is increasingly being recognised and used as a technique for obtaining information from subjects. Conversations are complex to analyse but may yield data which can be of considerable value to researchers.

Definition
An informal spoken exchange of thoughts and feelings

Example
Reason, P. (1981) An exploration in the dialectics of two person relationships. IN Reason, P. & Rowan, J. (eds) *Human inquiry: a sourcebook of new paradigm research.* Chichester: Wiley ISBN 0471279358 References Chapter 28 319-331

The researcher and a lesbian couple engaged in a three day workshop to explore the holistic view of the latters' relationships. The researcher felt the need to develop further skills as a facilitator (CR 2.11.5).

Annotations
2.80.1 Adelman, C. (ed) (1981) *Uttering, muttering: collecting, using and reporting talk for social and educational research.* London: Grant McIntyre ISBN 0862160421 References

Compilation of studies written by leading researchers which brings together the theory and practice of using talk in research. Details on how to gather, interpret and make use of talk in educational and cultural settings are given.

2.80.2 Graham, H. (1984) Surveying through stories. IN Bell, C. & Roberts, H. (eds) *Social researching, politics, problems and practice.* London: Routledge & Kegan Paul ISBN 0710098847 References 6: 104-124

Chapter explores the use of narrative in survey research by examining the experience of early motherhood (CR 2.1.5).

2.80.3 Jones, J.A. (1989) The verbal protocol: a research technique for nursing. *Journal of advanced nursing* 14(12) 1062-1070   20 References

Reports a pilot study undertaken to investigate use of the verbal protocol. It aimed to discover how nurses reach decisions about a patient's problems and how a nursing diagnosis is made. The theoretical background to the technique, its use in medical contexts and the analysis of such data is discussed.

2.80.4 Randell, R. & Southgate, J. (1981) Doing dialogical research. IN Reason, P. & Rowan, J. (eds) *Human inquiry: a sourcebook of new paradigm research.* Chichester: Wiley   ISBN 0471279358   References   Chapter 30   349-361

Project examined the psychodynamics of self-managed groups. A series of cartoons encapsulating the information gathered was presented back to the group to draw out the major contradictions (CR 2.11.5).

2.80.5 Tandon, R. (1981) Dialogue as inquiry and intervention. IN Reason, P. & Rowan, J. (eds) *Human inquiry: a sourcebook of new paradigm research.* Chichester: Wiley   ISBN 0471279358   References   Chapter 25   293-301

Presents a study where dialogue was used as inquiry and intervention simultaneously (CR 2.11.5).

2.80.6 Wardhaugh, R. (1985) *How conversation works.* Oxford: Blackwell   ISBN 0631139397   References

Book discusses the structure of conversation and describes what happens when people talk to each other.

Suggested textbook reading

	Pages	*Cross reference*
Silverman D. (1985)	118-137/145-148	2.36.14

Nursing research abstracts

Graham, H.	85/008

2.81 UNSOLICITED RESEARCH DATA

Many researchers find in the course of collecting their data, that additional information is given by their subjects. In many instances this is ignored in the final writing up process as it may prove to be 'messy'. However, these data may give additional insights into aspects of the research process, the tools which the researcher has used or developed, and the feelings of the participants.

Annotation
2.81.1 Cormack, D.F.S. (1981) Making use of unsolicited research data. *Journal of advanced nursing* 6(1) 41-49   11 References

Author believes that additional, unsolicited data which may be received during the data collection process, to be of value as it contributes to the understanding of nursing research in general, and the research subject in particular. 251 comments were obtained during a project which examined the role of the psychiatric nurse. These were analysed and highlighted some of the difficulties respondents were experiencing in thinking about nursing in specific terms. The role of trade unions in relation to gaining access to sites is also discussed.

DATA ANALYSIS, INTERPRETATION AND PRESENTATION

2.82   DATA ANALYSIS – GENERAL

Data analysis consists of examining, categorising, tabulating or otherwise re-combining the evidence, to address the initial propositions of a study (Yin 1984).

Definition
Application of one or more techniques to a set of data for the purpose of discovering trends, differences or similarities. The type of technique used is guided by the subject matter of the problem

Annotations
2.82.1   Downs, F.S. (ed) (1988) *Handbook of research methodology.* New York: American Journal of Nursing Company   ISBN 0937126756   References

Comprises a selection of articles originally published in the methodology corner of Nursing Research. Many of the major issues relating to effective procedures in research design and analysis are discussed. The book is intended to supplement existing texts.

2.82.2   Erickson, B.H. & Nosanchuk, T.A. (1979) *Understanding data: an introduction to exploratory and confirmatory data analysis for students in the social sciences.* Milton Keynes: Open University Press   ISBN 0335002528   References

Book is intended for professional sociologists and students who have always feared numbers. It utilises the techniques of exploratory data analysis developed by Tukey. The student is fully involved in the data and its analysis and it draws on their strengths and enables development of their own ideas. Suggestions for examination questions and homework are included (CR 2.82.5).

2.82.3   Goldstone, L.A. (1986) *Health and nursing management statistics.* Newcastle upon Tyne: Newcastle upon Tyne Polytechnic Products   ISBN 0906471427   References

Book is concerned with the improvement of managerial skills in handling, interrogating, understanding, presenting and utilising numbers. Actual examples of National Health Service data are used to illustrate each chapter.

2.82.4   Marsh, C. (1988) *Exploring data: an introduction to data analysis for social scientists.* Cambridge: Polity Press   ISBN 0745601723   References

Focuses on the problems of exploring data and seeks to close the gap between the technique and the problem. Some current major issues e.g. national income and welfare, education policies, health care, mortality and morbidity and unemployment are used to provide illustrative material upon which a wide range of techniques is discussed. These techniques, called Exploratory Data Analysis (Tukey 1977), seek to identify what the data is really saying, or decide if a particular result is spurious. Exercises are included which test an increasing number of variables and their inter-relationships. The use of Minitab is briefly discussed (CR 2.82.5, 2.88).

2.82.5 Tukey, J.W. (1977) *Exploratory data analysis.* Reading, Massachusetts: Addison-Wesley   ISBN 0201076160   References

Author advocates exploratory data analysis as the foundation stone necessary for analysing complex data. Worked examples are given to enable students gain confidence in handling data this way. Glossary contains terms particular to this method of analysis (pages 667-676).

Suggested textbook readings

	Pages	*Cross reference*
Adams & Schvaneveldt	331-377	2.1.2
Brink & Wood	200-221	2.1.7
Bulmer M. (DE 304) 2A	71-160	2.1.46
Bynner J. (DE 304) 5	5-37	2.1.51
Castles	110-125	2.1.15
Howard & Sharp	99-120	3.21.5
Kidder & Judd	315-391	2.1.30
Kovacs	115-145	2.1.31
LoBiondo-Wood	345-357	2.1.38
Mason D. IN Krampitz & Pavlovich	108-113	2.1.32
Miller D.C.	143-205	2.56.3
Nieswiadomy	267-279	2.1.43
Phillips L.R.F. (critique)	249-271	2.98.11
Roberts & Burke	272-303	2.1.59
Seaman	333-391	2.1.62
Senn S. IN Cormack	144-154	2.1.20
Smith H.W.	315-340	2.98.14
Sweeney & Olivieri	389-401	2.1.63
Thomas	245-276	2.1.64
Treece & Treece	401-453	2.1.65
Waltz & Bausell	101-116	2.21.4

Nursing research abstracts

Aaronson L.S.	90/010
Behi R.	90/111
Wu Y-W. & Slakter M.J.	90/011

2.83 STATISTICAL TEXTS

There are innumerable statistical texts on the market, many suitable for use by any discipline, and a few written with nurses in mind. The latter include examples related to health care so it may be easier for nurses to identify with these texts. A selection of books is included here, several of which were written to help students who have particular difficulties with handling numerical information.

Many texts include detailed information on how to do the necessary calculations but assume that understanding comes easily, and so do not always discuss how to select a test or what it actually means. Calculations can now be very speedily done by use of computer packages, and in view of this, several of the books included here concentrate on developing the students ability to understand.

Annotations

2.83.1 Castle, W.M. (1977) *Statistics in small doses.* 2nd edition Edinburgh: Churchill Livingstone   ISBN 0443014914

A programmed learning text covering topics in statistics needed by medical students and those in related professions. Learning is progressively assessed by questions with answers and each chapter is illustrated with a practical example and concludes with a short summary.

2.83.2 Chatfield, C. (1988) *Problem solving: a statisticians guide.* London: Chapman & Hall   ISBN 0412286807   References

Written for students and statisticians who feel unsure how to tackle a real problem where the data is 'messy' or the objectives unclear. Part 1 clarifies general principles; Part 2 presents a series of exercises to illustrate the practical problems of real data analysis; Part 3 contains a digest of statistical techniques; brief notes on two important packages − MINITAB* and GLIM**; useful addresses and statistical tables. Advice is given on choosing computer packages and about the consulting role of statisticians. Exercises are included throughout the text (CR 2.88).

*   MINITAB is a general purpose, interactive statistical computing system
** GLIM is a powerful programme for fitting generalised linear models

2.83.3 Cohen, L. & Holliday, M. (1982) *Statistics for social scientists: an introductory text with computer programs in BASIC.* London: Harper & Row   ISBN 0063182203   References

Text aims to help students understand statistical methods. The first part enables students to tackle research problems and later parts provide examples drawn from social science data. Interactive computer programs using an elementary subset of BASIC* (Revision 17). Appendices contain statistical tables. (CR 2.88)

* BASIC (Beginners All-purpose Symbolic Instruction Code) is a simple programming language.

2.83.4   Crocker, A.C. (1981) *Statistics for the teacher.* 3rd edition NFER-Nelson: Windsor, Berkshire   ISBN 0856332208

A primer in statistics which aims to be as non-technical as possible. Frequent questions enable consolidation of learning.

2.83.5   Hooke, R. (1983) *How to tell the liars from the statisticians.* New York: Marcel Dekker   ISBN 0824718178

Without using any mathematical calculations this guide spotlights the effects of statistical reasoning and its misuse. It highlights the fascination of statistics and its value in decision making. Seventy six mini-essays, on a very wide range of topics, point out statistically incorrect arguments and dubious inferences. Illustrations are included which feature key points.

2.83.6   Huff, D. (1973) *How to lie with statistics.* Harmondsworth, Middlesex: Penguin   ISBN 0140213007   (No references)

Discusses ways in which statistics are used to deceive. Everyday examples are used to expose 'the preposterous religion of our time'.

2.83.7   Irvine, J., Miles, I. & Evans, J. (eds) (1979) *Demystifying social statistics.* London: Pluto Press   ISBN 0861040686   References

Book comprises 22 essays written by social scientists for a variety of disciplines. It examines historical perspectives, the significance of statistics, official statistics, their uses and future applications.

2.83.8   Jaeger, R.M. (1983) *Statistics: a spectator sport.* Beverly Hills: Sage   ISBN 0803921721   References

Designed for those who want to understand rather than compute statistics. No equations are included which can sometimes obscure the meaning of the subject. Illustrations are provided from educational research and evaluation studies. Each chapter is summarised and contains problems to be worked through.

2.83.9   Johnson, P.R. & Wright, R.L.D. (1976) *Using statistics: a study guide to accompany R.L.D. Wright's Understanding statistics.* New York: Harcourt Brace Jovanovich   ISBN 0155928791

Study guide designed to give practice in all areas of statistical analysis discussed in the textbook. Each chapter contains objectives, questions on basic concepts, and short answer questions leading to more complex ones designed to test students' accumulating skills (CR 2.83.22).

2.83.10   Kapadia, R. & Andersson, G. (1987) *Statistics explained: basic concepts and methods.* Chichester: Ellis Horwood   ISBN 074580053X   References

A basic introduction to statistics using headlines, cuttings and figures from the mass media to provide systematic training in analysing statistical information. Examples chosen from everyday life emphasise fundamental ideas and underlying principles, while technical details are kept to a minimum. Book is intended for those who will be consumers of statistics rather than for those needing to develop mathematical skills. Exercises are included throughout the text.

2.83.11 Knapp, B.G. (1985) *Basic statistics for nurses.* 2nd edition New York: Wiley ISBN 0471875635 References

Book is intended for undergraduate nursing students as an introductory statistics text. The emphasis is on teaching students to be consumers of research and not statisticians. Each chapter includes an overview, detailed objectives, worked examples and solutions taken from many nursing settings, student exercises and a summary. A new chapter in this edition enables students to select the most appropriate statistical test in relation to the research question being asked (CR 2.87).

2.83.12 Moore, D.S. (1988) *Statistics, concepts and controversies.* 2nd edition New York: W.H. Freeman ISBN 0716717174

Presents statistical ideas to non-mathematical readers by teaching verbally rather than symbolically. Their relevance in public policy and human science is explored and many exercises are included.

2.83.13 Moroney, M.J. (1953) *Facts from figures.* Harmondsworth, Middlesex: Penguin ISBN 0140202366 References

Provides a 'tool-kit' of essential statistical techniques. Limitations and dangers of misuse are discussed and examples given.

2.83.14 Phillips, D.S. (1978) *Basic statistics for health science students.* San Francisco: Freeman ISBN 0716700506 References

Intended for use as a course textbook or quick reference book for students who have previously taken a course in statistics. Examples are taken from the health sciences field and some exercises are included. Appendices contain statistical tables.

2.83.15 Phillips, J.L. Jr. (1982) *How to think about statistics.* New York: Freeman ISBN 0716719231 References

Book is intended for those without prior statistical knowledge and may be suitable for use in courses with broad content domains. It may also be useful as a self-teaching tool for a course which focuses on statistics. It emphasises the logical structure of statistical thinking and de-emphasises techniques of data manipulation. Fundamental concepts are introduced using concrete examples. Sample applications and their solutions are included.

2.83.16 Reichmann, W.J. (1975) *Use and abuse of statistics.* London: Chapman & Hall ISBN 0412119803

Designed for the general reader and students to show the purposes for which statistics may be usefully employed and how they should not be used. It includes discussion on the application of mathematics and the position of the science and art of statistics and its relation to other branches of knowledge.

2.83.17 Rowntree, D. (1981) *Statistics without tears: a primer for non-mathematicians.* Harmondsworth, Middlesex: Penguin ISBN 0140223266 References

Intended for the non-mathematical reader and is a 'tutorial' in print. The basic concepts of statistics are illustrated by means of words and diagrams rather than by figures, formulae and equations. Questions are included at frequent intervals so the student can test understanding of the concepts.

2.83.18 Swinscow, T.D.V. (1983) *Statistics at square one.* 8th edition London: British Medical Association ISBN 0727901753 References

Compilation of revised and extended articles originally published in the British Medical Journal. The main statistical tests in common use are described with illustrations taken from clinical medicine.

2.83.19 Tashman, L.J. & Lamborn, K.R. (1979) *The ways and means of statistics.* New York: Harcourt Brace Jovanovich ISBN 0155951327 (No references)

'This book has been written in English and not in algebra'. A non-mathematical presentation which concentrates on developing understanding of statistical techniques. Illustrative examples are included throughout the text and the strengths and limitations of procedures are highlighted.

2.83.20 Volicer, B.J. (1984) *Multivariate statistics for nursing research.* Orlando: Grune & Stratton ISBN 0808916394 References

Text is orientated towards the non-mathematically minded reader and assumes no mathematical training beyond algebra. Its aim is to explain the meaning of advanced statistical techniques now widely used in health research, so that conclusions can be reached and judgements made, as to whether the appropriate methods have been used in any particular study.

2.83.21 Woodward, M. & Francis, L.M.A. (1988) *Statistics for health management and research.* London: Edward Arnold ISBN 034042009X References

Provides an introduction to the statistical methods most commonly used in health management and research. Only a basic mathematical knowledge is assumed, the concepts are introduced by example and worked through step by step. Formulae are clearly explained in terms of underlying assumptions and practical application. A comprehensive collection of exercises and solutions is provided.

2.83.22 Wright, R.L.D. (1976) *Understanding statistics: an informal introduction for the behavioural sciences.* New York: Harcourt Brace Jovanovich ISBN 0155928775

An introduction to statistics which uses words and visual imagery rather than mathematics to explain important basic concepts. Frequent examples are given throughout the text together with self-tests and end of chapter problems. Additional problems are given in a study guide accompanying the text (CR 2.83.9).

Nursing research abstracts

Bayliss D.	84/264
Munro B.H., Visintainer M.A. & Page B.B.	87/002

2.84 THE LANGUAGE OF STATISTICS

Statistics, like research, has a language of its own. As mentioned in section 2.2, the language of research, several research texts include both research and statistical terms in their glossaries so please also refer to this part of the book.

Annotation
2.84.1 Porkes, R. (1988) *Dictionary of statistics.* London: Collins ISBN 0004343549

Book is intended for the student and informed layman and is encyclopaedic in nature with 426 entries. The text contains definitions, with graphs, diagrams and worked examples of more advanced topics. Appendices include lists of symbols, formulae and statistical tables.

Suggested textbook readings

	Pages	Cross reference
Jaeger	329-339	2.83.8
Riegelman	255-264	2.87.1

2.85 DESCRIPTIVE STATISTICS

The aim of descriptive statistics is to summarise in precise, standard ways, the characteristics and measurements of a sample. They include measures of central tendency, dispersion and correlation co-efficients.

Definition
Statistics that summarise data generated from empirical observations and measurements by identifying frequencies, central tendencies and dispersion of scores

Suggested textbook readings*

	Pages	Cross reference
Bello A. IN LoBiondo-Wood & Haber	291-308	2.1.38
Jaeger	11-84	2.83.8
Kovacs	153-216	2.1.31
Lewis R.W. (DE 304) 2B	3-84	2.1.47
Polgar & Thomas	131-195	2.1.55
Polit & Hungler (1987)	370-393	2.1.56
Seaman	343-350	2.1.62
Sweeney & Olivieri	229-278	2.1.63
Williamson	233-250	2.1.67
Wilson H.S. (1989)	511-528	2.1.69
Woods & Catanzaro	385-395	2.1.72

* Note: Except for Jaeger (CR 2.83.8) only research texts are listed here, as most statistical books cover both descriptive and inferential statistics.

2.86 INFERENTIAL STATISTICS

In many instances in research there is a need to do more than just describe data, and inferential statistics provide a means for drawing conclusions about a sample drawn from the population. Researchers are then able to make judgements about, or generalise to, a large class of individuals based on the information gained from a limited number.

Definition
Statistics used for hypothesis testing and prediction

Suggested textbook readings*

	Pages	Cross reference
Grey M. IN LoBiondo-Wood & Haber	311-327	2.1.38
Jaeger	85-326	2.83.8
Nieswiadomy	309-332	2.1.43
Polgar & Thomas	199-241	2.1.55
Polit & Hungler (1987)	394-421	2.1.56
Seaman	361-380	2.1.62
Williamson	251-267	2.1.67
Wilson H.S. (1989)	528-549	2.1.69
Woods & Catanzaro	396-419	2.1.72

Nursing research abstracts
Weissfield L.A. & Butler P.M.   88/102

* Note: Except for Jaeger (CR 2.83.8) only research texts are listed here, as most statistical books cover both descriptive and inferential statistics.

2.87   CHOOSING A STATISTICAL TEST

Many of the research textbooks listed in 2.1 of this book include sections on descriptive and/or inferential statistics, but few actually give direct guidance on how to select an appropriate test. Because of the increasingly easy access to computer packages, students need more advice about which test to use, rather than how to undertake the calculations. Several texts included in section 2.83 also give some guidance: 2.83.2, 2.83.8, 2.83.12.

Annotations
2.87.1   Knapp, B.G. (1985) Selection of an appropriate statistical test. IN Author *Basic statistics for nurses.* 2nd edition New York: Wiley   ISBN 0471875635
References   Chapter 7   128-149

Chapter gives advice on choosing suitable statistical tests. Several examples with their solutions are provided, together with a flow chart (CR 2.83.11).

2.87.2   Riegelman, R.K. (1981) *Studying a study and testing a test: how to read the medical literature.* Boston: Little, Brown and Company   ISBN 0316745189
References   Part 4 Selecting a statistic 203-253

A framework for selecting a statistic is suggested and three questions are used to provide this.

1. What question is being asked by the statistical test being used?
2. Is the method appropriate to the type of data being collected?
3. Are the conclusions drawn from the statistical procedure appropriate?

A summary is included in the form of flow charts (CR 2.90.1).

Suggested textbook readings

	Pages	Cross reference
Brink & Wood	214-221	2.1.7
Polgar & Thomas	242-256	2.1.55

2.88   USING COMPUTERS TO ANALYSE DATA

With the advent of high powered computers, researchers are now able to handle much greater quantities of data, and this is of particular value in its analysis. Computers are fast, accurate and flexible and therefore are able to save much time.

Annotations

2.88.1 Boyle, C. (1986) *Mastering statistics with your computer.* Basingstoke: Macmillan Education ISBN 0333391721 References

A complete self-contained course on exploring and mastering statistics on a microcomputer. May be used by an individual or for a class and is intended for students undertaking Higher National Diploma courses or first degrees containing an element of statistics.

2.88.2 Cox, H.C., Harsanyi, B. & Dean, L.C. (1987) *Computers and nursing: application to practice, education and research.* Norwalk, Connecticut: Appleton & Lange ISBN 0838512240 References Section 2 The applications of computers 5 Computers and nursing research 61-92

Chapter focuses on the use of computers in nursing research by working through the research process and discussing application at each stage.

2.88.3 Dale, A., Arber, S. & Procter, M. (1988) Elements of computer technology. IN Authors *Doing secondary analysis.* London: Unwin Hyman ISBN 0043120423 References Chapter 6 98-133

A practical guide to choosing hardware and software for analysing secondary data. Chapter 7 outlines some of the major packages available for data analysis: MINITAB, p-STAT, SAS, SIR, SPSS*. Appendix to chapter gives software sources and documentation (CR 2.94.1).

* Please see Appendix B for sources of the above packages.

2.88.4 Francis, I. (1981) *Statistical software: a comparative review.* New York: North Holland ISBN 0444006583 References

Book presents a taxonomy of statistical software with broad comparisons being made rather than in-depth evaluations. Packages are grouped under the following programme headings: data management, editing, tabulation, survey variance estimation, survey analysis, general statistics, specific purpose interactive batch, multiway contingency table analysis, econometric and time series and mathematical sub-routine libraries. Each package is introduced and its capabilities listed. Its extensibility, proposed improvements, sample job, developers name and address, computer makes, interfaced language, source language, cost and documentation are all identified.

2.88.5 Hannah, K.J. (1987) Uses for computers in nursing research. *Recent advances in nursing* 17: 186-202 8 References

Discusses the basic structure and function of computers, together with their uses during particular stages in the research process. Chapter contains a table listing many of the literature data bases of interest to nurse researchers (CR 1.10.22).

2.88.6 Hedderson, J. (1987) *SPSS X made simple*. Belmont, California: Wadsworth ISBN 0534074588 (No references)

A concise handbook leading the reader through the major concepts, routines and functions of SPSS X. It is mainly intended for students with little background in statistics or programming. A single topic, the correlates of happiness, is used to illustrate the procedures and an easily conducted research project is incorporated into the text.

2.88.7 Heffernan, H.G. (ed) (1981) *Proceedings of the 5th annual symposium on the computer applications in medical care*. November 1st-4th Washington DC, New York: Institute of Electrical and Electronics Engineers Inc. IEEE Cat No 81 CH 1696-4 (No ISBN number found)

Section XII of this compilation covers nursing applications of computers and papers are included on nursing administration, research, practice and education (CR 3.26).

2.88.8 Hull, C.H. & Nie, N.H. (1981a) *SPSS pocket guide: release 9*. Chicago: McGraw Hill ISBN 0070465436

Provides a reference to the SPSS Batch system, Release system for readers who are familiar with this, the SPSS 2nd edition and SPSS Update 7-9. The guide is in two sections − one on procedure and the other on non-procedure commands.

2.88.9 Hull, C.H. & Nie, N.H. (1981b) *SPSS update 7-9: new procedures and facilities for releases 7-9*. New York: McGraw Hill ISBN 0070465428 References

10 new facilities are included in this update and there are several major revisions.

2.88.10 Klecka, W.R., Nie, N.H. & Hull, C.H. (1975) *SPSS primer: SP for the SS primer*. New York: McGraw Hill ISBN 007035023X

Book introduces the major features of SPSS in a simple, non-technical way. It may be used by students or more experienced researchers as a self study guide.

2.88.11 McCormick, K.A. (1981) Nursing research using computerised data bases. IN Heffernan, H.G. (ed) *Proceedings of the 5th Annual Symposium on Computer Applications in Medical Care*. November 1st-4th Washington, DC: New York Institute of Electrical and Electronic Engineers Inc. IEEE Cat No 81 CH 1696-4 (No ISBN number found)

Paper describes a taxonomy of research data available on hospital information systems that may be used for clinical nursing research (CR 2.88.7).

2.88.12 Morse, J.M. & Morse, R.M. (1989) QUAL: a mainframe program for qualitative data analysis. *Nursing research* 38(3) 188-189 2 References

Describes a computer programme which aimed to overcome the limitations of microcomputer packages when handling large data sets. Limitations of this programme are discussed.

2.88.13 Ryan, B.F., Joiner, B.L. & Ryan, T.A. Jr. (1985) *MINITAB handbook.* 2nd edition Boston: Duxbury Press ISBN 0871504707 References

Book is designed to be used with MINITAB, a general purpose statistical system. It emphasises aspects of statistics particularly suitable for computer use, and includes many examples and exercises which show step by step how to use the computer to explore data.

2.88.14 Saba, V.K. & McCormick, K.A. (1986) *Essentials of computers for nurses.* Philadelphia: Lippincott ISBN 039754457X References Chapter 14 Research applications 330-361

Six major uses of computers in nursing research are discussed: Information retrieval, data processing, statistical analysis, graphic displays, database management systems and text editing. Examples of computer usage in clinical nursing research are given, the issues which need to be considered and suggestions made for hands-on experiences. Objectives and study questions are included.

Book contains a glossary of computer terms, pages 409-415.

2.88.15 SPSS Inc. (1988) *SPSS X users guide.* 3rd edition Chicago: SPSS Inc. ISBN 0918469511

Provides detailed guidance on all aspects of this comprehensive, integrated system for managing, analysing and displaying data.

Suggested textbook readings

	Pages	Cross reference
Abdellah & Levine	245-248	2.1.1
Burns & Grove	409-432	2.1.12
Kovacs	217-249	2.1.31
Kovner C.T. IN LoBiondo-Wood & Haber	329-343	2.1.38
Polit & Hungler (1987)	454-480	2.1.56
Roberts & Burke	304-325	2.1.59
Seaman	381-391	2.1.62
Sweeney & Olivieri	297-388	2.1.63
Thomas	148-150	2.1.64
Wilson H.S. (1989)	584-615	2.1.69
Woods & Catanzaro	364-370	2.1.72

Nursing research abstracts

Abraham I.L., Nadzam D.M. & Fitzpatrick J.J.	90/004
Abraham I.L. & Schultz S.	86/456
Reed V.	86/454
Schultz S. & Abraham I.L.	87/004

2.89 ANALYSING QUALITATIVE DATA

Qualitative data are frequently expressed in words and the researcher must organise this material into groups and patterns in order to understand its meaning. Some qualitative data will also lend itself to description through the use of measures of central tendency, dispersion and correlation coefficients.

Definition

The non-numerical organisation and interpretation of observations for the purpose of discovering important underlying dimensions and patterns of relationships

Annotations

2.89.1 Ammon-Gaberson, K.B. & Piantanida, M. (1988) Generating results from qualitative data. *Image: the journal of nursing scholarship* 20(3) 159-161   4 References

Discusses the pitfalls commonly encountered by novice researchers and suggests strategies for avoiding or overcoming these difficulties. The importance of developing a line of reasoning to derive meaning from the data is stressed.

2.89.2 Bigbee, J.L. (1986) Beyond chi-square: log-linear analysis and related methods of qualitative analysis. *Advances in nursing science* 8(3) 70-79   12 References

Discusses the use of advanced statistical techniques – multivariate analysis as a means of analysing qualitative data. Steps are illustrated from a study of professional attitudes relating to practitioner prescribing.

2.89.3 Fielding, N.G. & Fielding, J.L. (1986) *Linking data.* Beverly Hills: Sage   ISBN 0803925182   References

Book concentrates on techniques for linking and analysing data obtained from both qualitative and quantitative research methods (CR 2.90).

2.89.4 Miles, M.B. (1983) Qualitative data as an attractive nuisance. IN Van Maanen, J. (ed) *Qualitative methodology.* Newbury Park: Sage   ISBN 0803921179 References 117-134

Addresses the issues and problems in analysing qualitative data through a review of experience in a 4 year study which investigated the process of developing new organisations in public schools (CR 2.36.15).

2.89.5 Miles, M.B. & Huberman, A.M. (1984) *Qualitative data analysis: a sourcebook of new methods.* Beverly Hills: Sage   ISBN 0803922744   References

A practical sourcebook for all researchers who make use of qualitative data. Strong emphasis is put on new types of data displays and each of 49 specific methods is described and illustrated with practical suggestions for their use. The authors' views of qualitative analysis are data reduction, data display, conclusion drawing and verification. They urge development and documentation of what is actually going on when data is analysed so that methods more generally replicable can be generated.

2.89.6 Riley, J. (1991) *Getting the most from your data.* Bristol: Technical and Educational Services   ISBN 0947885307

A practical text covering many ideas for the analysis of qualitative data.

2.89.7 Strauss, A.L. (1987) *Qualitative analysis for social scientists.* Cambridge: Cambridge University Press   ISBN 0521338069   References

A practical text written for all researchers in the social sciences and in such fields as education and nursing. It is designed to assist the teaching of qualitative analysis in a structured way with special emphasis on developing theory through such analysis. Tools for carrying out analyses are included and many examples are drawn from the author's varied research activities. Chapter 13 contains questions and answers commonly asked by students (pages 265-286). An overview is given of the main elements of grounded theory analysis (CR 2.46).

2.89.8 Youngman, M.B. (1979) *Analysing social and educational research data.* London: McGraw Hill   ISBN 007084089X   References

A reference book and manual for research students, designed to help those with little mathematical background understand the application of statistics to sociological data. The methods of choice of statistics, their assumptions and interpretation are discussed, and the authors own statistics package − Programmed methods for multivariate data (PMMD) is used to illustrate the processes.

Suggested textbook readings

	Pages	Cross reference
Brink & Wood	200-211	2.1.7
Bulmer (1984)	241-262	2.1.8
Burgess (1982)	177-184	2.1.9
Burns & Grove	544-566	2.1.12
Chenitz & Swanson	91-101	2.46.2
Fox	391-412	2.1.25
Holm & Llewellyn	157-197	2.1.26
Knafl K.A. & Howard B.J. IN Munhall & Oiler	265-278	2.1.42
Notter & Hott	107-124	2.1.44
Polgar & Thomas	131-195	2.1.55
Polit & Hungler (1987)	349-369	2.1.56

	Pages	Cross reference
Schroeder M.A. IN Phillips L.R.F. (critique)	249-262	2.98.11
Stern P. IN Morse (1989)	135-148	2.36.8
Thomas	127-151	2.1.64
Wilson H.S. (1989)	452-499	2.1.69
Woods & Catanzaro	437-456	2.1.72

2.90 ANALYSING QUANTITATIVE DATA

Statistical tests enable quantitative data to be made meaningful and intelligible. Having chosen the appropriate test and carried it out the researcher is then in a position to reduce, organise, evaluate, interpret and communicate the results. Descriptive and/or inferential statistics will be utilised depending on the problem and data obtained.

Definition

The manipulation of numerical data through statistical procedures for the purpose of describing phenomena or assessing the magnitude and reliability of relationships among them

Annotations

2.90.1   Riegelman, R.K. (1981) *Studying a study and testing a test: how to read the medical literature.* Boston: Little, Brown & Co.   ISBN 0316745189   References

Book provides a step by step approach to a clinical review of the medical literature and no prior knowledge of mathematics and statistics is assumed. The four parts explain how to evaluate the studies, tests, rates and statistics cited in journal articles.

2.90.2   Tufte, E.R. (ed) (1970) *The quantitative analysis of social problems.* Reading, Massachusetts: Addison-Wesley   ISBN 0201076101   References

A compilation of papers which includes many major quantitative studies of social problems and covers many aspects of quantitative analysis. Papers are grouped under five headings: statistical evidence and criticism, experimental and quasi-experimental studies, economic and aggregate analysis, survey data, data analysis and research design (CR 2.29, 2.35).

Suggested textbook readings

	Pages	Cross reference
Abdellah & Levine	261-278	2.1.1
Adams & Schvaneveldt	331-377	2.1.2
Brink & Wood	211-221	2.1.7
Burns & Grove	457-554	2.1.12

	Pages	*Cross reference*
Castles	110-125	2.1.15
Fox	291-390	2.1.25
Holm & Llewellyn	157-197	2.1.26
Miller D.C.	143-205	2.56.3
Polgar & Thomas	199-241	2.1.55
Schroeder M.A. IN Phillips L.R.F. (critique)	249-262	2.98.11
Thomas	152-244	2.1.64
Waltz & Bausell	101-116	2.21.4
Wilson H.S. (1989)	500-583	2.1.69

2.91 ANALYSIS OF DATA
Content analysis

Recorded words and sentences provide rich and varied sources of data about people and the contexts in which they live. In order to use these data objective and systematic procedures need to be employed to render them valid and reliable (Waltz, Strickland & Lenz 1984).

Content analysis involves creating a set of categories or statistically manipulable symbols that represent the presence, frequency, intensity or nature of selected characteristics (Markoff, Shapiro & Weitman 1977).

Definition
A technique for the objective, systematic and quantitative description of communication and documentary evidence

---

Example
Goddard, A. & Bowling, A. (1987) An international comparison of health education literature on breast disorders. *Health education journal* 46(3) 91-93   6 References

Content analysis was used to compare literature on breast disease and screening from six countries.

Annotations
2.91.1 Akinsanya, J. (1988) Complementary approaches. *Senior nurse* 8(5) 20-22   7 References

The use of content analysis as a means of bridging the gap between qualitative and quantitative approaches to research is discussed. The links are illustrated using a hypothetical study designed to identify the problems faced by the elderly in the community (CR 2.9).

2.91.2 Holsti, O.R. (1969) *Content analysis for social sciences and humanities.* Reading: Massachusetts Addison-Wesley   ISBN 0201029405   References

An introduction and guide to content analysis as an approach to documentary research for beginners as well as the more experienced. It integrates a model of the communication process, research designs and the techniques of content analysis. There is also an extensive discussion on the role of computers (CR 2.88).

2.91.3 Krippendorf, K. (1980) *Content analysis: an introduction to its methodology.* Beverly Hills: Sage   ISBN 0803914970   References

Intended for a fairly wide audience and can serve as a text and practical guide to content analysis in research contexts. An overview of the technique is given together with a comprehensive discussion of the key elements which need to be considered when it is used. Chapters on computer based content analysis techniques, reliability and validity are included (CR 2.24, 2.25, 2.88).

2.91.4   Rosengren, K.E. (ed) (1981) *Advances in content analysis.* Beverly Hills: Sage   ISBN 080391556X   References

Volume is one of the outcomes of the first Scandinavian conference on content analysis held in Sweden in 1979. Analytical perspectives are explored together with reports of various empirical studies in the field of communication.

Suggested textbook readings

	Pages	Cross reference
Adams & Schvaneveldt	305-308	2.1.2
Brink & Wood	203-205	2.1.7
Cohen & Manion	61-65	2.1.19
Fox	391-412	2.1.25
Kidder & Judd	306-309	2.1.30
Lin	217-219	2.1.37
Polit & Hungler (1987)	362-365	2.1.56
Seaman	81-82/334-339	2.1.62
Treece & Treece	348-350	2.1.65
Waltz, Strickland & Lenz	255-262	2.56.5
Wilson H.S. (1989)	469-476	2.1.69
Wiseman & Aron	113-125	2.66.1
Woods & Catanzaro	437-439	2.1.72

2.92   ANALYSIS OF DATA
Contextual analysis

Contextual analysis assumes that objects, and most obviously words, have more in common, the more the context they are in is alike. Context means the linguistic environment of words or within data surroundings of a recording unit (Krippendorf 1980). Both qualitative and quantitative analytical techniques may be used for these data.

Definition
Analysis which focuses on the individual's behaviour or attitudes, with reference to a group context

Example
Holzemer, W.L. & Chambers, D.B. (1988) A contextual analysis of faculty productivity. *Journal of nursing education* 27(1) 10-18   22 References

Study examined the contextual effects of the educational environment on faculty productivity of academic research. 25 doctoral nursing programmes were studied and the characteristics of the most productive are identified.

Annotations
2.92.1   Atkinson, J.M. & Heritage, J. (eds) (1984) *Structures of social action: studies in conversation analysis.* Cambridge: Cambridge University Press   ISBN 0521318629   References

Book reflects recent developments and current issues in the field of conversation analysis. The theoretical and methodological foundations are given together with preference and topic organisation. The integration of talk with non-vocal activities, aspects of response and everyday activities as social phenomena are also discussed (CR 2.80).

2.92.2 Boyd, L.H. Jr. & Iverson, G.R. (1979) *Contextual analysis: concepts and statistical techniques.* Belmont, California: Wadsworth ISBN 0534006930 References

Examines social contexts through multi-level analysis of individual and grouped variables and their statistical interactions. A working knowledge of multiple regression analysis is required. Statistical Package for the Social Sciences (SPSS) is used to illustrate the procedures. Issues surrounding contextual analysis are discussed in the final chapter (CR 2.80).

2.92.3   Hunt, M. & Robinson, K.M. (1987) Analysis of conversational interactions. *Recent advances in nursing* 17: 150-168   19 References

Describes ways in which talk can be interpreted using a technique called conversation analysis. Examples of talk from a health visitor and a sister from a symptom control team are discussed (CR 2.80).

2.92.4   Lindkvist, K. (1981) Approaches to textual analysis. IN Rosengren, K.E. (ed) *Advances in content analysis.* Beverly Hills: Sage ISBN 080391556X References   Chapter 1 23-41

Chapter compares different approaches with textual analysis − content analysis, analytical semantics, structuralism and hermeneutics. Non-textual ideas of interpretation and analysis are briefly discussed together with the possibility of synthesis between the approaches (CR 2.91.4).

2.92.5   Roger, D. & Bull, P. (1989) *Conversation: an interdisciplinary perspective.* Cleveland, Philadelphia: Multilingual Matters Ltd   ISBN 0905028864   References

Book covers concepts of interpersonal communication, methods of observation, transcription procedures, data analysis and research applications (CR 2.80).

Suggested textbook readings

	Pages	*Cross reference*
Benson & Hughes	154-191	2.43.3
Cohen & Manion	253-268	2.1.19
Krippendorf	109-118/169-180	2.91.3
Silverman D. (1987)	148-154	2.16.13

2.93   LEVELS OF DATA ANALYSIS
Primary

There are three levels of data analysis – primary, secondary and meta-analysis. Primary analysis in the health field usually involves examining archives such as personal or public health records.

Definition
The initial analysis of data, whether those data were collated originally for a research purpose or for other purposes

---

Example
Benoliel, J. (1978) *A care-cure problem: dying in teaching hospitals.* Final Report to the Division of Nursing, Bureau of Health Manpower, Health Resources Administration, Department of Health, Education and Welfare (unpublished manuscript).

'Author interested in the treatment trajectories of dying patients, studied data abstracted from their hospital records, to discover the types of medical and nursing treatments that were given to patients whose diagnosis indicated they were dying. The data in the medical records were recorded for clinical purposes yet Benoliel abstracted and analysed them to achieve her own research purposes' (Woods & Catanzaro 1988).

Suggested textbook reading

	Pages	*Cross reference*
Woods & Catanzaro	334-347	2.1.72

2.94   LEVELS OF DATA ANALYSIS
Secondary

The next level of data analysis is called secondary analysis. The data used for this may be raw data, statistical databases or archival material.

Definition
Any further analysis of an existing data set which presents interpretations, conclusions or knowledge additional to or different from those presented in the first report on the inquiry as a whole and its main results

---

Example
Munro, B.H. (1983) Job satisfaction among recent graduates of schools of nursing. *Nursing research* 32(6) 350-361   32 References

Study investigated the factors contributing to the job satisfaction of recently qualified graduate nurses. Level of responsibility and working conditions were found to be the major predictors.

Annotations
2.94.1   Dale, A., Arber, S. & Procter, M. (1988) *Doing secondary analysis.* London: Unwin Hyman   ISBN 0043120423   References

A detailed guide to all stages of secondary analysis. It includes a description of the hardware and software now available.

2.94.2   Hakim, C. (1982) *Secondary analysis in social research: a guide to data sources and methods with examples.* London: Allen & Unwin   ISBN 0043120164   References

Provides a guide to the secondary analysis of quantitative social data sets available in archives, and to the social data and statistics in published reports, on microfilm or as computer printouts. The practical and methodological problems and solutions developed by analysts are discussed, together with the range of secondary research currently being carried out. The two main data sets used are those carried out by the Office of Population Censuses and Surveys and the Social Science Research Council Archive.

2.94.3   McArt, E.W. & McDougal, L.W. (1985) Secondary data analysis: a new approach to nursing research. *Image: the journal of nursing scholarship* 17(2) 54-57   11 References

Defines secondary data analysis, discusses ways of conducting analyses and outlines its advantages and disadvantages. Data management issues and obtaining permission to use sources are discussed.

2.94.4 Stewart, D.W. (1984) *Secondary research information: sources and methods.* Beverly Hills: Sage ISBN 0803923392 References

Monograph designed as an introduction to locating, using, evaluating and integrating information which is available from printed materials. Book includes issues in evaluating research, information sources including computer assisted information searches, and integrating data from multiple sources. Exercises are included for each chapter and more relevant topic areas could easily be substituted for any particular discipline.

Suggested textbook readings

	Pages	*Cross reference*
Bulmer M. & Atkinson (DE 304) 2A	41-70	2.1.46
Polit & Hungler (1987)	173-176	2.1.56
Woods & Catanzaro	334-347	2.1.72

2.95 LEVELS OF DATA ANALYSIS
Meta-analysis

The third level of data analysis is meta-analysis which enables the researcher to summarise and integrate findings from several studies. It can be performed using either raw data from original studies or summary measures to generate effect sizes (Woods & Catanzaro 1988).

Definition
The statistical analysis of a large collection of results from individual studies for the purpose of integrating the findings

---

Example
Devine, E. & Cook, T. (1983) A meta-analysis of effects of psycho-educational interventions on length of post-surgical hospital stay. *Nursing research* 32(5) 267-274 72 References

Fourty nine studies of the relationships between brief psycho-educational interventions and the length of post-surgical hospitalisation were reviewed using meta-analysis. A reduction of 1 day was shown which may be cost effective with surgical patients of many kinds, as the length of hospital stay is reduced.

Annotations
2.95.1 Abraham, I.L., Shultz, S.II, Polis, N., Vines, S.W. & Smith, M.C. (1987) Research-on-research: the meta-analysis of nursing and health research. *Recent advances in nursing* 17: 126-147 24 References

Chapter introduces the theoretical and methodological aspects of meta-analysis and discusses its future in nursing.

2.95.2 Curlette, W.L. & Cannella, K.S. (1985) Going beyond the narrative, summarisation of research findings: the meta-analysis approach. *Research in nursing and health* 8(3) 293-301   67 References

There is full discussion of the advantages and disadvantages of meta-analysis over traditional literature review methods. Author also suggests that understanding the method, even if it is not adopted, can help to improve on the usual narrative approach.

2.95.3 Glass, G.V., McGaw, B. & Smith, M.L. (1981) *Meta-analysis in social research.* Beverly Hills: Sage   ISBN 0803916337   References

Book covers the problems of research review and integration. The characteristics of meta-analysis are explored, its development discussed and the processes involved in conducting this type of analysis are fully described.

2.95.4 Hunter, J.E., Schmidt, F.L. & Jackson, G.B. (1982) *Meta-analysis: cumulating research findings across studies.* Beverly Hills: Sage   ISBN 080391864X   References

Book reviews all the methods proposed for cumulating knowledge across studies including the narrative review, counting statistically significant findings, and the averaging of quantitative outcome measures.

2.95.5 Lee, K.A. (1988) Meta-analysis: a third alternative for student research experience. *Nurse educator* 13(4) 30-33   23 References

Discusses how topics may be appropriately identified for this type of procedure. Some examples of meta-analyses relevant to nursing are included and the steps involved are briefly outlined.

2.95.6 Massey, J. & Loomis, M. (1988) When should nurses use research findings? *Applied nursing research* 1(1) 32-40   45 References

Article sets out the use of meta-analysis as a research method. A study is described which aimed to determine if this technique could be used by nursing students to evaluate the readiness of research-based innovations for implementation in clinical practice. Authors concluded that it was useful for this purpose (CR 2.105).

2.95.7 O'Flynn, A.I. (1982) Meta-analysis. *Nursing research* 31(5) 314-316   12 References

A variety of techniques come under the title of meta-analysis and they generate different solutions. The following aspects are considered − the overall significance/probability of pooled data from combined studies being useful, the average effect across studies, and the interactions or relationships between variables. Some recommendations and implications of using this technique are made.

2.95.8 Smith, M.C. & Naftel, D.C. (1984) Meta-analysis: a perspective for research synthesis. *Image: the journal of nursing scholarship* 16(1) 9-13   83 References

A review of the literature on meta-analysis providing an introduction to its methodology together with evaluation of the technique by other authors.

Suggested textbook readings

	Pages	*Cross reference*
Polit & Hungler (1987)	176-178	2.1.56
Smith M.C. IN Sarter	77-91	2.1.61
Woods & Catanzaro	63/335	2.1.72

Nursing research abstracts

Lynn M.R.	90/009

2.96   INTERPRETING THE FINDINGS

The final steps in any research project are to interpret the data, so that it becomes meaningful within the context of this particular piece of research, and will also take its place in the literature. It is probably one of the most difficult parts of the research process and requires many different skills.

Annotations

2.96.1   Anderson, A.J.B. (1989) *Interpreting data: a first course in statistics.* London: Chapman Hall   ISBN 0412295709   References

Designed for students undertaking a statistics module, this book clarifies the basic requirements of data collection, examines the reliability of published data and the validation and analysis of data by computer. Examples are included from a wide range of disciplines and exercises conclude each chapter.

2.96.2   Walsh, M. (1988) Beyond statistical significance. *Applied nursing research* 1(2) 101-103   10 References

Article discusses the question of whether statistical significance is a necessary condition for clinical significance. When caring for people it is not so much the 'average' difference that is of interest, rather the individual's difference.

Suggested textbook readings

	Pages	*Cross reference*
Abdellah & Levine	279-297	2.1.1
Burns & Grove	567-578	2.1.12
Castles	117-125	2.1.15
Grady & Wallston	150-157	3.11.2
Marsh C. (DE 304) 6	41-94	2.1.52
Phillips L.R.F. (critique)	304-342/504	2.98.11
Polgar & Thomas	257-262	2.1.55
Williamson	269-288	2.1.67
Woods & Catanzaro	457-465	2.1.72

2.97 PRESENTING DATA

Once the data has been carefully analysed, the next step is to present it in the most clear way so that others who read it will have no difficulty in its interpretation. Depending on the type of research undertaken data may be presented in the form of tables, graphs, charts, figures, verbatim accounts or other means.

Annotations

2.97.1 Cardamone, T. (1981) *Chart and graph presentation skills.* New York: Van Nostrand Reinhold   ISBN 0442262868

Gives detailed guidance on how to design and use all types of graphs and charts.

2.97.2 Chapman, M. (1986) *Plain figures.* London: HMSO   ISBN 0114300011 References

Demonstrates and discusses ways of presenting numbers effectively so that their value can be realised. It also aims to help the reader interpret data more competently and confidently. No statistical tests are discussed and book concentrates on bringing together advice and research findings on statistical presentation.

2.97.3 Office of Health Economics (1987) *Compendium of health statistics.* 6th edition London: Office of Health Economics   (No ISBN number)

Provides a comprehensive statistical analysis of the functioning of the National Health Service in the UK. Book shows examples of different types of data presentation.

2.97.4 Open University (1985) Dealing with data. IN Author, *Studying health and disease.* (U 205) Milton Keynes: Open University Press   ISBN 0335150500 Chapter 4 21-34

Chapter is devoted to the interpretation and significance of data. Different visual means of presenting data are shown and explained using everyday examples. Activities are included for the reader to work through in order to assess their understanding. Commonly used terms are explained (CR 2.96).

2.97.5 Sprent, P. (1988) *Understanding data.* Harmondsworth, Middlesex: Penguin   ISBN 0140772065   References

A practical text which aims to develop skills in selection and presentation of numerical data. Data is discussed and presented in a number of different contexts and exercises to consolidate learning are interspersed throughout the text.

Suggested textbook readings

	Pages	*Cross reference*
Abdellah & Levine	245-260	2.1.1
Cormack	155-167	2.1.20
Nieswiadomy	335-347	2.1.43

	Pages	Cross reference
Polgar & Thomas	131-149	2.1.55
Sweeney & Olivieri	279-296	2.1.63
Wilson H.S. (1989)	512-515	2.1.69

Nursing research abstracts

Altman D.G. et al	84/1
Rehahn M.	81/285

2.98 EVALUATING RESEARCH FINDINGS

A research critique is an objective, systematic attempt to identify, appreciate and weigh the merits and demerits of, a particular piece of scientific research (Phillips L.R.F. 1986). There are many reasons for evaluating other's research and all nurses need to develop the necessary skills in order to enhance their practice.

Definition
A creative, constructive and positive process conducted for the purpose of identifying the strategies and limitations of a research project

Example
Ryden, M.B. (1985) Environmental support for autonomy in the institutionalised elderly. IN Castles, M.R. *Primer of nursing research.* Philadelphia: Saunders   ISBN 0721617131   Appendix – Critical Review Demonstrated 162-181

Article reviewed was published in Research in Nursing and Health 8: 363-371, and each stage of the research is analysed in detail and commented upon (CR 2.1.15).

Major text
Phillips, L.R.F. (1986) *A clinicians guide to the critique and utilisation of nursing research.* Norwalk, Connecticut: Appleton-Century-Crofts   ISBN 0838511627 References (CR 2.98.11)

Annotations
2.98.1   Alguire, P.C., Massa, M.D., Leinhart, K.W. & Henry, R.C. (1988) A packaged workshop for teaching critical reading of the medical literature. *Medical teacher* 10(1) 85-90   12 References

Describes the purpose, goals and format of a series of seminars whose aim was to teach students how to critically analyse the medical literature.

2.98.2   Barnard, K.E. (1985) *MCN keys to research.* New York: American Journal of Nursing Company   (No ISBN number)

A selection of articles from a column in the American Journal of Maternal/Child Nursing on aspects of research methodology. These were written particularly with practitioners in mind, together with those who will be generating small practice studies.

2.98.3 Chapman, C. (1984) Evaluating published research. IN Cormack, D.F.S. (ed) *The research process in nursing.* Oxford: Blackwell Scientific ISBN 0632010134 References 20: 207-214

Outlines the characteristics of a good critique and discusses points to be considered when reading research reports (CR 2.1.20).

2.98.4 Clark, E. (1991) *Evaluating research.* Research Awareness, Module 10, London: Distance Learning Centre, South Bank Polytechnic ISBN 0948250496

This is number 10 in a series of 13 modules, each of which deals with a different aspect of nursing research. It was developed to assist nurses, midwives and health visitors in understanding research in terms of their own professional practice. Modules can be used separately or as part of a programme. The reader is encouraged to work through a number of activities, self-assessment questions and answers and progress summaries. Some articles/book extracts referred to in the text are reproduced in full.

This module examines the skills necessary for critical evaluation of reported research. A step by step guide to the process is included (CR Appendix D).

2.98.5 Hawthorn, P.J. (1983) Principles of research: a checklist. *Nursing times* 79(23) August 31 41-43 12 item bibliography Occasional Paper

A checklist is presented which contains basic information about the research process. This can be used by those with little or no research experience to evaluate a research report or to assist those undertaking a small research project.

2.98.6 Heaney, R.P. & Barger-Lux, M.J. (1986) Priming students to read research critically. *Nursing and health care* 17(8) 421-424 4 References

Describes a course designed to equip nurses with skills for interpreting and reacting to research literature and for interacting with research intelligently and ethically. A series of goals was developed, which also proved suitable for students of other health disciplines, and enabled critical evaluation of qualitative research literature. Practical exercises facilitated students ability to understand and critique a research report.

2.98.7 Hutchings, M. (1981) A critique of Bendall's 'So you passed nurse'. *Journal of advanced nursing* 6(5) 405-408 1 Reference

It is suggested that Bendall's widely acclaimed book is seriously flawed by inappropriate statistical analysis, incomprehension of statistical principles, and failure to obtain information because of fragmentation of the evidence. Author believes that statistical standards must improve if nursing research is to have any credence.

2.98.8 Katzer, J., Cook, K.H. & Crouch, W.W. (1982) *Evaluating information: a guide for users of social science research.* 2nd edition Reading, Massachusetts: Addison-Wesley ISBN 0201047594 References

Only a small percentage of people will ever actually conduct research studies but they do need to be able to read critically research papers in their own field. This book is written from the consumer's point of view and focuses on the broad concerns common to all types of social science research. Thematic in approach, each chapter asks questions which form a step by step guide for evaluation of research reports. These are combined at the end of the book and used to analyse a published report.

Contains an extensive glossary of over 400 terms.

2.98.9   Light, R.J. & Pillemer, D.B. (1984) *Summing up the science of reviewing research.* Cambridge, Massachusetts: Harvard University Press   ISBN 0674854314 References

Discusses the art of combining information from several studies in a practical way. General guidelines and step by step procedures are included and examples given from several disciplines. A checklist for evaluating reviews is given. The book is written in non-technical language and is likely to become a methodological classic.

2.98.10   Ogier, M. (1989) *Reading research: or how to make research more approachable.* Harrow, Middlesex: Scutari   ISBN 1871364027   References

A small booklet which gives a brief, introductory step by step guide to reading research. It concentrates on examining quantitative research.

2.98.11   Phillips, L.R.F. (1986) *A clinicians guide to the critique and utilisation of nursing research.* Norwalk, Connecticut: Appleton-Century-Crofts   ISBN 0838511627   References

Book is designed to complement existing texts and aims to provide the information needed to conduct an objective research critique and to use this to make decisions about research utilisation. The three major units in the text focus on the current research-practice gap in nursing; development of critiquing skills and the utilisation of clinical nursing research Each chapter is summarised and includes additional learning activities and a bibliography. Two examples of published research are used to illustrate each aspect of the critiquing process.

2.98.12   Rose, G. (1982) *Deciphering sociological research.* London: Macmillan   ISBN 0333285581   References

This book, which complements existing texts, provides an approach to analysing sociological research. Systematic methods are given for deciphering reports in Part 1, and in Part 2 twelve selected examples, which are edited versions of articles originally published in sociological journals, provide the data for analysis. These illustrate a range of approaches to research and are chosen from three major areas of sociology; deviance, education and stratification. The link between theory and empirical evidence is thoroughly explored in the analyses and the degree of success achieved by the authors in 'translating' these.

2.98.13   Shipman, M. (1988) *The limitations of social research.*   3rd edition London: Longman   ISBN 058229729X   References

Four key questions are used to examine the stages of research and relate to reliability, validity, generalisation and clarity of overall methodology. Each chapter is introduced by a controversy which reflects a crucial issue in assessing research evidence in education. Various research studies are examined and methodological points explored. Readers are urged to read research reports critically and with scepticism as many issues in social research are contentious.

2.98.14 Smith, H.W. (1981) *Strategies of social research: the methodological imagination.* 2nd edition Englewood Cliffs, New Jersey: Prentice Hall ISBN 0138511543 References

Book, which is an Open University reader, comprises four major parts — sociology as a science; the production of data; improving data quality and the analysis and presentation of data. The emphasis is on evaluating research rather than doing it. Each chapter ends with readings for advanced students and suggested research projects. Case histories are used to illustrate ethical and moral problems in social research.

2.98.15 Trussell, P., Brandt, A. & Knapp, S. (1981) *Using nursing research: discovery, analysis and interpretation.* Wakefield, Massachusetts: Nursing Resources ISBN 0913654701 References

This is not a textbook, but is intended for consumers of research to assist in reading, undertaking and evaluating abstracts and research reports in the field of health care.

2.98.16 Ventry, I.M. & Schiavetti, N. (1980) *Evaluating research: speech pathology and audiology.* Reading, Massachusetts: Addison-Wesley ISBN 0201081946 References

Although written for advanced level students in speech pathology and audiology this book may also be useful to nursing students. It is not a 'how to do it' book, but rather shows how to read, understand and evaluate research done by others. Part 1 describes the underlying framework used to generate guidelines for evaluation; Part 2 covers the main sections of a research article and Part 3 contains two annotated articles to lead the reader through the process of evaluation.

2.98.17 Ward, M.J. & Fetler, M.E. (1979) What guidelines to be followed in critically evaluating research reports? *Nursing research* 28(2) 120-126 18 References

Response to a query in a 'question and answer' column about critically evaluating research reports. A checklist is given and each section elaborated upon.

Suggested textbook readings

	Pages	Cross reference
Abdellah & Levine	302-305	2.1.1
Burgess (1982)	209-220	2.1.9
Burns & Grove	609-624	2.1.12
Bynner J. (DE 304) 1	27-76	2.1.45

	Pages	*Cross reference*
Castles	139-181	2.1.15
Chenitz & Swanson	146-154	2.46.2
Duffy M.E. IN Strickland & Waltz	420-437	2.63.16
Fox	110-125	2.1.25
Heermann J.A. & Craft B.J.G. IN LoBiondo-Wood & Haber	381-413	2.1.38
Holm & Llewellyn	19-30	2.1.26
Kovacs	253-257	2.1.31
Meinert	272-277	2.29.11
Notter & Hott	143-149	2.1.44
Phillips L.R.F. (critique)	85-378/428-451	2.98.11
Polgar & Thomas	274-286	2.1.55
Polit & Hungler (1987)	498-506	2.1.56
Roberts & Burke	326-338	2.1.59
Romney D. (DE 304) 5	135-164	2.1.51
Seaman	153-162	2.1.62
Sweeney & Olivieri	50-64/402-430	2.1.63
Thomas	277-285	2.1.64
Treece & Treece	56-64	2.1.65
Walker	177-196	2.1.66
Williamson	289-299	2.1.67
Wilson H.S. (1989)	38-43/164-185	2.1.69
Woods & Catanzaro	469-478	2.1.72

Nursing research abstracts

Downs N.G.	79/200
Johnson M.	86/152
Long A.F.	85/378
Stephenson P.M.	86/009
Walker J.F.	85/010

2.99   RESEARCH PROPOSALS

A research proposal is a written document specifying what the investigator proposes to study. Proposals serve to communicate the research problem, its significance, and planned procedures for solving the problem (Polit & Hungler 1987)

Definition
The written plan and justification for a research project prepared before it begins. It is also used when applying for financial support to do the research

---

Example

Clinton, J. (1985) Couvade: patterns, predictors and nursing management; a research proposal submitted to the Division of Nursing. *Western journal of nursing research* 7(2) 221-248   77 References

Documents a successful grant proposal for a time-series field experiment which aimed to examine the experiences associated with being an expectant father. Details of the reviews and recommendations of the fund granting committee are also included.

Annotations

2.99.1   Davitz, J.R. & Davitz, L.L. (1977) *Evaluating research proposals in the behavioural sciences: a guide.* 2nd edition   New York: Teachers College Press ISBN 0807725447   References

Book designed for students who are planning or critically evaluating research studies. The points to be considered when evaluating research proposals are discussed and a series of questions accompanies each section.

2.99.2   Field, P.A. & Morse, J.M. (1985) The qualitative research proposal. IN Authors, *Nursing research the application of qualitative approaches.* Rockville, Maryland: Aspen   ISBN 0709910460   References   Chapter 3 33-49

Describes problems for the researcher considering qualitative research. The differences between qualitative and quantitative research proposals are described. The process of preparing to do research is discussed in detail and advice given on developing a qualitative research proposal (CR 2.1.24).

2.99.3   Holmes, S.B., Becher, M., Karande, U. & Riley, K. (1989) Research on every rung of the clinical ladder. *American journal of nursing* 89(2) 246,248,250   5 References

Describes the setting up of a nursing research committee whose aims were to review and approve research proposals, recommend changes in practice based on research findings, serve as a resource and co-ordinate research activities (CR 2.104, 2.105, 3.6).

2.99.4   Jacox, A.K. (1980) Nursing's statement: testifying in Washington. IN Davis, A.J. & Krueger, J.C. (eds) *Patients, nurses, ethics.* New York: American Journal of Nursing Company   ISBN 0937126845   References

A testimony presented on 3.5.1977 at a public hearing before the National Commission for the Protection of Human Subjects of Biomedical and Behavioural Research, National Institute of Health, Bethesda, Maryland. Presenter reports on the difficulties encountered in getting research proposals accepted by research committees. Author contends that committees are composed largely of physicians and representatives of the biomedical sciences. This creates a powerful pressure to encourage research designs that are experimental rather than non-experimental. The place and value of nursing research is explored and examples where permission has been refused are used illustrate these points. Physicians in their role as gatekeepers is discussed and the case for nursing representation on committees is outlined (CR 2.17).

2.99.5 Kalish, S.E., McCullum, T., Henry, Y., Schoenthaler, A. & Grady, S. (1984) *The proposal writer's swipe file: 15 winning fund-raising proposals ... prototypes of approaches, styles and structures.* Washington DC: Taft Corporation ISBN 0914756451

Provides a resource book of successful research proposals. Examples, covering a wide range of disciplines, were written by professional proposal writers and give insight into how fund-raising proposals should be constructed, organised, styled and presented.

2.99.6 Locke, L.F., Spirudoso, W.W. & Silverman, S. (1987) *Proposals that work: a guide for planning dissertations and grant proposals.* 2nd edition, Newbury Park: Sage ISBN 0803929862 References

Book comprises two major sections − the first gives practical advice on all aspects of writing research proposals, and the specimens show different designs and paradigms from several areas. These are analysed and points discussed. Appendices contain general standards for judging the acceptability of a thesis or dissertation proposal, an annotated bibliography and a sample form for informed consent.

2.99.7 National Board for Nursing, Midwifery and Health Visiting for Northern Ireland (1989) *Guidelines on writing a research proposal.* Belfast: National Board for Nursing References Occasional Paper OP/NB/1/89

Guidelines developed by the Board's research group which cover the major aspects to be considered when writing research proposals.

2.99.8 Richards, D. (1990) Ten steps to successful grant writing. *Journal of nursing administration* 20(1) 20-23 6 References

A step by step approach to writing a research proposal is given.

2.99.9 Sandelowski, M., Davis, D.H. & Harris, B.G. (1989) Artful design: writing the proposal for research in the naturalist paradigm. *Research in nursing and health* 12(2) 77-84 24 References

Describes the preparation of a research proposal for a five year study, the transition to parenthood of infertile couples. Parts of this are used to illustrate the article.

2.99.10 Sleep, J. (1989) *Writing a research proposal and applying for funding.* London: Royal College of Midwives (No ISBN number) References

Part 1 gives general guidelines on preparing research proposals, and Part 2 contains hints about applying for, and sources of, funding (CR 3.12).

2.99.11 Stewart, R.D. & Stewart, A.L. (1984) *Proposal preparation.* New York: Wiley ISBN 0471872881 References

Although largely aimed at business enterprises this book shows how to present the information required for successful research applications to funding bodies. It also describes how proposals are evaluated which gives clues about preparing a winning proposal.

2.99.12 Tornquist, E.M. & Funk, S.G. (1990) How to write a research grant proposal. *Image: the journal of nursing scholarship* 22(1) 44-51   1 Reference

Provides guidelines for writing all parts of a research proposal.

Suggested textbook readings

	Pages	Cross reference
Abdellah & Levine	343-354	2.1.1
Bond, S. IN Cormack	181-192	2.1.20
Brink & Wood	223-347	2.1.7
Burns & Grove	363-382	2.1.12
Chenitz & Swanson	39-47	2.46.2
Fox	126-133	2.1.25
Kovacs	109-114	2.1.31
Lauffer	230-251	3.12.10
Leedy	103-121/263-290	2.1.35
Munhall P.L. IN Morse (1989)	241-253	2.36.8
Polit & Hungler (1987)	507-523	2.1.56
Seaman	125-140	2.1.62
Tornquist	3-73	2.100.12
Treece & Treece	117-125	2.1.65
Wilson H.S. (1989)	619-654	2.1.69
Woods & Catanzaro	498-529	2.1.72

Nursing research abstracts

Cronenwett L.R.	87/221
Howie J.	79/302

2.100   WRITING RESEARCH REPORTS

Before a piece of research is complete the researcher is under an obligation to write about its results. The report may be written for different audiences, for example a thesis or dissertation, a paper for an employer who financed the project or as a journal article. Although the length may vary considerably, the content is very similar and will normally follow the steps of the research process.

2.100.1 Becker, H.S. (1986) *Writing for social scientists: how to start and finish your thesis, book or article.* Chicago: University of Chicago Press   ISBN 0226041085 References

An unusual book about how to improve writing skills. It focuses on the elusive work habits which contribute to good writing. It includes discussion on how to overcome others criticisms, how to revise again and again and develop the capacity to write clear prose. A chapter is included on the personal and professional risks involved in scholarly writing.

2.100.2   Berry, R. (1986) *How to write a research paper.* 2nd edition Oxford: Pergamon   ISBN 0080326803   References

Designed for students at all levels of higher education this book gives clear guidance on all stages of preparation of an academic paper. An example of a well researched, well written paper is included. A chapter on writing a paper for a learned journal is also included.

2.100.3   Cormack, D.F.S. (1984) *Writing for nursing and allied professions.* Oxford: Blackwell Scientific   ISBN 0632011297   References

Book is intended for those who wish to write for publication and for students who need to develop writing skills for course work and examinations. It includes guidance on all aspects of writing together with practical exercises. The roles of the author and publisher are explained to assist writers when preparing work for publication.

2.100.4   Cormack, D.F.S. (1986) Writing a research article. *Nurse education today* 6(2) 64-68   2 References

Summarises the major aspects of writing a research based paper and gives advice on selecting an appropriate journal for publication. An example of structure is given and guidance on the length and emphasis for each part. Mention is made of confidentiality, anonymity and other general issues. The importance of publishing research findings is stressed.

2.100.5   Daiute, C. (1985) *Writing and computers.* Reading, Massachusetts: Addison-Wesley   ISBN 0201103680   References

Book considers the benefits and problems of using computers in the writing process. It covers writing development from young children up to college students and discusses appropriate computer applications. A chapter is included which gives advice on the selection of hardware and software. Research findings are incorporated into the discussion and there is also a resource section listing programmes. A glossary of terms is included.

2.100.6   Fairfax, 'J. & Moat, J. (1981) *The way to write.* London: Elm Tree Books   ISBN 0241105579   (No references)

A practical guide for beginners which explains clearly how to evaluate ones own writing and then take steps to improve it. It covers every important aspect of writing from the blank page to the final manuscript.

2.100.7   Field, P.A. & Morse, J.M. (1985) Reporting qualitative research. IN Authors, *Nursing research: the application of qualitative approaches.* Rockville, Maryland: Aspen   ISBN 0709910460   References   Chapter 7   125-135

Gives specific advice on writing in general and for publication. Particular reference is made to the reporting of qualitative research (CR 2.1.24).

2.100.8   Figueroa, P.M.E. (1980) *Writing research reports.* 2nd edition Nottingham: University of Nottingham School of Education   ISBN 0853591237   References

A short practical guide intended primarily for Masters or PhD students although the general principles would be useful to anyone writing a research report for the first time. It contains advice on all aspects of a report together with practical points on style and strategy.

2.100.9   Lester, J.D. (1976) *Writing research papers: a complete guide.* 2nd edition Glenview, Illinois: Scott, Foresman & Co.   ISBN 0673079902   References

A guide to beginning researchers in all disciplines on how to write good research papers.

2.100.10   Poteet, G.W., Edlund, B.J. & Hodges, L.C. (1987) Promoting scholarship in graduate education. *Nurse education today* 7(3) 97-102   7 References

Author suggests that students on Masters degree programmes need to be taught both how to write well and how to write for publication. A course designed specifically to enhance writing skills is described. The important role which teachers play in fostering this development is stressed.

2.100.11   Stone, S. & Harris, C. (1984) *CRUS Guide 4. Writing research reports.* British Library Board, Sheffield: Centre for Research on User Studies, University of Sheffield   (No ISBN Number)

The importance of writing up research is stressed. Specific guidance is given for the inexperienced writer about tailoring the report for each audience, outlines what it should contain and suggestions are made about layout, writing style and organising the material. When to begin writing and presenting drafts and interim reports is also discussed.

2.100.12   Tornquist, E.M. (1986) *From proposal to publication: an informal guide to writing about nursing research.* Menlo Park, California: Addison-Wesley   ISBN 0201080125   References

Book is intended for both students and experienced researchers. It includes chapters on writing research proposals, theses, dissertations or research reports and articles. A concluding section covers other important aspects of writing and giving verbal presentations (CR 2.103).

2.100.13   Turabian, K.L. (1987) *A manual for writers of term papers, theses and dissertations.* 5th edition Chicago: University of Chicago Press   ISBN 0226816257 References

The first British edition of an American 'vade mecum' intended to assist all those preparing academic work for advanced level courses or presenting papers in scholarly journals. It gives comprehensive guidance on all aspects of style, presentation, examples of entries of reference styles, notes, bibliographical entries, annotated sample pages. Throughout, the needs of computer users are emphasised.

2.100.14   Turk, C. & Kirkman, J. (1982) *Effective writing: improving scientific, technical and business communication.* London: E.& F.N. Spon   ISBN 0419116702
References

Book gives clear, practical guidance on how to select, organise and present information in reports and papers. It is intended for college and university students.

2.100.15   Watson, G. (1987) *Writing a thesis: a guide to long essays and dissertations.* London: Longman   ISBN 0582494656   References

Gives practical guidance to students undertaking major written work for the first time. It covers the approach to scholarship, choosing and delineating a subject and techniques of writing and documentation.

2.100.16   Young, M. (1989) *The technical writers handbook: writing with style and clarity.* Mill Valley, California: University Science Books   ISBN 0935702601
References

Book includes examples and gives an introduction to technical writing. Much of it is in dictionary format and contains grammatical and technical terms, words and phrases, style, organisation, common errors and writing résumés.

2.100.17   Young, P. (1987) Writing for publication. *Nurse education today* 7(6) 285-288   3 References

The author suggests that nurses should be able to write for publication but lack the necessary skills which are identified and described. Advice is given on the use of language, presention of scientific papers, undertaking book reviews, writing letters and correct presentation of manuscripts. The stages in the publication process are explained.

Suggested textbook readings

	Pages	Cross reference
Abdellah & Levine	298-302	2.1.1
Adams & Schvaneveldt	379-394	2.1.2
Bell J.	124-135	3.21.3
Burns & Grove	579-605	2.1.12
Castles	139-144	2.1.15
Christensen	351-384	2.1.17
Fox	415-443	2.1.25
Holm & Llewellyn	201-210	2.1.26
Howard & Sharp	174-209	3.21.5
Kidder & Judd	427-451	2.1.30
Kovacs	259-276	2.1.31
Leedy	235-259	2.1.35
Notter & Hott	131-140	2.1.44
Phillips L.R.F. (critique)	101-106	2.98.11
Polgar & Thomas	265-273	2.1.55

	Pages	*Cross reference*
Polit & Hungler (1987)	487-497	2.1.56
Seaman	395-406	2.1.62
Smith H.W.	414-422	2.98.14
Tierney A. IN Cormack	168-180	2.1.20
Treece & Treece	467-483	2.1.65
Waltz & Bausell	117-124	2.21.4
Wilson H.S. (1989)	671-686	2.1.69

Nursing research abstracts

Chapman E.	86/007
Cheadle J.	79/79
Cormack D.F.S.	85/007
Figueroa P.M.E.	83/4
Murphy-Black T.	88/105
Willis P.	85/003
Wilson B.	84/404

Note: Most journals include instructions to authors regularly or periodically. This includes guidance on length, style of presentation, referencing and the use of illustrations and tables. Many journals have potential articles refereed by experts and editors are also available to give advice.

2.101   DISSEMINATING RESEARCH FINDINGS

One of the major responsibilities of researchers is to inform professional colleagues about the results of their research once it has been completed. This may be done in various ways, by writing for publication or presenting it verbally at a meeting or conference. This provides opportunities for others to examine the work in detail and helps to build on the body of nursing knowledge.

Annotations

2.101.1   Bergman, R. (1988) Omissions in nursing research: another look. *International nursing review* 35(6) 164,165-168   Issue 282   5 References

Article develops arguments in a previous paper (Bergman 1984) and poses some provocative questions about the non-doings and omissions in nursing research. These include inadequate communication between researcher and practitioner and nurses' lack of motivation to study findings or to do research themselves. The author advocates the development of a master plan for nursing research by a national or international organisation, and discusses the role of gatekeepers who provide access to research sites (CR 2.105.2).

2.101.2   Funk, S.G., Tornquist, E.M. & Champagne, M.T. (1989) Application and evaluation of the dissemination model. *Western journal of nursing research* 11(4) 486-491   2 References

Discusses the importance of ensuring that research findings are understandable and accessible to clinicians and that support mechanisms are available. The model developed by the authors has three major components: qualities of the research, characteristics of its communication and facilitation of its utilisation. Three mechanisms are suggested for accomplishing dissemination; topic focused, practice orientated research conferences, carefully edited and widely distributed volumes based on conference presentations and an information centre to provide ongoing support.

2.101.3 Hockey, L. (1987) Issues in the communication of nursing research. *Recent advances in nursing* 18: 154-167   6 References

Author discusses matters of concern regarding the communication of research findings. These include questions arising at various stages in the research process, between researchers themselves, between researchers and practitioners, other professionals and their sponsors. Further discussion is advocated.

2.101.4 Moody, L., Wilson, M.E., Smyth, K., Schwartz, R., Tittle, M. & Cott. M.L.V. (1988) Analysis of a decade of nursing practice research, 1977-1986. *Nursing research* 37(6) 374-379   22 References

Study analysed 720 articles for their research focus, theoretical basis, research designs, statistical methods and findings of nursing practice research. A secondary purpose was to assess the fit of the topics with the North American Nursing Diagnosis Association Taxonomy. Findings included 95% of the publications had nurses as first author; funded research had increased; multi-method and multi-site studies were more common. There was an increase in the use of sophisticated research methods and better reporting of reliability and validity.

2.101.5 O'Connell, K.A. (1983) Nursing practice: a decade of research. IN Chaska, N.L. *The nursing profession: a time to speak.* New York: McGraw Hill ISBN 0070106967   References   Chapter 15   183-201

Reports a replication study, and an extension of other research, which analysed research in nursing practice published in the journal Nursing Research. A comparison was also made with the first two volumes of Research in Nursing and Health. Many changes are noted which led to the conclusion that there was an improvement in the quality of research conducted (CR 2.13, 3.6.2).

2.101.6 Roberts, H. (1984) Putting the show on the road: the dissemination of research findings. IN Bell, C. & Roberts, H. (eds) *Social researching, politics, problems and practice.* London: Routledge & Kegan Paul   ISBN 0710098847 References 11: 199-212

Chapter is concerned with the problems of publishing for a wider readership, and disseminating research findings beyond academia (CR 2.1.5).

2.101.7 Thomson, A.M. & Robinson, S. (1985) Dissemination of midwifery research: how this has been facilitated in the UK. *Midwifery* 1(1) 52-53 (No references)

Paper describes the setting up and progress of the annual Research and the Midwife conferences in the UK.

Suggested textbook readings

	Pages	Cross reference
Abdellah & Levine	298-305	2.1.1
Grady & Wallston	157-162	3.11.2
Nieswiadomy	351-367	2.1.43
Polit & Hungler (1987)	487-495	2.1.56
Wilson H.S. (1989)	655-694	2.1.69
Woods & Catanzaro	479-497	2.1.72

Nursing research abstracts

Abdel-Al H. IN Harman E.	84/131
Australian Government	85/224
Gordon M.D.	81/404
Meadows A.J.	81/281
Perkins E.R.	81/407
Roberts H.	85/009
Schultz S.	87/004
Stodulski A.H.	83/488
Thomson A.M.	86/128

2.102 PUBLICATION PROCESSES

Many nurses in the United Kingdom are now writing for publication, and as more undertake advanced level studies the number will continue to rise. It is also the responsibility of all researchers to inform the profession about their work and this is most frequently done by publishing articles in nursing journals.

Annotations

2.102.1 American Psychological Association (1983) *Publication manual of the American Psychological Association.* 3rd edition, Washington DC: American Psychological Association ISBN 0912704578 References

Gives detailed guidance to authors on the content and organisation of a manuscript, expression of ideas, editorial style, typing instructions and a sample paper, submitting the paper, proof-reading and the journal programme of the association. Bibliography covers references to the history of the manual, references and suggested reading. Brief guidance is given on preparation of materials other than journal articles.

2.102.2 British Medical Association (1985) *How to do it.* 2nd edition, London: BMA ISBN 0727901869 References

A series of short articles from the British Medical Journal, several of which relate to publication processes, authorship, editing and writing.

2.102.3   Cohen, L.J. (1989) Reframing manuscript rejection. *Nurse educator* 14(2) 4-5   2 References   Guest editorial

Discusses how to rewrite an article which has been rejected for publication.

2.102.4   Cosgray, R.E., Davidhizar, R.E., Fawley, R. & Hann, V. (1989) Getting started on your first manuscript. *Hospital topics* 67(5) 28-32   16 References

Paper gives practical advice on some major factors involved in writing for publication: selecting a topic, consulting a subject expert, finding a writing mentor, finding a writing partner, selecting a journal, and developing an outline.

2.102.5   Downs, F.S. (1988) A cornerstone is in place. *Nursing research* 37(6) 323   Editorial

The quality of manuscripts presented to the journal over a ten year period is described. The acceptance rate is low at 13% but the editor believes this is because the level of research sophistication is so much greater and the problems more complex.

2.102.6   Ellis, H. (1985) Review a book. IN British Medical Association, *How to do it*. 2nd edition London: BMA   ISBN 0727901869   250-252

A personal account of the experience of reviewing medical books, usually textbooks and monographs of general surgery. Some of the problems and pleasures are described.

2.102.7   Fuller, E.O. (1983) Preparing an abstract of a nursing study. *Nursing research* 32(5) 316-317

Gives details of appropriate content for an abstract using an example for illustration.

2.102.8   Juhl, N. & Norman, V.L. (1989) Writing an effective abstract. *Applied nursing research* 2(4) 189-193   3 References

Describes how to write an abstract using two versions of one based on a particular study. Criteria for critiquing abstracts are given and the first version is revised according to these guidelines.

2.102.9   McElmurry, B.J., Newcomb, B.J., Barnfather, J. & Lynch, M.S. (1981) The manuscript review process in nursing publications. IN McCloskey, J.C. & Grace, H.K. (eds) *Current issues in nursing*. Boston: Massachusetts   ISBN 086542005X References   Part 2   Chapter 14   129-143   References

Reports a study which was designed to describe and clarify current organisational structures, policies and practices used in the review process by health-related journals to which nurses are likely to submit manuscripts.

2.102.10   Morris, S. (1988) Writing a book: some advice for new authors. *Nurse education today* 8(4) 234-238

Processes involved in publishing a book are discussed, from finding a publisher to its ultimate publication.

2.102.11   Nursing Mirror (1981) The publishing process. *Nursing mirror supplement* 152(19) May 7 39-51

A series of short articles written by the staff of the Nursing Mirror describing different facets of the journal. The publication process is fully described and advice given on how to submit a letter and prepare an article for publication. The importance of nurses contributing to the journal is stressed.

2.102.12   Pagana, K.D. (1989) Writing strategies to demistify publishing. *Journal of continuing education in nursing* 20(2) 58-63   26 References

Discusses publication processes and the steps necessary for manuscript preparation.

2.102.13   Peck, C. (1984) The publishing process. *Senior nurse* 1(25) 18, 20

An overview of the publishing process including discussion about what kind of nursing books are suitable, who the author should be and how the book should be promoted and sold.

2.102.14   Warner, S.D. & Schweer, K.D. (eds) (1982) *Author's guide to journals in nursing and related fields.* New York: Haworth Press   ISBN 0917724119

Profiles over 350 scholarly journals in nursing and related fields and is intended to assist writers in finding the appropriate journal for their articles. Each profile includes details of the types of articles usually selected, the percentage accepted, major content areas, preferred and inappropriate topics and in which indexing or abstracting services the information published will be listed (CR 1.6, 2.101).

2.102.15   Watson, C. (1984) What makes a good nursing book and how to write one. *Senior nurse* 1(25) 16-17

Describes the important characteristics of a nursing book. These are that they should be written by nurses, be research based, encourage research mindedness and be based on a nursing model. Simple advice is given to any nurse wishing to write a book.

2.102.16   White, J.H. (1987) The journal publication process: the perspective of the nurse author. *Journal of advanced nursing* 12(1) 121-127   19 References

Report of a study undertaken on 320 nurse authors in America. It focuses on their views about the steps in the publication process.

Suggested textbook readings

	Pages	Cross reference
Miller D.C.	484-513	2.56.3
Polgar & Thomas	269-271	2.1.55
Polit & Hungler (1987)	492-494	2.1.56
Tornquist E.M.	192-196	2.100.12
Treece & Treece	484-492	2.1.65
Wilson H.S. (1989)	686-692	2.1.69

Nursing research abstracts

Altman D.G.	84/1

[Note: Please also see section 2.100]

2.103   TALKING ABOUT RESEARCH

In addition to writing about research, opportunities arise for students or experienced researchers to present their work to colleagues verbally. This may be in the classroom, to a small group of interested people or a formal presentation at a conference. Presenting research findings orally is an additional skill which all who undertake research need to develop so that the profession may be informed of the findings.

Annotations

2.103.1   Beal, J.A., Lynch, M.M. & Moore, P.S. (1989) Communicating nursing research: another look at the use of poster sessions in undergraduate programmes. *Nurse educator* 14(1) 8-10   6 References

Reports on the use of the poster session as a teaching strategy in two undergraduate programmes.

2.103.2   Dixon, D. & Hills, P. (1981) *Talking about your research.* Leicester: Primary Communications Research Centre, University of Leicester ISBN 0906083192   References

Booklet is designed to assist those preparing for their first oral presentation to a professional audience.

2.103.3   Hawthorn, P.J. (1989) Presenting a paper. *Nurse education today* 9(2) 129-134   2 References

Gives practical advice on the various aspects of presenting papers to an audience.

2.103.4   Kirkpatrick, H. & Martin, M-L. (1991) Communicating nursing research through poster presentations. *Western journal of nursing research* 13(1) 145-148   4 References

Gives specific information on the presentation of poster sessions.

2.103.5 Lippman, D.T. & Ponton, K.S. (1989) Designing a research poster with impact. *Western journal of nursing research* 11(4) 477-485   3 References

Discusses all aspects of poster development and presentation.

2.103.6 Newble, D.I. & Cannon, R.A. (1984) How to make a presentation at a scientific meeting. *Medical teacher* 6(1) 6-9   3 References

A comprehensive guide to presenting a scientific paper. Advice given includes what needs to be prepared beforehand, how to use audio-visual aids, present yourself on the day and answer questions. Checklists are included for use on the day.

2.103.7 Sexton, D.L. (1984) Presentation of research findings: the poster session. *Nursing research* 33(6) 374-375   (No references)

Use of poster sessions for presenting research findings is discussed. The advantages are outlined together with practical aspects − content, materials, arrangement, visuals, displaying the poster and transporting it.

Suggested textbook readings

	Pages	*Cross reference*
Holm & Llewellyn	210-214	2.1.26
Polit & Hungler (1987)	494	2.1.56
Wilson H.S. (1989)	666-671	2.1.69

2.104 CREATING A RESEARCH UTILISATION ENVIRON-MENT

Creation of a research utilisation environment is a pre-condition to implementing appropriate research findings. Nurse managers, educators, researchers and clinicians all have responsibilities in relation to this. Creating support networks, providing opportunities for learning, communicating in a clear way and the willingness to participate in research are all required (Phillips L.R.F. 1986).

Definition
A process directed towards transferring specific research-based knowledge into actual clinical practice

Annotations
2.104.1 Davis, M.Z. (1981) Promoting nursing research in the clinical setting. *Journal of nursing administration* 11(3) 22-27   11 References

A nurse administrator describes her experiences in developing research knowledge and interest in clinical nurses. Focus is on the problems encountered and ways in which these were resolved. Introducing research values and activities to practising nurses are as much organisational and cultural as they are methodological and technical.

2.104.2 Hefferin, E., Horsley, J. & Ventura, M. (1982) Promoting research-based nursing: the nurse administrators role. *Journal of nursing administration* 12(5) 34-41   34 References

Reports on a survey of nurse administrators and nurse researchers in order to ascertain if, how and by whom research findings were implemented in practice. The role of the nurse manager in particular is examined and found to be pivotal.

2.104.3 Horsley, J.A., Crane, J. & Bingle, J.D. (1978) Research utilisation as an organisational process. *Journal of nursing administration* 8(7) 4-6   2 References

There is general discussion about why nursing research findings are not utilised in practice. A research utilisation project which ran for five years (1975-1980) in southern Michigan in the USA is described and the model used is discussed in detail (CR 2.105.14).

2.104.4 Krueger, J. (1978) Utilisation of nursing research: the planning process. *Journal of nursing administration* 8(1) 6-9   26 References

In an effort to bridge the research-practice gap a large scale project was undertaken in America in 1975. In a series of workshops nurses linked their identified problems with relevant research literature and were helped to plan how they might initiate change. The workshops and their evaluation are fully described.

2.104.5 Macguire, J.M. (1990) Putting research findings into practice: research utilisation as an aspect of the management of change. *Journal of advanced nursing* 15(5) 614-620   22 References

Identifies 10 areas of potential difficulty which need to be examined before research findings may be implemented in practice. These need to be addressed at all organisational levels, rather than putting blame on individuals for non-implementation of research findings.

2.104.6 Rizzuto, C. & Mitchell, M. (1990) Outcomes of a Research Consortium Project. *Journal of nursing administration* 20(4) 13-17   3 References

Gives a final report on the work of a unique collaborative model for facilitating the conduct of nursing research in service settings.

2.104.7 Stetler, C.B. (1984) *Nursing research in a service setting.* Reston, Virginia: Reston Publishing Co.Inc.   ISBN 083595045X   References

Describes a nursing studies programme which aimed to facilitate the involvement of clinical nurses in research at Massachusetts General Hospital. The book does not attempt to duplicate research texts, but consists of brief descriptions of the products and methods of programme operation, and exhibits which are the instruments, forms and policies used.

2.104.8 Tierney, A. (1987) Putting research to good use. *Senior nurse* 6(3) 10   12 References

Article stresses that research utilisation is a challenge to nursing and requires resources, further education and much time and effort by nurses.

2.104.9 Wright, S.G. (1989) *Changing nursing practice.* London: Edward Arnold ISBN 0713145811 References

Book explores the concept of change and discusses the complex skills which nurses need in order to become change agents. Many examples are included which illustrate 'how to' change nursing practice.

Suggested textbook readings

	Pages	Cross reference
Abdellah & Levine	5-6	2.1.1
Holm & Llewellyn	219-227	2.1.26
Phillips L.R.F.	406-411	2.98.11

Nursing research abstracts

Chonenwelt L.R.	87/219

2.105 IMPLEMENTING RESEARCH FINDINGS

It has been stated that historically 50 years intervene before research in any field is properly utilised (Johnson 1977). Because nursing practice today is in a state of rapid transition it is vital to keep pace with the technological changes, and conceptualise, synthesise and categorise the knowledge explosion. All nurses must therefore keep up to date in their own specialty in order to ensure the best possible care for patients and clients. We cannot afford to wait for 50 years!

Definition
To use in practice

Example
Dealey, C. & Berker, M. (1986) Action speaks louder than words. *Nursing times* 82(29) July 16 37-39 1 Reference

Describes how a specific research finding relating to the cleaning and correct storage of patients' wash bowls, was implemented in a hospital setting.

Annotations
2.105.1 Armitage, S. (1990) Research utilisation in practice. *Nurse education today* 10(1) 10-15 7 References

Discusses the findings of a working group set up to identify and explore the extent to which research findings were being used in practice. Criteria were developed to assist facilitators in their role of helping colleagues to learn about research. Author urges all nurses to develop critical reading skills.

2.105.2   Bergman, R. (1984) Omissions in nursing research. *International nursing review* 31(2)   Issue 254 55-56   5 References

Author identifies reasons why nursing research findings are not implemented throughout the world and suggests how the problems may be overcome. She believes omissions in nursing research are of ethical concern and may have more impact on patient care in the long term (CR 2.101.1).

2.105.3   Bircumshaw, D. (1990) The utilisation of research findings in clinical practice. *Journal of advanced nursing* 15(11) 1272-1280   39 References

Article reviews the literature from 1951-1988 on the utilisation of research findings in clinical nursing practice. It covers justification for the use of findings, whether they are used in practice, projects aimed at implementing findings, factors influencing nursing practice in relation to findings, research evaluation, implementation and change (CR 2.12).

2.105.4   Blair, J. (1983) The application of research findings: whose responsibility? *Nurse education today* 3(2) 42-43   5 References

Article is a précis of a prize winning essay by a student nurse. She stresses the need for research-based clinical practice and examines the roles of various grades of nurses. The original work provides a more extensive bibliography.

2.105.5   Bond, S. (1983) Promoting research utilisation through information services. IN Davis, B.D. *Research into nurse education.* London: Croom Helm ISBN 0709908253   References   Part 3   Chapter 10   188-201

Chapter describes the development of library and information services in the north region of England. Information workshops were held for ward sisters and nursing officers to enable them to become skilled in retrieving information and assist them in preparing and writing reports. A Nursing Topics Project also evolved and its purpose was to produce a resource of selected reports on topics relevant to nursing (CR 1.2).

2.105.6   Buckwalter, K.C. (1985) Is nursing research used in practice? IN McCloskey, J.C. & Grace, H.K. (eds) *Current issues in nursing.* 2nd edition, Boston: Blackwell Scientific   ISBN 086542019X   References   Part 2   9   110-123   52 References

Chapter, written in the form of a debate, examines issues related to the transfer of knowledge generated by nursing research. Factors which influence, and those which inhibit use of findings are outlined together with suggested strategies for increasing use of research in practice.

2.105.7   Chellel, A. (1987) Learned practice. *Nursing times* 83(21) May 27 64   1
Reference

Author suggests that research is often 'academic' and distant from the practicalities
of everyday care but the relationships between nurses and patients are equally
important.

2.105.8   Clark, E. (1989) *Using research findings: a guide for practitioners.*
Research Awareness, Module 11 London: Distance Learning Centre, South Bank
Polytechnic   ISBN 0948250380   References

This is number 11 in a series of 13 modules, each of which deals with a different
aspect of nursing research. It was developed to assist nurses, midwives and health
visitors in understanding research in terms of their own professional practice. Modules
can be used separately or as part of a programme. The reader is encouraged to work
through a number of activities, self-assessment questions and answers and progress
summaries. Some articles/book extracts referred to in the text are reproduced in full.
    This module discusses the research-practice gap, the reasons for it and possible
remedies. Positive suggestions are made of ways in which practising nurses could
become more research aware, better able to disseminate research findings and utilise
them in practice. A chapter is devoted to the management of change (CR Appendix
D).

2.105.9   Clarke, M. (1985) The use of research reports in planning continuing
education for trained nurses. *Journal of advanced nursing* 10(5) 475-482   27
References

Author suggests that there are now a number of studies with similar findings which
could be implemented in practice. The available research in the following areas is
reviewed; continuing education from the recipients point of view, management
training for ward sisters, teaching and learning in the ward and clinical nursing.

2.105.10   Downs, F.S. & Fleming, J.W. (1979) *Issues in nursing research.* New
York: Appleton-Century-Crofts   ISBN 0838544363   References

Book discusses some of the problems related to developing nursing research and
its implementation. Chapters cover trends and historical perspectives; educational
issues; support for an emerging institution; clinical and theoretical research;
development of theoretical frameworks; ethical issues and the future of nursing
research.

2.105.11   Edwards-Beckett, J. (1990) Nursing research utilisation techniques.
Journal of nursing administration 20(11) 25-30   44 References

A review of the literature from 1978-1988 which identifies techniques for facilitating
nursing research utilisation, using nine general themes to organise the materials.
Examples are given of research themes which may be implemented by individuals,
small groups or by organisations and professions (CR 2.12, 3.23.7).

2.105.12   Gould, D. (1986) Pressure sore prevention and treatment: an example of nurses' failure to implement research findings. *Journal of advanced nursing* 11(4) 389-394   32 References

The failure of nurses to implement long established research findings is examined. One of the main reasons postulated is that nurse educationalists have failed to incorporate findings into basic and post-basic teaching programmes.

2.105.13   Hakel, M.D., Sorcher, M., Beer, M., & Moses, J.L. (1982) *Making it happen: designing research with implementation in mind.* Beverly Hills: Sage   ISBN 0803918666   References

Monograph focuses on designing and executing research when implementation is the prime objective. Exercises are included together with a case study which illustrates some of the difficulties which may be encountered.

2.105.14   Horsley, J.A. (1983) *Using research to improve nursing practice: a guide.* CURN Project.* Orlando: Grune & Stratton   ISBN 080891510X   References

* Conduct and Utilisation of Research in Nursing Project, Michigan Nurses Association

Book attempts to move research and practice closer together by describing the processes involved in incorporating research-based knowledge into practice. Emphasis is put on the activities undertaken by the organisation involved in change rather than in individuals; these are creating a climate for practice change, planning, implementing and then evaluating the processes (CR 2.104.3).

2.105.15   Hunt, J. (1981) Indicators for nursing practice: the use of research findings. *Journal of advanced nursing* 6(3) 189-194   19 References

Relevant research findings are available for some nursing practices, but not all, the author suggests. Five reasons why findings are not used by practitioners are discussed.

2.105.16   Hunt, J. (1984) Why don't we use these findings? *Nursing mirror* 158(8) February 22 29   7 References

Reasons are given as to why nurses do not use research findings. Author stresses that it is part of nurses' professional responsibility to do so.

2.105.17   Hunt, M. (1987) The process of translating research findings into nursing practice. *Journal of advanced nursing* 12(1) 101-110   74 References

Paper describes an action research study undertaken to encourage nurse teachers to use research critically as the basis for their teaching. Librarians conducted searches for research-based practice literature. The information obtained was collated, reviewed and policies and procedures altered accordingly (CR 2.37).

2.105.18 Jennings, B.M. & Rogers, S. (1988) Merging nursing research and practice: a case of multiple identities. *Journal of advanced nursing* 13(6) 752-758   49 References

Possible explanations are given for the limited progress in merging nursing research findings with practice. The multiple identities taken on by nurses of administrator, clinician, educator and researcher create different responsibilities and orientations, and may stifle the desired merger. The common factor is that all are nurses, each with their own contribution to nursing, and a combination of these skills can lead to innovations in practice.

2.105.19 Ketefian, S. (1975) Application of selected nursing research findings into nursing practice: a pilot study. *Nursing research* 24(2) 89-92   25 References

Describes a study undertaken to ascertain whether research findings relating to a specific, widely used nursing task, taking temperatures, were being used by practising nurses. The findings were not being used and some reasons for this are discussed. Questions are raised about post-graduate nursing education.

2.105.20 Larson, E. (1989) Using the CURN project to teach research utilisation in a baccalaureate program. *Western journal of nursing research* 11(5) 593-599   4 References

Clinical issues selected from the Conduct and Utilisation of Research in Nursing Project (CURN Project) provided the basis for examination of the research process. Evaluation showed a positive attitude to research but limitations are the age of the data base used, and some were based on medical rather than nursing research. Students also had some difficulty in working on group assignments (CR 2.105.14).

2.105.21 LeLean, S.R. (1982) The implementation of research findings in nursing practice. IN Lerheim, K. (ed) *Collaborative research and its implementation in nursing*. 4th Conference of European Nurse Researchers, Oslo: Norwegian Nurses Association   35 References

Reasons for non-implementation of research findings are discussed. Author suggests there are many challenges to overcome if nursing is to have a firm scientific base. Some of the initiatives being set up in England to bridge the research-practice gap are described (CR 3.26).

2.105.22 Luker, K. (1986) Who's for research? *Nursing times* 82(52) December 31 55-56   3 References

The difference between research and common sense is defined. Author suggests that all research is useful and outlines ways it may be used to fuller effect.

2.105.23 Myco, F. (1981) The implementation of nursing research related to the nursing profession in Northern Ireland. *Journal of advanced nursing* 6(1) 51-58   30 References

Reports the findings of a survey in Northern Ireland which aimed to assess the degree to which those most concerned with administering, managing and teaching patient care were implementing information gained from nursing research. Author concludes that the personnel involved had not yet begun to identify to any great extent the importance of research to nursing practice, or with identifying processes through which research may be implemented and evaluated.

2.105.24 Robinson, J. (1987) The relevance of research to the ward sister. *Journal of advanced nursing* 12(4) 421-429   18 References

Article gives an overview of how research impinges on the role of the ward sister, with particular reference to paediatrics. Mention is made of funding issues and the difficulties of applying research findings to practice. The author stresses that nursing should look to the sociological, rather than just the technical model of research, in order to better understand childrens' needs and the world in which they live.

2.105.25 Tanner, C.A. & Lindeman, C.A. (1989) *Using nursing research.* New York: National League for Nursing   ISBN 088737414X   References

Book focuses on evaluating research for use in practice. Three introductory chapters discuss the idea of research in practice and Part 2 contains articles chosen for their continuing relevance to practice. A critique of each of these is included (CR 2.98).

2.105.26 Walsh, M. & Ford, P. (1989) *Nursing rituals, research and rational actions.* Oxford: Heinemann Nursing   ISBN 0433000805   References

Book highlights key areas of nursing practice where research evidence is available but which in many instances is not being used. Rituals of clinical practice and organisation are explored and recommendations for good practice given.

2.105.27 White, J. (1984) The relationship of clinical practice and research. *Journal of advanced nursing* 9(2) 181-187   15 References

This specific case study, which examined client attrition at an obesity clinic, shows how nurse practitioners can make use of research skills to identify problems, investigate them and then implement their findings. The practice/research relationship is explored.

2.105.28 Wilson-Barnett, J.& Batehup, L. (1988) *Patient problems: a research base for nursing care.* London: Scutari   ISBN 1871364108   References   Chapter 1 1-7

The introduction to this book discusses directions for nursing research, approaches to it and applications to practice. The remainder of the book covers research relating to particular patient problems.

2.105.29 Wright, D., Goodman, C. & Hall, D. (1986) Pressure to act. *Senior nurse* 5(1) 12-13   4 References

The progress made by a 'service based' nursing research unit towards implementing research findings is shown. The kind of problems encountered are demonstrated by an example relating to the use of solutions on superficial skin breaks over pressure areas. The research team persuaded staff of all disciplines to stop using these lotions.

Suggested textbook readings

	Pages	*Cross reference*
Abdellah & Levine	298-299	2.1.1
Burns & Grove	625-668	2.1.12
Holm & Llewellyn	215-219	2.1.26
Kidder & Judd	395-426	2.1.30
Levin R.F. IN LoBiondo-Wood & Haber	359-379	2.1.38
MacLachlan L.W. IN Phillips L.R.F.	379-405	2.98.11
Roberts & Burke	46-79	2.1.59
Treece & Treece	494-497	2.1.65
Wilson H.S. (1989)	48-53	2.1.69
Woods & Catanzaro	479-497	2.1.72

Nursing research abstracts

Barnett D.E.	82/283
Blair J.M.	84/132
Copcutt L.	85/0298
Goode C.J.	87/357
Hinshaw A.S.	87/217
Hockey L.	83/5, 84/136
Hunt J.M.	82/66, 83/231, 84/138
Kratz C.R.	83/111, 83/232
Marks-Maran D.	82/8
McFarlane J.K.	82/293
Myco F.	81/284
Richardson A.M.	81/134

Part 3

**THE BACKGROUND TO
RESEARCH IN NURSING**

DEVELOPMENT OF NURSING RESEARCH

3.1 DEVELOPMENT OF NURSING RESEARCH – AUSTRALASIA/OTHER COUNTRIES

The history of nursing research development in Australasia shows a similar pattern to that of various European countries. Opportunities are being created for nurses to undertake research in order to base practice on sound foundations.

Annotations

3.1.1 Chick, N.P. (1987) Nursing research in New Zealand. *Western journal of nursing research* 9(3) 317-334   65 References

Provides an overview of the development of nursing research in New Zealand. This includes its history, progress in educating nurses for research, research as a career pathway, avenues for publication, information retrieval systems, consumership, funding, policy and research priorities.

3.1.2 Olade, R.A. (1990) A survey of nursing research in Nigeria. *International nursing review* 37(4) 299-302   11 References

Reports a survey which examined the status of nursing research in Nigeria. The background is discussed, as are infra-structural facilities, funding, the climate, nursing practice, education, services and the future.

3.1.3 Pittman, E. (1989) Making the most of new opportunities: clinical nursing research in the 1990's. IN Gray, G. & Pratt, R. (eds) *Issues in Australian nursing 2*. Melbourne: Churchill Livingstone   ISBN 0443040338   References 26 393-407

Examines three major research issues in Australia: wider recognition of the value of clinical nursing research, collaboration between academic and clinical nurses and building institutional bases for nursing research.

3.1.4 Smith, M.G. & Shadbolt, Y.T. (eds) (1984) *Objects and outcomes: New Zealand Nurses Association 1909-1983*. Wellington: New Zealand Nurses Association   ISBN 0908669097

Documents the development of the association, its structure and functions, professionalism and unionism, nursing services, basic and post-basic education, politics and power, the international idea and the New Zealand Nursing Journal. Mention is also made of the Nursing Education Research Foundation (CR 3.15).

Suggested textbook readings

	Pages	Cross reference
Angerami E.L.S. IN Bergman R.	87-100	3.27.1
Bennett M. IN Bergman R.	145-161	3.27.1
Clark M.R., Moore P.J. & Wang E.Y.N. IN Bergman R.	162-182	3.27.1
Hirschfield M.J. & Krulik T. IN Bergman R.	101-111	3.27.1
Marshall-Burnett S. IN Bergman R.	53-71	3.27.1
Searle C. IN Bergman R.	183-194	3.27.1

3.2 DEVELOPMENT OF NURSING RESEARCH – EUROPE

The development of nursing research in Europe is at several different stages, with some countries having much experience and expertise, while others are beginning to create an appropriate structure within which it may start to flourish.

Annotations

3.2.1 Abraham, I.L. (1986) Chronological analysis of nursing research content in an international context. IN Stinson, S.M. & Kerr J.C. (eds) *International issues in nursing research.* London: Croom Helm ISBN 0709944373 References Part 4 Chapter 15 259-288

Chapter discusses the development of the European nursing research movement and the major issues which surround it. Results of a study are reported which examined the content of 5035 articles published between 1976 and 1980 in four European countries. Its aim was to define the current state of nursing and future directions as seen in the literature. Evidence showed that nursing research investigation was being promoted and facilitated and attention given to the dissemination and utilisation of research findings (CR 2.101, 2.105, 3.27.7).

3.2.2 Hamrin, E.K.F. (1990) Nursing research in Sweden. *International journal of nursing studies* 27(2) 149-157 41 References

Discusses the development of interest in nursing research, new opportunities, the relationship of nursing education to research, research training, significant accomplishments, funding, interest groups and prospects for the future (CR 3.12, 3.18).

3.2.3 Lanara, V.A. & Raya, A.A.C. (eds) (1981) *Collaborative research and its implementation in nursing.* 3rd Conference of European Nurse Researchers Athens: Hellenic National Graduate Nurses Association ISBN 02514753

Reports the development of nursing research in 16 European countries. Also contains a keynote speech by Baroness McFarlane of Llandaff entitled 'Standards of nursing care, can research help the nurse manager?' (CR 2.15, 3.26).

3.2.4 Lauri, S. (1990) The history of nursing research in Finland. *International journal of nursing studies* 27(2) 169-173   15 References

Outlines the history of nursing research in Finland and discusses the aims and activities of the Research Institute of Nursing, university level nurse education and research, nurse researchers and publication of studies and prospects for the future.

3.2.5 LeLean, S.R. (1981) Collaborative research in nursing in Europe. *Nurse education today* 1(4) 21-23   9 References

The developments in nursing research in Europe over the last five years are discussed. Particularly noted are the World Health Organisation Medium Term Programme in Nursing/Midwifery in Europe and the formation of the Workshop of European Nurse Researchers (CR 2.15, 3.2.7).

3.2.6 Lerheim, K. (1990a) Nursing research developments in Norway. *International journal of nursing studies* 27(2) 139-147   28 References

Discusses the origins of nursing research in Norway, research in the 1970's and 1980's, the influence of nursing organisations on nursing research, funding and the future.

3.2.7 Lerheim, K. (1990b) Workshop of European Nurse Researchers, a historical review: WENR 1978-1988. IN Christensen, E.H. & Lerheim, K. (eds) *Proceedings of the 10th and 11th Workshop of European Nurse Researchers*. Copenhagen: Danish Nurses Organisation   ISBN 8772660635   4-11

Provides an overview of the development of the Workshop of European Nurse Researchers, how and where it links with other associations and institutions, the venues and broad subject areas of its 11 conferences, what has been accomplished over this period and a glimpse of the the the future (CR 3.26.2).

3.2.8 Lorenson, M. (1990) Research resource development in Denmark. *International journal of nursing studies* 27(2) 159-168   72 References

Discusses the development of nursing research in Denmark, the work of the Danish Nurses Organisation and the Danish Medical Research Council, educational opportunities for nursing research and future prospects.

3.2.9 Poletti, R. (1984) Obstacles and hopes for nursing research in southern Europe. IN *Nursing research — does it make a difference?* Proceedings of the 7th Workgroup Meeting, 2nd Open Conference of the Workgroup of European Nurse Researchers: 10-13th April 1984, London: Royal College of Nursing   ISBN 0902606891   References 115-125

The development of nursing research in different countries is compared and contrasted. The reasons for these differences are examined, as are the means by which research development could be enhanced (CR 3.26.4).

3.2.10 to 3.2.25 Workshop of European Nurse-Researchers (1984) Developments in nursing research. IN *Nursing research — does it make a difference?* Proceedings of the 7th Workgroup Meeting, 2nd Open Conference: 10-13th April, London: Royal College of Nursing ISBN 0902606891 Section 1: (CR 3.26.4).

[Please note that this entry differs in format and articles have not been annotated]

[Reports from each country are given under the following headings: introduction, education for/in nursing research, completed and ongoing research in nursing, dissemination of research findings, funds available for nursing research and perspectives for the future. Some include references]

3.2.10 Bengtsson-Agostino, M. Nursing research in Italy 1983/1984. 58-59

3.2.11 Bjorn, A. Nursing research in Denmark 1983/1984. 32-35

3.2.12 Dwyer, M. Nursing research in Ireland. 52-54

3.2.13 EK, A-C. Nursing research in Sweden 1983/1984. 68-71

3.2.14 Finnsdottir, M. Nursing research in Iceland. 50-51 3 References

3.2.15 Hirschfield, M. Nursing research in Israel 1983/1984. 55-57

3.2.16 Hunt, J. Nursing research in the United Kingdom 1983/1984. 75-78

3.2.17 Jacquerye, A. Nursing research in Belgium 1982/1984. 21-31 42 References

3.2.18 Krohwinkel, M. Nursing research in the Federal Republic of Germany 1983/1984. 39-45 5 References

3.2.19 Lerheim, K. Nursing research in Norway 1983/1984. 64-66 4 References

3.2.20 Lima Basto, M.H. Nursing research in Portugal 1983/1984. 67

3.2.21 Poletti, R.A. Nursing research in Switzerland 1983/1984. 72-74 11 References

3.2.22 Raya, A. Nursing research in Greece 1983/1984. 46-49 3 References

3.2.23 Seidl, E. Nursing research in Austria 1983/1984. 17-20 4 References

3.2.24 Sorvettula, M. Nursing research in Finland 1983/1984. 36-38

3.2.25 Van der Bruggen, H. Nursing research in the Netherlands 1983/1984. 60-63

Suggested textbook readings

	Pages	Cross reference
Bernal M.O. IN Bergman R.	72-86	3.27.1
Farrell M. & Christenson B.W. IN Bergman R.	11-19	3.27.1

Nursing research abstracts

Hamrin E.	84/134

3.3 DEVELOPMENT OF NURSING RESEARCH – UNITED KINGDOM

In the United Kingdom nursing research began in the 1960's, about 80 years after Florence Nightingale had laid the foundations. Since that time, after a fairly slow beginning, the number of nurses who have had research training has continued to increase, and the volume of literature is continuing to grow all the time.

Annotations

3.3.1 Chapman, C. (1989) Research for action: the way forward. *Senior nurse* 9(6) 16-18   5 References

The development of nursing research over the last 25 years is described. Research is still not implemented in practice and there is some discussion as to the reasons why, and how this might be rectified. Mention is made of the responsibilities of the researcher.

3.3.2 Dunn, A. (1979) Research at the Joint Board. *Nursing times* 75(37) September 13 1562-1563

A description of some of the research projects undertaken by professional and research staff of the Joint Board of Clinical Nursing Studies. The importance of the involvement of professional researchers and the need for research is stressed (CR 3.3.10).

3.3.3 Gardener, M.G. (1977) The history, philosophy and evaluation on the work of the Joint Board of Clinical Nursing Studies. *Journal of advanced nursing* 2(6) 621-632   12 References

Describes the establishment, philosophy, organisation and evaluation of the work of the Joint Board of Clinical Nursing Studies. Mention is made of the small research department whose programme was to assist with the aims of establishing and maintaining a national standard. Projects included an examination of the methods of continuous practical assessment, and simulation in the testing of certain skills (CR 2.54, 3.3.10, 3.18.24).

3.3.4 Goodman, C. (1989) Nursing research: growth and development. IN Jolley, M. & Allan, P. (eds) *Current issues in nursing*. London: Chapman & Hall   ISBN 041232850X   References 5 95-114

259

Chapter discusses the growth of research in nursing, the research/practice debate, research that is ready for practice, problems of implementation, future trends and issues (CR 2.9, 2.105, 3.7).

3.3.5 Hayward, J.C. (1982) Nursing research. IN Allan, P. & Jolley, M. (eds) *Nursing, midwifery and health visiting since 1900.* London: Faber & Faber References ISBN 0571118399 Chapter 15 196-214

Describes the development of nursing research in the UK and the educational facilities available for nurses. The setting up of nursing research units is outlined and ways in which research findings may be disseminated. Some studies into aspects of clinical nursing and nursing education are mentioned and future directions for research (CR 2.101, 3.13).

3.3.6 Hockey, L. (1979) Expanding the nursing horizon. *Nursing mirror* 149(17) October 25 32-35

Author believes that the misunderstanding of what research is, i.e. the rules of the game, its objectives and outcome can be the greatest barrier to its development. The commitment to and roles of teachers, administrators and practitioners are explored. Her hopes for the future are outlined (CR 3.16).

3.3.7 Hockey, L. & Clark, M.O. (1984) Nursing research in Scotland. IN Werley, H.H. & Fitzpatrick, J.J. (eds) *Annual review of nursing research.* Volume 2 New York: Springer ISBN 0826143512 References Chapter 13 307-324

Chapter discusses Scotland's policy on nursing research, the structure and early development of the Nursing Studies Research Unit, Department of Nursing Studies, University of Edinburgh. The application of Donabedian's evaluative framework to the Women in Nursing study is outlined together with the unit's core programme of research (CR 3.13).

3.3.8 Hockey, L. (1986) Frontiers of nursing research: real or imagined. IN *New frontiers in nursing research.* Proceedings of the International Nursing Research Conference, Edmonton, Alberta, Canada 7-9th May 1986 Faculty of Nursing, University of Alberta 20-24

Discusses the conventional territory of nursing research and the origins of its frontiers. The properties of frontiers are identified and author asks if they are real or imagined. Nurses are urged to build bridges between disciplines so that nursing research can move forward (CR 3.26).

3.3.9 Hunt, J. (1982) Nursing research in the United Kingdom. IN Lerheim, K. (ed) *Collaborative research and its implementation in nursing.* 4th Conference of Nurse Researchers, Oslo: Norwegian Nurses Association 73-77 6 References

An overview of progress being made in the UK including courses available, development of nursing research units, current projects, lectures, publications and funding. Mention is made of the involvement of the Royal College of Nursing in nursing research (CR 3.12, 3.13, 3.15.14, 3.26, Appendix A).

3.3.10 Joint Board of Clinical Nursing Studies (1980) *Review of the work of the Joint Board of Clinical Nursing Studies 1970-1980.* London: JBCNS (No ISBN number)

Describes the background, structure, finances, philosophy and work of the Joint Board in connection with post-basic clinical courses. The future of these courses is also discussed.

Part 4 outlines the projects undertaken by the research staff which included, assessment in relation to clinical nursing skills, the planning and execution of Joint Board courses and a follow up study on nurses holding the Board's certificates. A course evaluation package, and one designed to assist teachers in introducing research into courses were developed by professional and research staff (CR 3.3.3, 3.18.24).

3.3.11 Keith, J.M. (1988) Florence Nightingale: statistician and consultant epidemiologist. *International nursing review* 35(5) Issue 281 147-150   16 References

Article explores a lesser known aspect of the work of Florence Nightingale, her expertise and use of statistics and epidemiology. A major health problem in New Zealand in 1860 is used for illustration.

3.3.12 King's Fund Centre (1986) *Scholarship and the growth of nursing knowledge.* Report from a symposium held at the King's Fund Centre, 18th February 1986 London: King's Fund Centre (No ISBN number)   References

Chapman, C.M.	1-5	The contribution of the Journal of Advanced Nursing to the body of nursing knowledge
Clarke, M.	7-22	Scholarship and nursing education
Cox, A.M.	23-37	Scholarship and nursing management
Pembrey, S.	39-52	Scholarship and nursing practice
Wilson-Barnett, J.	53-66	Research: its relationship to practice and representation in the Journal of Advanced Nursing

Symposium was held to celebrate the first 10 years of the Journal of Advanced Nursing. Papers cover the contribution of the journal to the body of nursing knowledge.

3.3.13 LeLean, S.R. (1980a) Research in Nursing: an overview of DHSS initiatives in developing research in nursing − 1. *Nursing times* 76(2) January 17 5-8 Occasional Paper

The need for, and the history of the development of nursing research is described with particular reference to the work of the Department of Health and Social Security. Amongst the items discussed are introducing research in basic nurse education, the Nursing Research Liason Group scheme, research courses and fellowships. The evolution of the Index of Nursing Research and the role of librarians in relation to it is outlined (CR 3.3.14, 3.17, 3.19, Appendix A).

3.3.14 LeLean, S.R. (1980b) Research in nursing: an overview of DHSS initiatives in developing research in nursing − 2. *Nursing times* 76(3) January 24 9-12   35 References   Occasional Paper

An overview is given of some research commissioned by the Nursing Research Liason Group. The problems in undertaking research in nursing are identified and suggestions made for future development (CR 3.3.13).

3.3.15 LeLean, S.R. & Clarke, M. (1990) Research resource development in the UK. *International journal of nursing studies* 27(2) 123-138   72 References

Traces the development of nursing research in the United Kingdom over the last three decades. Its origins are outlined and the following areas covered: the role of government departments, the National Health Service, professional organisations, the higher education sector, research funding, training for research, the present position and future prospects (CR 3.8, 3.12, 3.17, 3.18).

3.3.16 Norton, D. (1987) A veterans view of research in nursing. IN Hawthorn, P.J. (ed) *Proceedings of Royal College of Nursing Research Society Annual Conference* Nottingham: University of Nottingham 137-140   7 References

A former Nursing Research Liason Officer looks back over her career and the developments in nursing research. She discusses changes in nursing literature, research funding, research education, the worlds of academia and practice, and ways in which the communication gaps may be closed (CR 3.12, 3.16, 3.19, 3.26).

3.3.17 Oguisso, T. (1990) How ICN is promoting research. *International nursing review* 37(4) Issue 292 295-290   9 References

Examines the role of the International Council of Nurses in promoting research. Its historical background is discussed, together with study seminars held and the statement and guidelines published on research. Health research was the theme for discussion at the World Health Assembly and the ICN statement is included in the article. The Task Force was given a mandate to provide for each country a history of nursing research; up to date figures of nursing researchers and where they were prepared; types of education programme; research being undertaken; funded posts available; number of nurses employed to undertake research; the greatest needs, trends and priorities for nursing research.

3.3.18 Scott-Wright, M. (1982) The contribution of research to nursing. IN *Research − a base for the future.* Proceedings. Edinburgh: Nursing Studies Research Unit, University of Edinburgh   ISBN 0950782408   References 6-14

Documents some highlights of past developments in nursing research history, including the creation of the Nursing Research Unit in Edinburgh and activities in Canada. Three pointers for the future are identified and discussed (CR 3.4, 3.13, 3.26).

3.3.19 Simpson, M. (1971) Research: the first steps. *Nursing mirror* 132(22) March 12 22-27   64 References

Documents the early history of nursing research in the UK. Author discusses the influence of Florence Nightingale and medical practice, the weaknesses and strengths of nursing research, matters hindering its progress and the value of interdisciplinary teams.

3.3.20 Simpson, M. (1981) Issues in nursing research. IN Hockey, L. (ed) *Current issues in nursing.* Recent Advances in Nursing 1: Edinburgh: Churchill Livingstone   ISBN 0443021864   References   Chapter 2 19-32

The growth and development of nursing research, training and funding of nurse researchers, and the foundation of nursing research units are all discussed. The importance of research to the profession and for policy making is described, and the roles of both the Department of Health and Social Security and the Joint Board of Clinical Nursing Studies discussed (CR 3.3.10, 3.8, 3.10).

3.3.21 Smith, J.P. (1979) Is the nursing profession really research-based? *Journal of advanced nursing* 4(3) 319-325   11 References

Discusses the early development of nursing research in the United Kingdom, contrasting it with its much earlier introduction into nurse education programmes in the United States. Although there was a considerable increase in interest in the 1970s, a dearth of research minded nurses and apparent lack of findings which could be implemented, placed much responsibility on nurse teachers. The introduction into curricula for basic and post-basic courses and the first research guide published by the Joint Board of Clinical Nursing Studies were seen as milestones in developing research awareness (CR 3.18.24).

3.3.22 Smith, J.P. (1986) The end of the beginning. *Senior nurse* 5(1) 14-15   9 References

Discusses the developments in nursing research in the UK including growth of the Royal College of Nursing Research Society, nursing research departments and research fellowships. It is suggested that much nursing research needs to be replicated and that nurses should document their innovations and develop the ability to analyse their work and roles (CR 2.13, 3.13, 3.15, 3.17).

3.3.23 Stacey, M. (1984) Future directions in health care research. IN Proceedings from the 7th Workgroup Meeting, 2nd Open Conference of the Workgroup of European Nurse Researchers: *Nursing research — does it make a difference?* 10-13th April 1984, London: Royal College of Nursing   ISBN 0902606891   References 126-148

The growth of nursing research over the last 30 years is described. The problems encountered by nurses when trying to implement research findings, although they were not involved in the research, is demonstrated by reference to the report of the Platt Committee in 1959. Difficulties experienced by nurses trying to combine their jobs with day release studies are described. The future of health care research in the UK is discussed particularly with regard to funding and complex social relationships and roles (CR 2.105, 3.11, 3.12, 3.16, 3.26).

Suggested textbook reading

	Pages	*Cross reference*
Altschul A. IN Cormack	11-20	2.1.20

3.4 DEVELOPMENT OF NURSING RESEARCH – UNITED STATES OF AMERICA/CANADA

The development of nursing research is at its most advanced in the United States, and so much of the available literature comes from there. Nurses in other countries have much to build upon and perhaps adapt for use within their own countries.

Annotations

3.4.1 Baer, E.D. (1987) 'A cooperative venture' in pursuit of professional status: a research journal for nursing. *Nursing research* 36(1) 18-25   64 notes and references

Describes the origins and purpose of the journal, Nursing Research. Themes explored are educational issues, establishing the editorial process, defining and developing nursing research, centralising research in nursing, the search for a theory base and financing the journal.

3.4.2 Brimmer, P. (1986) The American Nurses Association: its role in nursing research. IN Stinson, S.M. & Kerr, J.C.A. (eds) *International issues in nursing research*. Beckenham: Croom Helm   ISBN 0709944373   References   Chapter 16 289-312

Documents the role of the American Nurses Association and the development of nursing research since 1978. Its structure, policies, financing and programmes are discussed. Because of legislative difficulties preventing the ANA from undertaking some types of research the American Nurses Foundation was established. Its aims are to fund research projects, analyse health policy and identify issues of concern to nursing, and assist the educational and research aims of the ANA. The work of the American Academy of Nursing is also described and its aims are to advance new concepts in nursing and health care; identify and explore issues in health; examine the dynamics within nursing and identify and propose solutions (CR 3.27.7).

3.4.3 Brown, J.S., Tanner, C.A. & Padrick, K.S. (1984) Nursing's search for scientific knowledge. *Nursing research* 33(1) 26-32   19 References

The characteristics of nursing research today are described and trends and changes over the past three decades are outlined. A sample of 137 studies published between 1952 and 1980 were analysed. The conclusions drawn were that nursing research had increased substantially in amount; become more clinically focused; demonstrated a higher theoretical orientation and was more sophisticated and sound in the methods employed. Limitations noted were insufficient conceptualisation and the failure to build a cumulative science.

3.4.4 Canadian Nurses Association (1984) *The research imperative for nursing in Canada: a 5 year plan towards year 2000.* Ottawa: Canadian Nurses Association ISBN 0920381030

Documents a plan for the development of nursing research under three major headings: development of nurse researchers, nursing research and nursing research reality (establishment of a general expectation among nurses, governments and the public of nursing research as the basis for care within the discipline). The plan includes goals, objectives, detailed strategies and recommended actions.

3.4.5 Fitzpatrick, J.J., Taunton, R.L. & Benoliel, J.Q. (eds) (1988) *Annual review of nursing research.* Volume 6 New York: Springer ISBN 0826143555 References

Part of an ongoing series which contains reviews of research literature under five major headings – nursing practice, care delivery, nurse education, the profession of nursing and other research.

3.4.6 Fitzpatrick, M.L. (1986) A historical study of nursing organisation: doing historical research. IN Munhall, P.L. & Oiler, C.J. *Nursing research: a qualitative perspective.* Norwalk, Connecticut: Appleton-Century-Crofts ISBN 0838570488 References Chapter 11 195-225

Chapter describes the history of American nursing during the 20th century through the development of its organisations. The development of the American Nurses Association, among others, is described (CR 2.1.42, 2.47).

3.4.7 Hinshaw, A.S. & Merritt, J. (1988) Moving nursing research to the National Institutes of Health. IN *Perspectives in nursing 1987-1989.* New York: National League for Nursing ISBN 0887373844 References 93-103 [based on presentations at the 18th biennial convention].

Discusses the history of the National Centre for Nursing Research, its mission in relation to that of the National Institute of Health, the current structure, research programmes and future initiatives (CR 3.4.9).

3.4.8 Jamieson, E.M., Sewall, M.F. & Suhrie, L.B. (1966) *Trends in nursing history: their social, international and ethical relationships.* 6th edition Philadelphia: Saunders (No ISBN number) References Chapter 14 323-357

Documents the development of the American Nurses Association, the National League for Nursing, the National Student Nurses Association and the Canadian Nurses Association. The early development of nursing research is outlined.

3.4.9   Merritt, D.H. (1986) The National Centre for Nursing Research. *Image: the journal of nursing scholarship* 18(3) 84-85

Outlines the origins of this centre, its program activities, support and funding mechanisms, present plans and future directions (CR 3.4.7).

3.4.10   O'Connor, A. (1989) Nursing research in Canada: progress, problems and prospects. *Canadian journal of nursing research* 21(1) 1-2   3 References   Editorial

Highlights some of the difficulties of assessing progress because of lack of information. The problem of minimum funding is mentioned.

3.4.11   Stevenson, J.S. (1987) Forging a research discipline. *Nursing research* 36(1) 60-64   30 Notes and References

Article reports the history of nursing research over the last 35 years in the USA. Aspects discussed are its development in the military and Veterans Administration, funding, centralisation of resources, national and regional associations, conference networks and networking through journals. Suggestions for the future are also made.

3.4.12   Stinson, S.M. (1977) Central issues in Canadian nursing research. IN LaSor, B. & Elliot, M.R. (eds) *Issues in Canadian nursing*. Scarborough, Ontario: Prentice Hall   ISBN 0135062381   References   Section 1:1 3-42

Examines questions relating to what is nursing research, why nursing research, how should it and researchers be organised and funded, and what are the priorities for study?

3.4.13   Stinson, S.M., Lamb, M. & Thibaudeau, M-F. (1990) Nursing research: the Canadian scene. *International journal of nursing studies* 27(2) 105-122   51   References

Provides an overview of the development of nursing research in Canada. Sections cover the national factors governing science policy, key national nursing organisations, provincial/territorial nursing organisations and how this affects nursing research. Research literature, libraries, nursing research manpower, networking, funding and the future are also discussed.

3.4.14   Thurston, N., Tenove, J., Church, J. et al (1989) Nursing research in Canadian hospitals. *Canadian journal of nursing administration* 2(1) 8-10   7 References

Describes a 1986 survey of Canadian teaching hospitals which aimed to provide a historical record, and identify the status and stage of nursing research studies in order to provide comparative data for current endeavours. 43% of hospitals did not respond, but those which did showed that nursing research is in its infancy and that clinical nurses are involved in undertaking research.

Suggested textbook readings

	Pages	*Cross reference*
Abdellah & Levine	28-37	2.1.1
Flaherty M.J. IN Bergman R.	38-52	3.27.1
Hinshaw A.S. & Heinrich J.A.		
IN Bergman R.	20-37	3.27.1
LoBiondo-Wood & Haber	6-18	2.1.38
Notter & Hott	3-18	2.1.44
Phillips L.R.F.	416-427	2.98.11
Polit & Hungler (1987)	5-12	2.1.56
Sweeney & Olivieri	3-31	2.1.63
Thomas	2-9	2.1.64
Williamson	13-19	2.1.67
Wilson H.S. (1989)	22-28	2.1.69

3.5 THE STATE OF THE ART

The development of nursing research has taken place over varying periods of time in different countries, but reported progress is ongoing and exciting. The need for such research does not now have to be continually justified as the profession and governments recognise its importance alongside medical research.

Annotations
3.5.1 to 3.5.8 *Advances in nursing science* (1987) 10(1) State of the art
[Please note this entry differs in format and articles have not been annotated]

3.5.1 Agan, R.D. Intuitive knowing as a dimension of nursing. 63-70   19 References

3.5.2 Allen, D.G. The social policy statement: a reappraisal. 39-48   34 References

3.5.3 Fulton, J.C. Virginia Henderson: theorist, prophet and poet. 1-9   13 References

3.5.4 Ramos, M.C. Adopting an evolutionary lens: an optimistic approach to discovering strength in nursing. 19-26   39 References

3.5.5 Rew, L. & Barrow, E.M. Intuition: a neglected hallmark of nursing knowledge. 49-62   36 References

3.5.6 Schutlz, P.R. When client means more than one: extending the foundational concept of person. 71-86   44 References

3.5.7 Thompson, J.L. Critical scholarship: the critique of domination in nursing. 27-38   30 References

3.5.8 **Watson, J.** Nursing on the caring edge: metaphorical vignettes. 10-17 15 References

3.5.9 **Fawcett, J.** (1984) Hallmarks of success in nursing research. *Advances in nursing science* 7(1) 1-11 36 References

Identifies three hallmarks of success in nursing research − identification of its boundaries; explication of the types of research required by the discipline and delineation of research activities according to educational preparation. Three major issues are identified − elimination of obstacles; acceptance of multiple methods of inquiry and utilisation of research findings in clinical practice (CR 2.105).

3.5.10 **Hockey, L.** (1986) Nursing research in the United Kingdom: the state of the art. IN Stinson, S.M. & Kerr J.C. (eds) *International issues in nursing research.* Beckenham: Croom Helm ISBN 0709944373 References Part 4 Chapter 13 216-235

A wide-ranging chapter covering a personal view on the position of nursing research in Britain in relation to seven requirements: individual academic curiosity, research education, research activity, appropriate research climate, research finance, dissemination of information and research utilisation. Focus is also put upon research activities in nursing education, practice and management. The chapter concludes with an appraisal of past performance and a glimpse of the future (CR 3.27.7).

3.5.11 **Larson, E.** (1984) The current state of nursing research. *Nursing forum* 21(3) 131-134 11 References

Discusses the state of research in the USA and outlines some studies undertaken by nurses. The late entry of nursing into politics is discussed and the paucity of funds currently available. The Institute of Medicine report on nursing and nursing education advocates the development of a federally sponsored centre for nursing research (CR 3.12).

3.5.12 **Sheehan, J.** (1986) Nursing research in Britain: the state of the art. *Nurse education today* 6(1) 3-10 41 References

Compares the development of medical and nursing research. The discussion on nursing research includes the development of nursing units, chairs in nursing, funding, available literature and application of findings (CR 2.105, 3.12, 3.13).

3.5.13 **Silva, C.P.** (1986) Research testing nursing theory: state of the art. *Advances in nursing science* 9(1) 1-11 20 References

62 studies, in which the nursing models of Johnson, Roy, Orem, Rogers and Neuman were used as a framework, were examined to determine the extent to which nursing theories had been tested through empirical research. Nine of the studies specified evaluation criteria for the explicit testing of nursing theory. The implications of this are discussed (CR 2.7).

A PROFESSION'S RESPONSIBILITY

3.6 RESEARCH AND PROFESSIONAL RESPONSIBILITY

'Many of us in nursing simply accept our professional status is based on tradition. Examination of the literature reviewing professionalisation of occupations leads one to the conclusion that nursing must continue to grow to meet the professional ideal ... professional practice is based on a systematic body of theoretical knowledge and application of this will lead to improvements in client care' (Roberts & Burke 1989).

Annotations

3.6.1 Ashworth, P. (1987) Nursing research: academic exercise or professional necessity. IN Hawthorn, P.J. (ed) *Proceedings of the Royal College of Nursing Research Society Annual Conference 1985.* Nottingham: University of Nottingham (No ISBN number) References 1 1-5

Discusses the value of research as an academic exercise and the reasons for it being a professional necessity. It can be cost-effective and give credibility and confidence. Author believes that both elements are important so that research can inform professional practice (CR 3.26).

3.6.2 Chaska, N.L. (1983) *The nursing profession: a time to speak.* New York: McGraw Hill ISBN 0070106967 References

A compilation of writings by many major figures in nursing under the headings of professionalisation, nursing education, research, theory, practice, administration, nursing service and the future of nursing. Introductory comments are made on each chapter by the editor, together with questions for discussion.

3.6.3 Clark, E. (1987) Research awareness: its importance in practice. *The professional nurse* 2(11) 371-373 12 References

It is suggested that all practitioners could and should become research aware. The importance of using research findings in practice is discussed and some resources available to nurses are mentioned. Contains an annotated bibliography.

3.6.4 Clark, E. (1988) *Nursing research in professional development.* Research awareness, Module 1 London: Distance Learning Centre, South Bank Polytechnic ISBN 0948250348 References

This is number 1 in a series of 13 modules, each of which deals with a different aspect of nursing research. It was developed to assist nurses, midwives and health visitors in understanding research in terms of their own professional practice. Modules can be used separately or as part of a complete programme. The reader is encouraged to work through a number of activities, self-assessment questions and answers and progress summaries. Some articles/book extracts referred to in the text are reproduced in full.

This module explores the place of research in nursing, research and professional responsibility and local research networks. It also provides an introduction to the whole series (CR Appendix D).

3.6.5 Clark, E. (1990) Research and common sense. IN *The professional nurse, The ward sister's survival guide*. London: Austen Cornish   ISBN 1870065123 References   Part 54 284-289

Section examines the differences between common knowledge derived from experience and that derived from research. An example is given to illustrate the points.

3.6.6 Hardy, L. (1982) Nursing models and research: a restricting view? *Journal of advanced nursing* 7(5) 447-451   19 References

The use of nursing models by practioners is reviewed. It is suggested that no one model is ideal for all situations and there should be discussion and adaptation of those in use. Concern is expressed that research may be regarded in a similar way, thus limiting its potential.

3.6.7 MacGuire, J. (1990) Nursing practice research and the advancement of nursing. *Nursing practice* 3(3) 2-5   15 References

The changing nature of nursing research is explained and examples from cancer nursing are used to examine the notion of a research-based profession. Author believes that practitioners should be involved in doing research as well as being consumers.

3.6.8 Minckley, B.B., Anderson, R. & Sands, D. (1989) Collaborative research: the Arizona experience. *Journal of continuing education in nursing* 20(5) 228-234   12 References

Describes a project whose aim was to develop an on-going dialogue and network of nurse faculty and nurse clinicians in order to use each others expertise. Examples of collaborative research are given and ways of developing skills discussed. Authors believe this model of research development to be advantageous to all involved (CR 2.15).

3.6.9 Moody, M. (1987) Illuminating research. *Nursing times* 83(39) September 30 62   1 Reference

Discusses the nurses responsibility in taking up the challenge of basing practice on research findings.

3.6.10 Roper, N. (1977) Justification and use of research in nursing. *Journal of advanced nursing* 2(4) 365-371   19 References

Report of a study day organised by the Nursing Research Advisory Group for Scotland. Its main aim was to generate interest in published research, encourage critical thinking and activity in practice. Various factors which were felt to justify the use of research were discussed.

3.6.11   Skeet, M. (1988) Issues in accountability: accountability in nursing research. *Recent advances in nursing* 19: 1-20   29 References

It is suggested that nursing research highlights many questions about nurses responsibilities and their accountability. These are outlined briefly.

3.6.12   Stephenson, P. (1985) Getting the message across. *Senior nurse* 2(9) 17-19   11 References

Theory, research and practice are cyclical and inter-dependent the author suggests. Nurses expectations of research are discussed and whether it is comprehensible to practising nurses. The image of the researcher and the availability of research findings are mentioned.

3.6.13   Wells, J. (1983) A survey of uptake by senior nursing staff of nursing literature on research and effects on nursing practice. IN Davis, B.D. *Research into nurse education.* London: Croom Helm   ISBN 0709908253   References   Part 3 Chapter 8 146-169

Chapter, based on an MA thesis, reports on a survey of senior nursing staff to determine their attitudes to nursing practice research. Sisters, nurse managers and educationalists were questioned about ways in which they kept their knowledge up to date and what attempts they had made to utilise research findings. Author suggests that the introduction of innovations should be carefully co-ordinated following development of an integrated local policy.

3.6.14   White, J.H. (1984) The relationship of clinical practice and research. *Journal of advanced nursing* 9(2) 181-187   15 References

Paper demonstrates the process, using a case study approach, whereby nurses can move from a clinical problem through the research process and back to the application of findings. The respective roles of practitioner and researcher are discussed, together with factors facilitating joint projects (CR 2.15, 3.16).

3.6.15   Wright, S.G. (1986) *Building and using a model of nursing.* London: Edward Arnold   ISBN 0713145137   References   Chapter 6 129-135

It is suggested that nursing research is an important component of a nursing model. There is brief discussion of the importance of research awareness in clinical nursing. Five items are identified as necessary for this change to occur: research awareness to be included in all objectives, skilled research nurse support to be available, ease of access to nursing literature, resources to be available at clinical level and peer support groups to be fostered by managers.

Suggested textbook readings

	Pages	Cross reference
Crow R. IN Cormack	215-223	2.1.20
Holm & Llewellyn	247-260	2.1.26

Nursing research abstracts

Alderton J.	84/263
Clarke B.	86/051
Crow R.	82/285, 82/286 & 82/422
Hamrin E.	84/134
Hockey L.	83/5
Hunt J.	85/018
Hunt M.	83/6
Luker K.A.	87/003
Pank P.	85/013
Perkins E.R.	85/526
Ray G.	85/0235
Roux B. Le	88/106
RCN Research Society	83/233
Thomson A.	85/655
Walton J.G	86/150
Wells J.C.A.	82/429

3.7 RESEARCH/PRACTICE GAP

'Professional accountability demands that nurses utilise the findings of research to perform their roles' (Polit & Hungler 1987). One of the most challenging and complex problems found in nursing today is the gap between research and practice. Despite studies carried out over the last decades, initially in the USA and now increasingly in the UK, the results of clinical nursing research are not being used. Although disturbing, this is not surprising as research and practice are not the same. At one level they are intimately connected, at another far apart because they arise from different philosophical positions. Some major attempts have been made in the USA to overcome this and a beginning has been made in the UK (Conway 1978; Dracup & Bruce 1977; Horsley et al 1978, 1983; Krueger et al 1978; Lindeman & Krueger 1977; & Stetler & Marram 1976).

Definition

The lag between the rate at which research results are produced and ... utilised

---

Example

Pritchard, A.P. & David, J.A. (eds) (1988) *The Royal Marsden Hospital, Manual of clinical procedures*. 2nd edition London: Harper & Row ISBN 0063184044 References

Aim of this book is to link available research findings with practical policies and procedures. Each policy/procedure includes reference material (where available), the procedure itself and a nursing care plan.

Annotations

3.7.1 Clark, J. (ed) (1990) *Clinical nursing manual*. Hemel Hempstead: Prentice Hall ISBN 0131378112 References

A compilation of nursing procedures which aims to provide broad guidelines rather than prescriptive detail, reflect the stages of the nursing process and gives a rationale for the principles given. Where available, research findings are referred to and guidance given for further reading.

3.7.2 Hunt, J. (1984) Nursing research − does it make a difference? IN *Nursing research − does it make a difference?* Proceedings of the 7th Workgroup Meeting, 2nd Open Conference of the Workgroup of European Nurse Researchers. 10-13th April, London: Royal College of Nursing ISBN 0902606891 99-114 25 References

Six definitions of nursing research are given which highlight some of the disagreements about what it really is. The development of nursing research in the UK is briefly described, together with the different roles which nurses adopt. Author suggests that although a considerable amount of nursing research has been done it has made little difference to practice, and the reasons for this are discussed (CR 3.3, 3.16, 3.26).

3.7.3 Phillips, L.R.F. (1986) Elements of the research-practice gap. IN Author, *A clinicians guide to the critique and utilisation of nursing research*. Norwalk, Connecticut: Appleton-Century-Crofts ISBN 0838511627 References Unit 1 1-84

Unit provides the philosophical and social/political background necessary to understand the research/practice gap. The benefits of closing this are explored from the nurses and clients point of view. The areas where communication and co-operation between researchers and practitioners can best flourish are explored (CR 2.98.11).

3.7.4 Thomas, E. (1985) Attitudes towards nursing research among trained nurses. *Nurse education today* 5(1) 18-21 14 References

Report of a survey of trained nurses which aimed to examine their attitudes towards research. Some reasons for the research/practice gap are explored and suggestions made for the future.

Nursing research abstracts

Hamer S.	87/352
Hayward J. & LeLean S.R.	82/423
Hunt J.	82/426, 85/014
Slack P.	81/286
Smith L.	84/401

THE ROLE OF GOVERNMENT

3.8 GOVERNMENT AND NURSING RESEARCH – UNITED KINGDOM

The Department of Health (formerly the Department of Health and Social Security) has played a leading role in the development of nursing research in England and Wales by establishing a Nursing Research Department, initially funding a few regional posts, funding research units and awarding a small number of scholarships for nurses to receive research training.

The Scottish Home and Health Department offer research training fellowships, mainly for nurses from Scotland, and in Northern Ireland their Nursing Research Studentship is at present under review.

Annotations
3.8.1 Department of Health (1990) *Department of Health Yearbook of Research and Development 1990*. London: HMSO ISBN 0113213204

Provides the annual record of Department of Health sponsored research for 1989/1990. Abstracts are included for individual projects and the progammes currently in progress include: Health and Personal Social Services programme, NHS Information Technology research and Procurement Directorate research. Priority themes are research into AIDS and Child Care. Book will be of value to those seeking funding (CR 3.12, 3.23).

3.8.2 Gordon, M.D. & Meadows, A.J. (1981) *The dissemination of findings of DHSS funded research: a final report.* Leicester: Primary Communications Research Centre, University of Leicester ISBN 0906083184

Examines factors affecting the dissemination of findings arising from DHSS funded research. The role of the Index of Nursing Research and Nursing Research Abstracts in disseminating both published and unpublished work is outlined. The main limitations to dissemination were the fixed-term nature of funding with consequences for researchers careers, and the fact that researchers tend to publish in specialist journals, so other practitioners may be omitted from the communication networks. Feedback given to researchers was felt to be generally inadequate, and there was a lack of clarity in the delineation of responsibilities related to completed reports. Suggestions are made as to how communication networks could be improved (CR 1.12.6, 2.101, 2.102, 3.12, 3.23).

Index of Nursing Research – section 7.23 230-232
Nursing Research Abstracts – section 7.32 238-240

3.8.3 House of Lords (1971) *A framework for government research and development.* London: HMSO Cmnd 4814 (Includes The organisation and management of government research and development [Rothschild Report]) SBN 101481403

Examines the problems raised by this complex government activity and makes suggestions about improving its role, structure, organisation, personnel and financing (CR **3.8.4**).

3.8.4 Kogan, M. & Henkel, M. (1983) *Government and research: the Rothschild Experiment in a Government Department.* London: Heinemann Educational ISBN 0435825089 References

Book describes research undertaken into the research management system installed following the Rothschild Report in the Department of Health and Social Security. The context for the relationship between government and science are discussed, together with the organisation of the DHSS and the purposes of DHSS research units. The processes of peer and customer review, functions and outcomes of research and the commissioning system are discussed (CR **3.8.3, 3.13**).

3.9 GOVERNMENT AND NURSING RESEARCH – UNITED STATES OF AMERICA/CANADA

Although medical research has taken precedence in the past, nurses are now in the forefront of making governments aware of the importance of investing in nursing research. Governments in both the USA and Canada have contributed to the development of nursing research in various ways, for example by providing funding, establishing research centres and responding to leads from the profession.

Annotations

3.9.1 Brown, B.J. (1985) Past and current status of nursing's role in influencing governmental policy for research training in nursing. IN McCloskey, J.C. & Grace, H.K. (eds) *Current issues in nursing.* 2nd edition Boston: Blackwell Scientific ISBN 086542019X References Part 7 Chapter 51 697-712

History of nurses involvement in legislation in the USA is reviewed together with their current influence. The benefits of involvement, ways in which this may be increased, and the goals for influencing legislation are discussed.

3.9.2 Department of Health and Human Services, Public Health Service, National Institutes of Health (1989) *Report of 1989 NIH Task Force on nursing research.* Bethesda, Maryland: NIH Publication no. 89-487

Report outlines the creation and functioning of the National Centre for Nursing Research, the characteristics of nursing research and the development of a national nursing research agenda. The main part of the report covers extra-mural grant application and award data and intra-mural project data, the implementation plan and update of the 1984 Task Force recommendations, statements of nurse consultants and conclusions and recommendations of the NIH Task Force (CR **3.4.7, 3.4.9**).

3.9.3 Fondiller, S.H. (1986) The American Nurses' Association and National League for Nursing: political relationships and realities. IN White, R. (ed) *Political issues in nursing: past, present and future.* Volume 2 Chichester: Wiley ISBN 0471909130 References Chapter 7 119-143

Chapter documents the history of the ANA and NLN, examines collaboration and conflicts, new structural arrangements, the question of entry to the profession, political activities and the future (CR 3.4.2).

3.9.4 Gortner, S.R. (1986) Impact of the Division of Nursing Research. IN Stinson, S.M. & Kerr, J.C. (eds) *International issues in nursing research.* Beckenham: Croom Helm ISBN 0709944373 References Part 2 Chapter 7 113-130

Chapter describes the historical development of the Division of Nursing Research, support for research, research training, institutional resources, the development of a scientific base for practice and scientific communication through conferences (CR 3.27.7).

3.9.5 Wilmot, V. (1986) Health science policy and health research funding in Canada. IN Stinson, S.M. & Kerr, J.C. (eds) *International issues in nursing research.* Beckenham: Croom Helm ISBN 0709944373 References Part 2 Chapter 5 76-96

Discusses the evolution of science policy in Canada and the problems experienced in health science research. As in the UK bio-medical research commands popular support and the major share of funds. This position is being hotly contested and the passing in 1984 of the Canada Health Act may have important implications for change. Federal expenditure management systems are discussed, as it is change within these which would enable financial support for nursing research to take place (CR 3.10, 3.12, 3.27.7).

3.10 RESEARCH AND POLICY MAKING

Research is essential to the policy makers within governments, and others, who are responsible for planning health care facilities. The nature of research into nursing, with all its complexities, and in the United Kingdom its comparatively short history, has meant that appropriate information has not always been available.

Annotations
3.10.1 Allen, T.H. (1978) *New methods in social science research: policy sciences and futures research.* New York: Praeger ISBN 0275236307 References

Book is written for academics and policy makers and aims to help solve social problems through better policy making which results from new advances in social science methodology. The philosophical groundwork for embarking on novel approaches to social science research is discussed together with new methodologies for effective policy making. These include policy sciences, futures research, the DELTA chart, Delphi technique, cross-impact analysis and policy making with scenarios (CR 2.5, 2.68).

3.10.2   Booth, T. (1988) *Developing policy research.* Aldershot: Avebury   ISBN 0556052164   References

Book serves three purposes, as a textbook on policy research, a sourcebook of examples of the use of social research in the making of policy and as a series of essays on social planning.

3.10.3   Bulmer, M. (ed) (1980) *Social research and Royal Commissions.* London: Allen & Unwin   ISBN 0043510558   References

Aim of this collection of studies is to bring understanding and enable generalisations to be made about the part social science can play in the formulation of public policy. Various reports published following Committees of Inquiry or Royal Commissions are examined in relation to the extent to which they utilised research to inform each project.

3.10.4   Heller, F. (ed) (1986) *The use and abuse of social science.* London: Sage   ISBN 0803980175   References

Book addresses the issue of social science and its uses. A series of successful and unsuccessful applications of research are discussed. Studies have shown that social science research can lead to important developments in policy and practice.

3.10.5   Hinshaw, A.S. (1988) Using research to shape health policy. *Nursing outlook* 36(1) 21-24   11 References

Discusses strategies for using nursing research to shape policy and influence practice.

3.10.6   MacPherson, K.I. (1987) Health care policy, values and nursing. *Advances in nursing science* 9(3) 1-11   40 References

Discusses the major flaws in American health care policy creation which contribute towards inequalities in the system. Nurses are urged to examine their own values when helping to shape policies.

3.10.7   Nuffield Provincial Hospitals Trust (1985) *A fresh look at policies for health services research and its relevance to management.* London: Nuffield Provincial Hospitals Trust   ISBN 0900574526   References

With the increasing complexity of health issues and the necessity to contain expenditure the need to develop objectives is becoming urgent. Without these, adequate and appropriately directed research are unlikely to be achieved. This report is directed mainly at the NHS Management Board which it is hoped will take steps to ensure adequate funding and competent research management.

3.10.8   Pollitt, C., Lewis, L., Negro, J. & Patten, J. (eds) (1979) *Public policy in theory and practice.* Sevenoaks: Hodder and Stoughton in association with the Open University Press   ISBN 0340247797   References

[A reader for Open University Course No. D336 - Policies, People and Administration]

A book of readings which examines the stages in the policy making cycle – formulation, implementation and evaluation. Both theoretical articles and case studies are included and strategic and more local issues are explored.

3.10.9 Robinson, J. & Elkan, R. (1989) *Research for policy and policy for research: a review of selected DHSS funded nurse education research 1975-1986.* Coventry: Nursing Policy Studies Centre, University of Warwick References Nursing Policy Studies 5

Report examines 20 selected studies commissioned by the DHSS into nurse education. The policies relating to commissioning practices at the time are examined to put the studies in context. The reports are examined broadly in terms of the area researched, methods used, their strengths and weaknesses and detailed summaries are included in an appendix. The studies are put in their historical context and the difficulties of the relationship of research to policy is explored. The future of nurse education research is discussed and main issues highlighted (CR 3.8).

3.10.10 Sippert, A. (1981) What makes good research? *British journal of addiction* 76: 9-12   (No references)

A medical administrator in the Department of Health and Social Security examines the ingredients of 'good' research from a policy makers point of view.

3.10.11 Walker, J.F. (1989) Toward a policy for nurse education. *Nurse education today* 9(4) 217-218   2 References   Editorial

Editorial comments on definitions of policy and outlines the findings of a recent review (Robinson & Elkan 1989) of selected DHSS funded nurse education research from 1976-1986. Findings included the lack of a policy orientated research programme (CR 3.10.9).

3.10.12 Walker, R. (1989) We would like to know why: qualitative research and the policy maker. *Research, policy and planning* 7(2) 15-21   48 References

Discusses qualitative research as part of the policy making process. Some objections to this mode of research have been overcome and the contributions it can make are outlined. Policy makers can also be involved in research teams and the advantages of this are discussed.

3.11 RESEARCH IN HEALTH CARE

Health services research is an area where governments spend a considerable amount of money, albeit far less than that spent on defence. The demand for care is undiminished and it is important that nurses play their part in trying to obtain funding to undertake relevant research.

Annotations

3.11.1 Butler, J.R. & Boddy, F.A. (1983) The evolution of health services research in Britain. *Community medicine* 5(3) 192-199   28 References

A historical view of health services research over the last 20 years. In England there has been lack of consistent policies for commissioning and funding research and a system which would allow government to acquire the research it needs (CR 3.8, 3.12).

3.11.2 Grady, K.E. & Wallston, B.S. (1988) *Research in health care settings.* Newbury Park: Sage   ISBN 0803928750   References

Book focuses on the substantive area of research application in health care settings. It aims to increase collaboration between social scientists and practising health care professionals and real life examples are used for illustration. Each chapter concludes with exercises.

3.11.3 Gray, A.M. (1987) *The economics of nursing: a review of the literature.* Coventry: Nursing Policy Studies Unit, University of Warwick   (No ISBN number)   Nursing Policy Studies 2

A comprehensive review of health economics research in nursing. Both historical and contemporary research is covered, much of it from North America together with British and European studies. The calibre of research was frequently found to be poor so works have been selected which are of reasonably high quality (CR 2.12).

3.11.4 Styles, M.M. (1990) A common sense approach to research. *International nursing review* 37(1) 203-206, 218   9 References

Article aims to start a debate about the political significance of knowledge, appropriate paradigms, the presentation of knowledge, power brokers, professional priorities and evaluation.

3.11.5 Taylor, D. (1981) *Health research in England: a topic for debate.* London: Office of Health Economics   References   (No ISBN number)
[Based on the proceedings of a symposium at the Royal College of Obstetricians and Gynaecologists on 11.9.1980]

Discusses the historical background to scientific research in England, the present arrangements, defining health services research and choices for the future. An appendix examines economics and health service research.

3.11.6 Warren, M.D. (1983) Health services research — contracting, conducting and communicating. *Community medicine* 5(3) 200-207   22 References

Discusses the funding of health services research, training and career prospects of researchers, processes of communicating, ensuring the maintenance of standards and the dissemination and utilisation of results. Author suggests that regional and district health authorities should become more involved.

3.11.7 Williams, A. (1983) The practice of health services research. *Community medicine* 5(4) 317-320   No references

An overview of how research is and could be used in the health service. The issue of whether health service research is an academic, political or management activity is addressed as are questions about funding, commissioning research and whether it influences policy making (CR 3.10, 3.12).

3.12 FUNDING FOR RESEARCH

Probably the most crucial issue relating to research is that of the funding which is available. Governments, private institutions, industry and individual donors all have many calls on the funds which they are able and willing to allocate to any particular form of research. Nursing has frequently been fairly low on the list of priorities.

Annotations

3.12.1 Bell, C. (1984) The SSRC:* restructured and defended. IN Bell, C. & Roberts, H. (eds) *Social researching: politics, problems and practice.* London: Routledge & Kegan Paul   ISBN 0710098847   References

Discusses the changes within the Social Science Research Council which affected research funding (CR 2.1.5).

*Now Economic and Social Research Council

3.12.2 Cahoon, M.C. (1987) Nursing research and industry: some current issues. *Recent advances in nursing* 18: 142-153   9 References

Article identifies some of the background to the development of links between nursing research and industry. The implications of this are explored.

3.12.3 Economic and Social Research Council (1986) *Postgraduate studentships in the social sciences.* London: ESRC   ISBN 0862261716

Gives advice on ESRC subjects, eligibility, types of studentships, application procedures for students and departments, terms and conditions, assessment of award and details of relevant forms.

3.12.4 Fineman, S. (1981) Funding research: practice and politics. IN Reason, P. & Rowan, J. (eds) *Human inquiry: a sourcebook of new paradigm research.* Chichester: Wiley   ISBN 0471279358   References   Chapter 40   473-484

Chapter illustrates what has happened to some researchers whose declared epistemology did not meet the usual expectations of 'orthodox' research requirements. Author speculates on the implications of these experiences for research funding (CR 2.11.5).

3.12.5 Hardy, M.A. (1987) The American Nursing Associations influence on federal funding for nursing education, 1941-1984. *Nursing research* 36(1) 31-35   4 Notes and references

Study aimed to identify factors contributing to the enactment of federal funding for nursing education, to describe the development of the ANA legislative programme from 1896-1984, identify the goals and strategies in its attempt to influence funding legislation and examine the results (CR 3.4.2).

3.12.6 Hayward, J.C. & LeLean, S.R. (1986) Research training and funding in the United Kingdom. IN Stinson, S.M. & Kerr, J.C. (eds) *International issues in nursing research.* Beckenham: Croom Helm   ISBN 0709944373   References   Part 3   Chapter 10 168-181

Chapter outlines the initial difficulties nursing experienced in gaining access to universities which hindered the development of a research base. The main sources of research funding are briefly examined − the dual support system, government departments and private sources. An overview of research training is given and the means by which nurses have been enabled to develop these skills − the Study of Nursing Care Project at the Royal College of Nursing, DHSS Research Fellowships and Research Assistantships (CR 3.17, 3.27.7).

3.12.7 Institute of Nursing (1991) *Directory of funding for nurses.* 2nd edition Oxford: Institute of Nursing   References

This directory, which is the first comprehensive publication of its kind, is specifically designed to assist individual nurses seeking funding for research or further education. Information was obtained by questionnaire from grant-making organisations. Those willing to consider giving financial assistance are listed and the following information is included for each entry: purpose of award/grant, eligiblity, projects considered, application and selection procedure, how the grant is administered, the amount of award per annum, restrictions or exclusions and general information.

[Note: The above annotation has kindly been provided by Sharon Withnell, former Administrator at the Institute of Nursing in Oxford. It is anticipated that the directory will be updated annually. The Oxfordshire edition of this book will be of value locally. It is not included in this publication].

3.12.8 Kerr, J.C. (1986) Structure and funding of nursing research in Canada. IN Stinson, S.M. & Kerr, J.C. (eds) *International issues in nursing research.* London: Croom Helm   ISBN 0709944373   References   Part 2   Chapter 6   97-112

Chapter discusses the growth of graduate education and research, federal support, funding for nursing research and the development of research supported by university schools of nursing in Canada (CR 3.27.7).

3.12.9 Kratz, C. (1987) In search of funds. *Nursing times* 83(29) July 22 18-19   1 Reference

Author suggests there is a scarcity of funds available for nursing research although the situation is improving. Some of the organisations which might provide funds are identified.

3.12.10 Lauffer, A. (1984) *Grantmanship and fund raising.* Beverly Hills: Sage   ISBN 0803922345   References

Book covers general fund raising strategies, grantsmanship programme design and resource development. Each chapter begins with a vignette and ends with references and further reading. Although sources mentioned are American it covers useful material for fund seekers in any country.

3.12.11 Lerner, C.A. (ed) (1988) *The grants register.* 1989-1991 11th edition London: Macmillan   ISBN 0333366875

Intended for students at or above graduate level and all who require further professional or advanced vocational training. The following are listed: scholarships, fellowships, research grants, exchange opportunities, grants-in-aid, grants for scientific projects, professional and vocational awards and special awards.

3.12.12 Margolin, J.B. (1983) *The individual's guide to grants.* New York: Plenum Press   ISBN 0306413094   References

Book is designed to assist individual grant seekers to obtain funding and it covers all aspects of the process. Although written for an American audience it would also be useful for those in other countries.

3.12.13 *Maws midwives research scholarship*, in conjunction with the Royal College of Midwives

Scholarship is awarded for research into any aspect of midwifery practice, education or management within the midwifery service. It may be used towards the cost of a course which includes research methodology and a project.

[Source: Information leaflet from the Director of Education, The Royal College of Midwives Trust, 15, Mansfield Street, London W1M 0BE].

3.12.14 National Centre for Nursing Research (1989) *Facts about funding.* Bethesda, Maryland: Office of Information and Legislative Affairs   ISSN 3014960207

Document, which is based on a range of frequently asked questions, provides information on the types of research training supported by the National Centre for Nursing Research. The structure and application procedures within the National Institutes of Health are explained (CR 3.4.7, 3.4.9, 3.9.2).

3.12.15 National Florence Nightingale Committee of Great Britain and Northern Ireland (no date) *Chairman's annual report*, List of donations and statement of accounts 1989   8-13

Lists holders of 1989 awards and their topics of study.

3.12.16 Office of Health Economics (1986) *Crisis in research.* London OHE ISSN 04738837

Expresses concern about the UK government's funding of research. It is noted, for example, that 50% of available funding is allocated to defence. Comparisons are made with funds available in other countries. There is specific discussion about funding given to the Medical Research Council. A résumé of progress made in drug research over the last 50 years is included.

3.12.17 Parahoo, K. (1988) Funding nursing research. *Senior nurse* 8(9/10) 12-14   16 References

Nursing research is under threat due to shortage of available funds as it seems unable to compete for the dwindling resources. Nurses, it is suggested, need to become more politically and financially pro-active in order to secure the future development of nursing research and hence nursing itself.

3.12.18 Peden, H. & Hills, P. (1983) *Sources of funding for research and publication.* Leicester: Leicester University of Primary Communications Centre   ISBN 0906083249

Booklet provides information on organisations giving grants for writing, publication and research. Includes organisations giving funds for other means of disseminating research findings.

3.12.19 Salter, B. (1985) The funding market for nursing research. *Journal of advanced nursing* 10(2) 155-163   20 References

Nursing research relies too heavily on government funding and it is suggested that other sources of financial support should be explored. Seven possible sources are mentioned and advice is given on how nursing might compete in the funding marketplace.

3.12.20 Tierney, A.J. (1989) Grantsmanship: resources for nursing research. *Senior nurse* 9(2) 9   5 References

The art of successful fund raising is discussed and nurses are urged to develop the skill of writing good research proposals.

Suggested textbook readings

	Pages	Cross reference
Abdellah & Levine	309-354	2.1.1
Burns & Grove	383-408	2.1.12
Hakim	156-170	2.21.1
Locke, Spirduso & Silverman	109-119	2.99.6
Miller D.C.	461-480	2.56.3
Payne et al	253-276	2.36.10
Tripp-Reimer & Cohen IN Morse (1989)	225-238	2.36.8

Nursing research abstracts

Association of Researchers
  in Medical Science   81/280
Brittain R.D.   81/130
Hockey L.   82/424
Rogers J. & Scott E.   82/427

3.13 NURSING RESEARCH UNITS/CENTRES/DEPARTMENTS

Probably one of the major ways in which a consistent research programme can be carried out is for units, centres or departments in colleges, polytechnics or universities to establish their priorities, and obtain private funding or be financed by government sources. Staff members will usually be engaged in research as well as having teaching commitments, and students will be in the process of receiving research training, frequently for higher degrees.

Annotations

3.13.1 Carr, P. (1981) The centre for research into psychiatric nursing. *Nurse education today* (5)1 11   8 References

Briefly explains why the centre for research into psychiatric nursing was established and outlines its staffing, philosophy and purpose.

3.13.2 Cox, C. (1979) The Nursing Education Research Unit: the early days. *Nursing times* 75(18) May 3 747-749

Describes the early development of the Nursing Education Research Unit at Chelsea College, University of London in terms of its structure, policies and projects (CR 3.13.3, 3.13.13, 3.13.23).

3.13.3 Cox, C. (1981) The pros and cons of having a nurse education research unit in a university. *Journal of advanced nursing* 6(3) 237-238   Janforum

Former director of the nursing research unit in London University highlights the factors which encourage the development of research, and outlines the different nature of research work which necessitates much support from colleagues. The problem of fixed-term contracts is noted (CR 3.13.2, 3.13.13, 3.13.23).

3.13.4 Daphne Heald Research Unit (1989) *Report for 1989.* London: Royal College of Nursing of the United Kingdom

Briefly describes development of the unit, its organisation, staff development and chosen focus, which is the care received by patients and ways of assessing this outcome. Studies carried out include two relating to the work of clinical nurse specialists in stoma care and diabetes; the care of patients with sickle cell disease; the effects of early discharge of patients following surgery and some methodological studies. The future of the units programme and staff in relation to the Royal College of Nursing are briefly outlined. A list of publications and conference papers is included.

3.13.5   Department of Nursing, University of Manchester (1990) *Departmental Research Activities.* Manchester: University of Manchester

Publication provides a report on research work being undertaken by the Department of Nursing at the University of Manchester. A Departmental profile is given, staff activities, publications and details of the research being undertaken. Contracted research comes under the following broad areas: education, human resources and practice activities; families, health and illness; AIDS/HIV and research associated with international matters. Research scholarships are included together with associated developments (CR 3.13.15, 3.13.16).

3.13.6   Dienemann, J. (1987) Nursing research centres: a survey of their prevalence, functions and school characteristics. *International journal of nursing studies* 24(1) 35-44   28 References

Reports a survey conducted to establish the number of research centres in schools of nursing with graduate programmes, their functions and productivity. Comparisons were made with schools with no research centres and the implications of this discussed.

3.13.7   Goodman, C., Wright, D., Hall, D. & McLoughlin, C. (1984) Luxury or necessity? *Senior nurse* 1(30) October 24   11-12   7 References

Describes the setting up of a nursing research unit within a district health authority which was not linked to an academic department. The unit's staffing and function is described and examples of projects given. The financial viability and usefulness of such a unit is discussed.

3.13.8   Gortner, S.R. (1982) Researchmanship: structures for research productivity. *Western journal of nursing research* 4(1) 119-123   9 References

Resources for research, time, money, tools and personnel are discussed. The organisational structure within one university is described.

3.13.9   Hinshaw, A.S. (1988) The new National Centre for Nursing Research: patient care research programmes. *Applied nursing research* 1(1) 2-4   3 References

Outlines the functions of the National Centre for Nursing Research established in 1986 and gives details of the major research areas within its programmes. These are health promotion/disease prevention; acute and chronic illness research and nursing systems/special programmes. Discusses future initiatives of the centre including the development of a national research agenda, and ways in which interdisciplinary collaboration can be fostered (CR 3.4.7, 3.4.9, 3.9.2, 3.28).

3.13.10   Hockey, L. (1981) The pros and cons of having a nursing research unit in a university. *Journal of advanced nursing* 6(3) 235-237   Janforum

A personal view of the difficulties and potential of research in a university setting. The importance of including health service staff in discussion and educational programmes is stressed.

3.13.11   International Council of Nurses (1984) Survey of nursing research units. *International nursing review* 31(4) 116-121

Survey identified resources available for nursing research throughout the world and highlighted three major problem areas – funding, staff/faculty/students and general factors which hinder development.

3.13.12   International Council of Nurses (1990) *Directory of nursing research units.* 2nd edition Geneva: ICN   (No ISBN number)   ICN/89/202

Directory cites 115 nursing research units worldwide which were identified by national nurses associations in membership with the International Council of Nurses. Information included is unit name and address, contact person, type of setting, number of professional staff, disciplines included, research activities and support, and conducted research. The latter are reported under the following categories: recipients of care, nursing practice, theory, education, research on nurses, organisations, management and administration and research methodology. Also included are methodological approaches used, additional research activities, and whether consultancy is provided to outside professionals with or without fees (CR 1.4.12, 3.24).

3.13.13   King's College, University of London, Nursing Research Unit (1989/ 1990) *Research programme.* (Personal communication – Letter from Dr S.J.Redfern, Director of Nursing Research Unit, King's College, University of London 23.4.1990)

Papers include details of the Unit's approach to research, the projects which are being undertaken, the use of computers and other activities of the staff. The 1990 research programme includes a study relating to the role and education of the nurse in relation to the prevention and management of violence; career patterns of midwives, career patterns of nurses and midwives; the relationship between the system of ward organisation and the practice of individualised nursing care and the reliability of quality assessment measures (CR 3.13.2, 3.13.3, 3.13.23).

3.13.14   Journal of Advanced Nursing (1989) Foundation of Nursing Studies: major new resource for nursing in the UK. *Journal of advanced nursing* 14(10) 803-804   Editorial

Outlines the aims of this charity set up to validate and act upon research findings which will be used to improve patient care in the UK. Brief details are given of the first project to be undertaken.

[Note: Investigations have shown that this organisation no longer exists]

3.13.15   McFarlane of Llandaff, Baroness, J. (1980) Nursing as a research-based profession. *Nursing times* 76(13) May 15 57-59   Occasional Paper   15 References

A strong case is made for nursing practice to be research based. The growth of studies with a clinical focus is discussed together with ways in which nurses may learn how to develop research awareness. Activities based in the Department of Nursing at the University of Manchester are described which assist in its development as a resource centre (CR 3.13.5).

3.13.16 McFarlane of Llandaff, Baroness, J. (1981) The contribution of research to the understanding of nursing. *Journal of advanced nursing* 6(3) 231-235   7 References   Janforum

Discusses some of the ways in which the Department of Nursing at Manchester University has tried to deepen the understanding of nursing through various research activities (CR 3.13.5, 3.13.15).

3.13.17 Nursing Policy Studies Centre (1988) *Quadrennial report 1985-1988.* Coventry: Nursing Policy Studies Centre, University of Warwick NPSU   Reference 3 (28)

Describes work of the centre in its first quadrennium which concentrated on examining major nursing policy issues. These included studies related to the Griffiths Report, literature reviews on the economics of nursing and an examination of selected DHSS commissioned nursing education research from 1975 to 1986. A further study examined the role of the support worker in the ward health care team. Report lists publications, other consultancies and conference papers given by staff (CR 3.10.9, 3.11.3).

[The Nursing Policy Studies Centre ceased to exist in September 1989 and the tradition has been transfered to the University of Nottingham]

3.13.18 Nursing Practice Research Unit (1987) *Nursing Practice Research Unit, Report on development, January 1984–December 1986.* Guildford: University of Surrey

Report describes overall direction of the research programme which examined pressure sores, urinary tract infections and the measurement of nursing care. Also included are a statisticians report, supplementary research activities and other unit programmes. Publications and other papers given are listed.

  Research programme's remit has been widened and these are hospital acquired infection, prevention and treatment of chronic wounds, the organisation and delivery of nursing care, focussing on primary nursing, and clinical decision making. The financial and other costs of patient care are being examined and ways of targetting resources appropriately.

[Update of unit's activities − material as yet unpublished (Personal communication − Letter from Professor Rosemary Crow, Nursing Practice Research Unit, University of Surrey, Guildford March 1990)]

3.13.19 Nursing Research Unit, Department of Nursing Studies, University of Edinburgh (1988) *Ninth biennial report 1987-1988.* Edinburgh: Nursing Research Unit

Report includes information on the staff, their appointments and memberships, the units core programme, other research projects, educational activities, reports/papers presented, international visitors and visits. A list of reports from the core research programme is included (CR 3.13.20).

3.13.20 Prophit, P. (1984) Another chapter. *Nursing mirror* 159(20) November 28 26-28   No references

The 7th report of the Nursing Research Unit at the University from January 1983 to August 1984 documents the work undertaken by unit staff and students. This comprises a major project to establish clinical nursing research priorities in Scotland using the Delphi technique. The courses run by the unit are noted together with staff changes (CR 2.68, 3.13.19, 3.23).

3.13.21 University of Newcastle upon Tyne, Health Care Research Unit (1990) *Report: January 1989 to December 1989.* Newcastle upon Tyne: Health Care Research Unit

Describes the work of this unit and includes information on its staff, publications, current and proposed Department of Health funded projects, and other activities undertaken.

3.13.22 White, D.L. & Hamel, P.K. (1986) National Centre for Nursing Research: how it came to be. *Nursing economics* 4(1) 19-22   7 References

Describes the strategies adopted by a group of nurses to get nursing research on the national agenda in the USA. This resulted in legislation being amended and the establishment of a national centre for nursing research (CR 3.4.7, 3.4.9).

3.13.23 Wilson-Barnett, J. & Robinson, S. (eds) (1989) Developments in nursing research at King's College, London University. IN Wilson-Barnett, J. & Robinson, S. *Directions in nursing research: ten years of progress at London University.* London: Scutari Press   ISBN 1871364213   Chapter 1   1-7

Chapter outlines the developments in nursing research conducted at King's College since 1977 in the Department of Health funded Nursing Research Unit and Department of Nursing Studies. Research directions and strategies are outlined together with information on studies included in the book. These come under four major headings – the delivery of care, the consumers perspective, preparation for practice, aspects of basic and post-basic education and career paths of nurses and midwives (CR 3.13.2, 3.13.3, 3.13.13).

Nursing research abstracts

Alderman C.	82/281
Altschul A.T.	82/282
Goodman C. et al	85/0234
Hockey L.	82/3, 82/54

ROLE OF THE UNITED KINGDOM STATUTORY BODIES IN RESEARCH

3.14 ROLE OF THE UNITED KINGDOM STATUTORY BODIES IN RESEARCH

The United Kingdom Central Council and the four National Boards of England, Northern Ireland, Scotland and Wales were set up under the Nurses, Midwives and Health Visitors Act of 1979. The Central Council is required to establish and improve standards of training and professional conduct and to maintain a register of qualified practitioners. The National Boards are required to make provision for training in their respective countries. Research provides a vital underpinning to all nursing activities and each body has developed strategies for this.

Annotations
3.14.1 **English National Board for Nursing, Midwifery and Health Visiting** (1983) *The end of the beginning September 1980 — September 1983.* London: English National Board   Part 3   10   Research policy

Outlines the deliberations of the ENB Research Working Group in terms of its strategy, research programme, funding and the future of the Board's research activities.

3.14.2 **English National Board for Nursing, Midwifery and Health Visiting** (1989) *Annual Report 1988-1989.* London: English National Board   12

Briefly reports on the projects in which the Board is involved. These are open/distance learning materials for Enrolled Nurse conversion courses, the effect on learning and teaching on the movement of care from institutions to the community and the evaluation of Project 2000 implementation.

3.14.3 **National Board for Nursing, Midwifery and Health Visiting for Northern Ireland** (1989) *Sixth annual report.* Belfast: The National Board   2.19 31-32

Reports activities of the Research Group which included guidelines for nurses undertaking research and research ethical committees, interim report on a project which aimed to establish attitudes towards research, first and second line priorities, higher education related to research needs, annual awards for students of nursing/midwifery, the research element in Project 2000 nurse training and liason with the Health and Social Services Board (CR 2.17, 3.12, 3.17, 3.19).

3.14.4 **National Board for Nursing, Midwifery and Health Visiting for Scotland** (1989) *Annual report 1988-1989.* Edinburgh: National Board for Scotland   23

Reports the deliberations of one meeting where the Research Advisory Group clarified its role and reviewed its remit. A new allocation procedure for awarding funds has been agreed (CR 3.12).

3.14.5 United Kingdom Central Council (1983) *Nursing research: the role of the UKCC.* London: United Kingdom Central Council

Booklet outlines the role of the UKCC in relation to research and a series of recommendations are made by its Research Committee. The ideas were provisional and aimed to facilitate the work of others.

3.14.6 United Kingdom Central Council (1990) *Nurse selection project.* Leeds: School of Education, University of Leeds (Personal communication from project director, Senior Research Fellow, Dr Carol Borrill 10.5 1990)

The UKCC are currently funding two main projects. The first is a validation study of the DC Test Series which compares the performance of DC Test and O level entrants to nursing throughout their training. The second project is examining alternative entry routes to nursing.

3.14.7 Welsh National Board for Nursing , Midwifery and Health Visiting (1989) *Annual report 1988-1989.* Cardiff: Welsh National Board   2:1 (i)   17

Reports on one meeting of the Research Advisory Group during which members considered the lack of statistics relating to the outcome and use of nursing graduates in Wales. The Welsh National Board validated research course was discussed, together with reports of study days and conferences. The group also discussed its own future.

PROFESSIONAL ASSOCIATIONS/SOCIETIES/GROUPS

3.15   PROFESSIONAL ASSOCIATIONS/SOCIETIES/GROUPS

Professional associations, societies and groups have played many important roles in the development of nursing research, and continue to do so both locally, nationally and internationally.

Annotations

3.15.1   Allen, D.G. (1987) The social policy statement: a reappraisal. *Advances in nursing science* 10(1) 39-48   34 References

A statement by the American Nurses Association has emerged as a pivotal document in nursing. This article explores and analyses many of the assertions made. It examines the definition of nursing and discusses whether nursing may want to support the view it portrays (CR 3.4.2).

3.15.2   Clinical Nurses Association (no date) *Aims and organisation.* (Personal communication from Mary Walker, Association Secretary − 20.6.1990)

Paper briefly outlines the role of the association, its aims, membership, organisation and conferences.

3.15.3   College of Nursing, Australia (1989) *Annual report 1988.* Melbourne: College of Nursing   15

Reports the development of a national nursing research network which consists of a database, and nurses who are willing to advise less experienced colleagues.

3.15.4   Commonwealth Nurses Federation (1989) *Commonwealth Nurses Federation newsletters* 9 & 10 March and November 1989   ISSN 02684063 1(4)   6

Federation does not itself hold funds for research, but encourages member states to 'support the development of research on more efficient and effective methods of using nursing and midwifery resources, including training in research methodology'.

3.15.5   Houston, M. & Weatherson, L. (1986) Creating change in midwifery: integrating theory and practice through practice-based research groups. *Midwifery* 2(2) 65-70   12 References

Discusses the links between practice, education and research in midwifery. The processes involved in the development of two midwifery research and discussion groups in the United Kingdom and Canada are outlined.

3.15.6   International Council of Nurses (1985) *Guidelines for nursing research development.* Geneva: International Council of Nurses

Booklet offers guidelines for national nurses associations and other institutions about the development of nursing research. These come under the major headings of appraisal of the organisational climate for research, organisation, resources, research programmes and the role of national nurses associations. Appendices A and B give brief guidance on the development of research proposals (CR 2.99).

3.15.7   King Edward's Hospital Fund for London (1990) *Annual report 1989.* London: King Edward's Hospital Fund   (No ISBN number)

Report includes information on the Grant's Committees allocations of money for various projects, including research. The Fund's priorities are listed (CR 3.12).

3.15.8   LeLean, S.R. & Clarke, M. (1990) Research resource development in the UK. *International journal of nursing studies* 27(2) 123-138

Amongst other developments, this article briefly traces the history of the Royal College of Nursing Research Society from a research interest discussion group to an active society. It has prepared ethical guidelines and a paper on research-mindedness, and holds an annual conference (CR 2.17.42, 3.15.13, 3.18.40, 3.26).

3.15.9 Queens Nursing Institute (1990) *Annual report 1989.* London: Queens Nursing Institute

Reports that the Queens Nursing Institute in Scotland awarded two research fellowships, and agreed to fund the Institute's centenary Readership in District Nursing at Glasgow College.

3.15.10   Royal College of Midwives (1990) *Annual report 1989.* London: Royal College of Midwives

Reports college activities related to research. These include a research and midwifery conference; evidence given to the Royal College of Physicians on research on patients; committee involvement in other bodies and publication of a booklet on writing research proposals and applying for funding (CR 2.99.10).

3.15.11   Royal College of Nursing History of Nursing Society (1989) *Information leaflet.* London: Royal College of Nursing

Members of this group aim to promote the study of nursing history and provide a forum for interested nurses. They also give help and guidance to other researchers. The preservation of historical material is actively encouraged together with the creation of oral history archives.

3.15.12   Royal College of Nursing Research Advisory Group (1991) *Activities.* (Source − RCN Diary 1991 35-36)

Group formed in 1989 as a move on from the Royal College of Nursing Research Society which was founded in 1959. It provides assistance to nurses without research skills and a forum for discussion of methodological and other issues. The group organises two colloquia a year and an annual research conference. Two special interest groups are computers in nursing and pain research.

3.15.13 Royal College of Nursing Research Society (Scotland) *Activities.* (Personal communication - letter from Dr.Alison Tierney, Chairman of the Society 19.3.1990)

Society was set up in 1983 and its main activity was to organise an annual symposium. In 1989 a symposium was held to relaunch the society and plans are being made for activities which will promote research in nursing in a variety of ways.

3.15.14 Simpson, M. (1985) The place of the Royal College of Nursing Research Discussion Group/Society in the development of research in nursing. IN Proceedings from the 7th Workgroup Meeting, 2nd Open Conference of the Workgroup of European Nurse Researchers: *Nursing research − does it make a difference?* 10-13th April 1984 London: Royal College of Nursing ISBN 0902606891 References 91-95

Briefly documents the history of the society to date and discusses the role of government, education for research, funding, publication of research results, and its relationship with the Royal College of Nursing (CR 2.101, 3.8, 3.12, 3.15.11, 3.26.4).

3.15.15 Whyte, L. (1984) For all those interested. *Senior nurse* 1(30) October 24 12-13

Describes the establishment of a research interest group for trained and student nurses within Leeds Eastern Health Authority. Its aims and objectives are described, as are the methods used to advertise the group and the staff's responses.

Nursing research abstracts
Fairbrother C.   83/3

RESEARCH ROLES/CAREERS

3.16 RESEARCH ROLES/CAREERS

There are a variety of roles which exist in relation to research and all are important to ensure that professional practice is based on firm foundations. Some nurses will conduct research themselves, others will facilitate this process and most nurses will be informed consumers.

Annotations

3.16.1 Armitage, S. (1987) Research liason in Wales. *Senior nurse* 7(5) 46-47   1 Reference

The establishment of the post of research liason nurse in Wales is described. The role, major responsibilities and the difficulties are outlined, as are the developments and progress made towards finding solutions to some of the problems.

3.16.2 Bishop, V. (1984) A caring way to research. *Nursing mirror* 159(4) August 8 26-27

The research sister in an anaesthetic department writes about her role, professional history and how her research interests were kindled.

3.16.3 Closs, J. (1990) Regrading: how do nurse researchers fit in? *Senior nurse* 10(5) 8   2 References

Discusses some of the problems nurse researchers face in the recently introduced clinical grading structure where such skills are regarded as only a minor component within the job.

3.16.4 Cormack, D.F.S. (ed) (1990) *Developing your career in nursing.* London: Chapman & Hall   ISBN 0412321300   References

A practical text giving advice on how to plan one's career. Several sections in the book cover aspects of nursing research and nurse researchers.

3.16.5 Dennis, K.E. & Strickland, O.L. (1987) The clinical nurse researcher: institutionalising the role. *International journal of nursing studies* 24(1) 25-33   6 References

Study examined the implementation of the role of clinical nurse researcher in the clinical setting. three types of roles are identified − dual, collaborative and functional. Ways of generating support for such nurses is discussed together with future directions of these roles.

3.16.6   Flitton, D. (1984) *Nurse researchers in the UK in 1980: research activity in relation to employment.* Edinburgh: Nursing Research Unit, Department of Nursing Studies, University of Edinburgh   (No ISBN number)   References

Reports a survey undertaken as part of a core programme of research which explored various aspects of communication in nursing. Its aims were to describe the location of nurse researchers geographically and area of employment; to compare their activities; the presence or absence of a job description requiring research activity; their involvement in research; academic qualifications; whether they were working alone or in a team and the sources of funding. The study also examined the adequacy of communicating research findings and gave suggestions for improvement.

3.16.7   Hamilton, G. (1986) Two faces of nurse faculty: teacher and researcher. *Journal of advanced nursing* 11(2) 217-223   31 References

Author suggests that nurse educators occupy multiple roles, practitioner, teacher and researcher. The latter two are examined in detail, in particular the reasons why little research is carried out by teachers (CR 3.19).

3.16.8   Harrison, L.L. & Kitchens, E.K. (1989) Implementing the research facilitator role. *Nurse educator* 14(5) 21-26   28 References

Reviews the literature relating to research facilitation and describes the author's experiences in planning, implementing and evaluating this role in two schools of nursing. The implications of this are also discussed.

3.16.9   Hockey, L., Johnson, R. & Laing, E. (1983) Look, learn, listen. *Nursing mirror* 157(2) July 13 21-22   2 References

Describes a survey which aimed to replicate one undertaken in Canada. It examined the role of nurse researchers in establishing communication networks for informing the profession about research findings (CR 2.13, 2.101).

3.16.10   Hollshwander, C.H., Kinsey, D. & Paradowski, M. (1984) Teacher-practitioner-researcher. *Nursing and health care* 5(3) 144-149   7 References

Describes the processes undertaken in a development programme for the creation of posts where the roles of teacher, practitioner and researcher are combined.

3.16.11   Hoyt, D.P. & Spangler, R.K. (1976) Faculty research involvement and instructional outcomes. *Research in higher education* 4: 113-122   13 References

Investigates the dual role of teacher and researcher and seeks to identify whether this is supportive or incompatible.

3.16.12   Jordan, S. (1990) Look before you leap: becoming a nurse researcher. *Nursing times* 86(11) March 14-20 42   (No References)

Discusses some aspects of the role of a clinical nurse researcher.

3.16.13 Kirchhoff, K.T. (1988) Nurse researchers in clinical settings. IN National Centre for Nursing Research, State of the science invitational conference: *The delivery of patient care.* 18-19 February 1988 Bethesda, Maryland: National Institute of Health NIH Publication Number 89-3008 35-37

Reports a study which aimed to document the range of activities, funding and responsibilities currently associated with the role of clinical nurse researchers. Other elements of their role were explored and comparisons made with those of chief nurse executives.

3.16.14 Lambert, C.E. & Lambert, V.A. (1988) Clinical nursing research: its meaning to the practical nurse. *Applied nursing research* 1(2) 54-57   18 References

Clinical nursing research is examined, together with its meaning, significance, who does it and how it is utilised by clinical nurses.

3.16.15 Lancaster, A. (1977) The Nursing Research Liason Officer scheme. *Nursing times* 73(45) November 10 1759-1761   3 References

A description of how and why the scheme was started and the role of the liason officer.

3.16.16 Mayer, G.G. (1983) The clinical nurse-researcher: role-taking and role-making. IN Chaska N.L. *The nursing profession: a time to speak.* New York: McGraw Hill   ISBN 0070106967   References   Chapter 17 216-224

The role of the clinical nurse-researcher is explored and suggestions made about its further development. Strategies for obtaining support are put forward as well as ways in which role ambiguity may be reduced. A suggested job description is included (CR 3.6.2).

3.16.17 Medical Research Council (no date) *The Medical Research Council's General Practice Research Framework.* London: Medical Research Council

Paper describes the Medical Research Council's General Practice Framework which was set up originally for a mild hypertension trial, but may also be used for other studies. The advantages and disadvantages of the framework are discussed. Mention is made of the role of practice research nurses.

3.16.18 Oberst, M.T. (1985) Integrating research and clinical practice roles. *Topics in clinical nursing* 7(2) 45-53   22 References

Paper argues the need for more clinical specialists to undertake research in order to improve the quality of care. It discusses the attitudes and abilities necessary, the organisational climate and resources, obstacles and strategies for overcoming them and progress towards an integrated model (CR 3.7).

3.16.19 Sweeney, M.A. (1985) Clinical nursing research: exposing the myths. IN McCloskey, J.C. & Grace, H.K. (eds) *Current issues in nursing.* 2nd edition Boston: Blackwell Scientific   ISBN 086542019X   References   Part 2   Chapter 13 161-181

Chapter challenges some of the assumptions made about the role of clinical nursing researcher and who should be engaged in doing it. Artificial distinctions between different types of research has led to the compartmentalisation of ideas which have the potential to limit progress. The following are briefly discussed: research is a must for everyone; doctorates will solve everything; beware of collaborative projects; publication is the be-all and end-all and quantitative studies and experimental designs are the only way to go (CR 2.15).

3.16.20   Wilson-Barnett, J., Corner, J. & DeCarle, B. (1990) Integrating research and practice: the role of the researcher as teacher. *Journal of advanced nursing* 15(5) 621-625   20 References

Two recent studies are examined to show how researchers can assist practitioners in developing some research skills by working in close co-operation. This model is suggested as the way forward for increasing research based practice.

EDUCATION FOR RESEARCH

3.17 GOVERNMENT/STATUTORY BODIES TRAINING FELLOWSHIPS, STUDENTSHIPS AND AWARDS

Each year there are a few opportunities for nurses to obtain funding to undertake research from government sources, or in Scotland from the National Board. These are advertised nationally in the professional press, local newspapers or notified via government Health Circulars.

Funding agencies differ in their requirements for acceptance and nurses should write directly to the body concerned for detailed information.

[Permission has kindly been granted from the Department or Board concerned to include the information in this section.]

Annotations
3.17.1 Department of Health and Social Security (now the Department of Health) (1988) *Management services: arrangements for locally organised and clinical research in the NHS*. Health Circular (88)6

Circular describes arrangements for locally organised research in the NHS and Health Authorities responsibilities regarding clinical research promoted by the Medical Research Council.

Nurses may apply to their Regional Nursing Department for further information.

3.17.2 Department of Health and Social Security (now the Department of Health) (1990) *Nursing Research Studentship and Post-Doctoral Nursing Fellowship.* (Personal communication – Letter from E.J.C. Scott, Research Management Division, Department of Health, London – 1.3.1990)

'In 1967 the DHSS established the Nursing Research Fellowship scheme with the primary objective of assisting the development of a research expertise within the nursing profession. Over the years the organisation of these awards has been modified to meet changing needs in both the nursing and research communities. Currently two types of awards are made annually, these are:

Post-doctoral nursing fellowship
Nursing research studentship

The aim of both these schemes is to promote the development of individual nurse's experience of and expertise in health services research'

The advertisements inviting applications for these awards are published during November/December each year in the professional press. Detailed information on the application procedure may be obtained by writing to Research Management

Division, Department of Health, Alexander Fleming House, Elephant and Castle, London SE1 6BY.

3.17.3 Department of Health and Social Services, Northern Ireland (1990) *Clinical research grants*. (Personal communication — letter from W.J. Allen, Deputy Chief Nursing Officer in the Department of Health and Social Services, Northern Ireland — 8.3.1990).

The Nursing Research Studentship Scheme is at present under review, and it is likely that a new scheme offering a more flexible mode will be introduced for the next academic year.

Detailed information may be obtained from The Admissions Officer, University of Ulster, Cromore Road, Coleraine BT52 1SA

3.17.4 National Board for Nursing, Midwifery and Health Visiting for Northern Ireland (1989) *Annual report*. Belfast: The National Board 2.19   Research Group 5

The Research Group of the Board offer an annual award for students of nursing/midwifery which takes the form of a prize essay competition on research related topics.

3.17.5 National Board for Nursing, Midwifery and Health Visiting for Scotland (1990) *General Nursing Council for Scotland (Education) Fund 1983: Guidelines to applicants for awards for research projects and study tours*. Edinburgh: NBS (Personal communication — Letter from M.C. Grubb, Professional Adviser (Nursing) 21.3.1990)

Awards are available to qualified nurses resident in Scotland and these are advertised annually in the nursing press in October/November.

The Board wishes to offer the awards for the following purposes:

(i)   innovative, small scale research projects related to nurse and midwife education, or clinical practice
(ii) pilot studies possibly leading to further full scale research studies
(iii) study tours resulting in a report of relevance to the National Board
(iv) study tours undertaken for the purpose of gathering data to facilitate the development of a pilot programme at a later date.

Detailed information may be obtained from Miss K. Reynolds, Records Officer and advice for non-experienced researchers from Mrs. M. Grubb, Professional Adviser, National Board for Nursing, Midwifery and Health Visiting for Scotland, 22 Queen Street, Edinburgh EH2 1JX.

3.17.6 Scottish Home and Health Department (1990) *SHHD Research Training Fellowships*. Edinburgh: SHHD (Personal communication — Letter from Dr. M.O. Clark, Chief Scientist Office 12.3.1990.)

The aim of this scheme is to provide opportunities for all health professions to learn about and gain experience in research by undertaking a supervised study. General priority areas have been designated by the Chief Scientist Committee although any subject relevant to health or the health services will be considered.

The advertisements for these awards usually appear in late December/January and detailed information may be obtained from Dr. M.O.Clark, Scottish Home and Health Department, St. Andrew's House, Edinburgh EH1 3DE.

3.17.7 Welsh Office (1991) (Personal communication from Dr D.M. Keyzer, Nursing Division, Welsh Office, Cathay's Park, Cardiff CF1 3NQ 17.4.1991).

'The Nursing Division commissions research studies through the Welsh Office's call on the Department of Health's Health and Personal Social Services research budget. Similarly, nurses in Wales can apply for the Department of Health's scholarships/fellowships' (CR 3.17.2).

3.17.8 Welsh Scheme for the Development of Health and Social Research (1991) Notes for applicants.

The aims of this scheme are to provide opportunities for individuals to undertake studies relevant to every-day practice, or enable the development of research expertise. All health care professionals, including nurses, who are in contract with a health authority may apply for funding.
Information and application forms may be obtained from: The Secretary, Welsh Scheme for the Development of Health and Social Research, University of Wales College of Medicine, Heath Park, Cardiff CF4 4XN.

3.18 TEACHING NURSING RESEARCH

The process of teaching nursing research is best begun during basic training, in order that students can link it with practice right from the beginning. Some students initially find it difficult to see its relevance to nursing practice but the teacher's skills should help to overcome this.

Annotations
3.18.1 Akinsanya, J.A. (1988) Nursing research: a demystifying process. *Nurse education today* 8(5) 284-288   21 References

Paper describes attempts made to introduce nurses to the research process at basic and post-basic levels. Learners followed the process through to publication and dissemination. Tutors are urged to bring research to the centre of all learning activities.

3.18.2 Allen, M. (1986) The relationship between graduate teaching and research in nursing. IN Stinson, S.M. & Kerr, J.C. (eds) *International issues in nursing research.* Beckenham: Croom Helm ISBN 0709944373 References Part 3   Chapter 9   151-167

Chapter examines the relationship between graduate teaching and the growth of nursing science. The development of nursing research in Canada is described and the conditions which need to be created to ensure the growth of practice related studies (CR 3.27.7).

3.18.3 Altschul, A.T. (1981) The problems of safeguarding the community's interest if students are doing research. *Journal of advanced nursing* 6(3) 239 Janforum

Discusses the problems of allowing access to patients for collecting data. Author suggests that undergraduate students can use each other as subjects and collect data during the course of their practice which can subsequently be used in class exercises. Masters students are required to develop an extended research proposal for their dissertation (CR 2.17).

3.18.4 Armitage, S. & Rees, C. (1988) Student projects: a practical framework. *Nurse education today* 8(5) 289-295   13 References

Guidelines are given to enable teachers and students avoid some of the pitfalls which may be experienced when undertaking project work. A practical framework is suggested based on each major stage within any project.

3.18.5 Bamisaiye, A. (1986) A short course in research methods. *International nursing review* 33(3) Issue 267 74-75

The first short course for senior nurses in West Africa is described. Its particular focus was on health services research in primary health care.

3.18.6 Beck, C.T. (1988) Review of strategies for teaching nursing research 1979-1986. *Western journal of nursing research* 10(2) 222-225   26 References

Reviews column in Western Journal of Nursing Research entitled 'Strategies for Teaching Nursing Research'. It is presented in chart form for easy reference.

3.18.7 Beckingham, C. (1988) Nursing research: some guidelines for practitioners. *International nursing review* 35(6) Issue 282 169-171,174

Author identifies the divisions which exist within the nursing profession in relation to nurses preparation. She believes that research based on an area of practice could be a uniting factor particularly in the search for cost cutting programmes.

3.18.8 Bond, S. (1982) The research component in SRN education. *Nurse education today* 2(2) 5-10   8 References

Results of a survey of the research element in basic nursing courses are presented. The findings from two regions are compared and discussed, one of which had a Nursing Research Liason Officer (NRLO). The importance of this aspect of the curriculum, suggestions for its development, education of nurse teachers and the role of the NRLO are discussed (CR 3.16).

3.18.9 Bzdek, V.M. & Ganong, L.H. (1986) Teaching the research process through participatory learning. *Nurse educator* 11(6) 24-28   13 References

A method of teaching is described which introduced basic research concepts and the research process. It was found to compare favourably with previous methods.

3.18.10   Centre for Applied Health Studies, University of Ulster (1989) *Attitudes towards nursing research: report of a survey of the views of nursing service and education staff in Northern Ireland.* Belfast: The National Board for Nursing, Midwifery and Health Visiting   Occasional Paper OP/NB/1/90

Study commissioned by the National Board for Northern Ireland which examined nurses experience of research, their attitudes towards it and the level of interest in research training. Over 1000 service and education staff took part. Results showed there is much work to be done in further educating staff.

3.18.11   Coppens, N.M.C. (1988) The newspaper as a tool for introducing research. *Western journal of nursing research* 10(5) 677-679   3 References

Method of introducing students in various disciplines to research through use of health related articles from newspapers is described. Students reported sessions as being helpful and interesting.

3.18.12   Cox, C. (1984) Learning through research. *Senior nurse* 1(18) 8-9   9 References

Provides a brief overview of the developments in research relating to nurse education. Mention is made of student stress iherent in encouraging clinical research-based practice.

3.18.13   Downs, F. (1980) Teaching nursing research: strategies. *Nurse educator* 5(1) 27-29,34   7 References

Article suggests numerous teaching approaches to enable students to understand the principles of research and the research process at baccalaureate, masters and doctoral levels.

3.18.14   Duffy, M.E. (1987) The research process in baccalaureate nursing education: A ten year review. *Image: the journal of nursing scholarship* 19(2) 87-91   24 References

Reviews the literature over a ten year period relating to teaching nursing research in the USA. Headings used are research related to nursing research; placement of research in the undergraduate programme and strategies for research content. Although great strides have been made the author believes there is still much to do.

3.18.15   Eckerling, S., Bergman, R. & Bar-Tal, Y. (1988) Perceptions and attitudes of academic nursing students to research. *Journal of advanced nursing* 13(6) 759-767   36 References

Perceptions of nursing research activities of Tel Aviv university students were examined. The research concentrated on attitudes, role perception, ability and intentions to perform research themselves after graduation. The best predictors were perception of their own ability and the importance of research as part of the nursing role.

3.18.16   English National Board for Nursing, Midwifery and Health Visiting (1987) The nurse teachers role IN *Managing change in nursing education.* London: English National Board   ISBN 0946810109   Section 2 2:10 Research 58-67   20 References

Unit explores the implications of becoming research minded. Sections are included on promoting the use of research findings, fostering a spirit of enquiry in students and asking questions about ones own teaching. Twenty questions useful for self assessment are included, together with relevant sources. A list of further reading is included and brief information on courses available (CR 3.16).

3.18.17   Fontes, H.C. (1986) Stratifying research curricula: the logical next step. *Nursing and health care* 7(5) 259-262   17 References

It is suggested that there should be standardisation of the level for the research component of undergraduate and higher degree programmes. Author questions at what level of education nurses should become researchers rather than research consumers. The importance of the preparation of faculty members for research teaching is stressed.

3.18.18   Guice, R.T. (1986) Learning nursing research: a preliminary survey. *Australian journal of advanced nursing* 3(4) 18-29   8 References

An evaluation of small group research projects, other key aspects of research and statistics in a Victorian degree programme is reported. The seven major areas covered were broad course structure, statistical content, nursing seminar topics, class notes, handouts, textbooks, assessment, quality of course lecturers and the research project.

3.18.19   Heaney, R.P. & Barger-Lux, M.J. (1986) Priming students to read research critically. *Nursing and health care* 7(8) 421-424   4 References

Describes the development of a multidisciplinary course designed to enable graduates to critically evaluate research.

3.18.20   Heerman, J.A. & Craft, B.J.G. (1986) Teaching an introductory research course on and off campus. *Journal of nursing education* 25(3) 129-130   4 References

Describes the content, methodology and evaluation mechanisms of an off-campus research programme in Nebraska which enabled registered nurses working throughout the state to work towards the bachelors degree in nursing.

3.18.21   Hunt, M. & Hicks, J. (1983) Promoting research awareness in post-basic nursing courses. *Nursing times* 79(6) March 30 41-42   4 References   Occasional Paper

Difficulties experienced in teaching research mindedness to nurses are discussed. Authors describe an alternative method which was tried with positive results.

3.18.22   Irvine, J. & Miles, I. (1979) Statistics teaching in social science: a problem with a history. IN Irvine, J., Miles, I & Evans, J. *Demystifying social statistics.*

London: Pluto Press   ISBN 0861040686   References   Chapter 2   11-26

Chapter discusses problems experienced over many years in teaching the subject of statistics (CR 2.83.7).

3.18.23 Jamann-Riley, J.S. (1990) Nursing research education IN Fitzpatrick, J.J., Taunton, R.L. & Benoliel, J.Q. (eds) *Annual review of nursing research.* Volume 8 New York: Springer   References   Chapter 8   177-191   ISBN 0826143571

Chapter focuses on current practices in research education and identifies trends that can shape nursing in the 1990's. The following headings are used to discuss the literature: undergraduate and graduate content, teaching strategies, curriculum structure, doctoral education, research education in action and future directions.

3.18.24   Joint Board of Clinical Nursing Studies (1977) *The research objective in Joint Board courses: an introductory guide.* London: JBCNS   Occasional Paper 1

First UK publication designed to assist nurse teachers in introducing research into post-basic curricula. Suggestions are made as to how this may be achieved. Appendices contain an outline of the research process, a glossary and reference materials (now outdated) (CR 3.3.2, 3.3.3, 3.3.10).

3.18.25   Kim, H.S. (1984) Critical contents of research process for an undergraduate nursing curriculum. *Journal of nursing education* 23(2) 70-72   5 References

Article describes the development of a framework to examine the types and levels of the knowledge base necessary for the creation of scientists.

3.18.26 Ludeman, R. (1980) Strategies for teaching nursing research: the language and importance of nursing research. *Western journal of nursing research* 2(1) 432-434   (No References)

Describes a tool developed to familiarise students with research terminology and concepts. Students work through existing research reports and complete the tool which then forms the basis for detailed discussion (CR 2.2).

3.18.27   Ludeman, R. (1982) Strategies for teaching nursing research: coping with the 'dry well' syndrome. *Western journal of nursing research* 4(4) 445-447   9 References

Briefly discusses the theory behind creativity and makes suggestions as to how ideas for research may be generated.

3.18.28   Mander, R. (1988) Encouraging students to be research minded. *Nurse education today* 8(1) 30-35   14 References

Paper discusses how and why research should be taught to student nurses, who should teach it, and what the role of newly qualified nurses is with respect to research. The question of why research is not used in practice is also discussed (CR 3.7).

3.18.29 McGhee, M. (1986) Nursing research and nursing practice: implications for undergraduate research IN Stinson, S.M & Kerr, J.C. (eds) *International issues in nursing research.* Beckenham: Croom Helm   ISBN 0709944373   References Part 3   Chapter 8   131-150

Examines the factors distinguishing the research process and the clinical problem solving process. Four levels of research models are identified and a suggested learning programme discussed (CR 3.27.7).

3.18.30 Morle, K. (1990) We need more research. *Nursing* 4(3) January 25/February 7 13-15   6 References

Discusses the teaching of research in nursing courses and some particular difficulties are identified.

3.18.31 Muhlenkamp, A.F. (1981) Desensatisation of research phobia: instructor as therapist. *Western journal of nursing research* 3(3) 305-309   8 References

Selected classroom exercises are described which can help students to overcome research phobia. Operational definitions are generated; sampling techniques learnt; research instruments and techniques are introduced and data generated by the class. A standard test is completed on the students attitudes to self and methods of content analysis are described (CR 2.91).

3.18.32 Munro, B. (1985) Promoting enthusiasm for research amongst undergraduate students. *Journal of nursing education* 24(9) 368-371   12 References

Ways in which student nurses might be stimulated to be more aware of research and its relevance to clinical practice are suggested. Teachers are asked to examine their own attitudes as they are the role models for students. The importance of research-based clinical practice is stressed.

3.18.33 Murphy, J.R. (1977) Research Q & A − how can statistics be introduced effectively into the undergraduate nursing curriculum? *Nursing research* 26(5) 391-392

Describes a course for undergraduates at the University of Colorado School of Nursing which deals practically and unmathematically with the problems involved in collecting, presenting and interpreting data which nurses use every day. Students also learn to critically evaluate these elements within the research literature (CR 2.83).

3.18.34 Myco, F. (1980) Nursing research information: are nurse educators and practitioners seeking it out? *Journal of advanced nursing* 5(6) 637-646   15 References

The author investigates whether nurse teachers, ward sisters and nursing officers were obtaining information on nursing research. Their reading of nursing journals and use of specialist libraries is examined and compared.

3.18.35 National Board for Nursing, Midwifery and Health Visiting for Northern Ireland (1986) *Training requirements and guidelines for the research element in first level curricula.* Belfast: The National Board Circular number NBNI/86/10 17th July 1986 and enclosure NBNI/86/10/A

Gives details of training requirements and guidelines for the research element in first level curricula. It includes a rationale, broad objectives, organisation of this element, content of programmes and evaluation.

3.18.36 National Board for Nursing, Midwifery and Health Visiting for Northern Ireland (1989a) *The branch programme in nursing: curriculum requirements and guidelines.* Belfast: The National Board Circular number NBNI/89/6, and enclosure 89/6/A (adult branch), 89/6/B (child branch), 89/6/C (mental health branch) and 89/6/D (mental handicap branch) Programme objectives (ii) Nursing research

Board's requirements for Project 2000 programmes are given.

3.18.37 National Board for Nursing, Midwifery and Health Visiting for Northern Ireland (1989b) *The common foundation programme in nursing curriculum: requirements and guidelines.* Belfast: The National Board Circular number NBNI/89/4 and enclosure NBNI/89/4A Part A (ii) Nursing research

Outlines the Board's requirements for this part of the syllabus.

3.18.38 Overfield, T. & Duffy, M.E. (1984) Research on teaching research in the baccalaureate nursing curriculum. *Journal of advanced nursing* 9(2) 189-196   22 References

Paper reviews published research relating to teaching undergraduates about nursing research. The teaching methods advocated by various authors are discussed and compared, as are the findings of the research studies. Authors describe their own teaching strategies and make suggestions for further research.

3.18.39 Pinch, W.J. (1989) Integrating research into practice. *Nurse educator* 13(3) 30-33   16 References

Active involvement of students in research projects during clinical experiences encourages implementation of research in practice. Examples are given where students used or collected data related to adolescents and the elderly. A third method used was the writing of a research abstract.

3.18.40 Royal College of Nursing of the United Kingdom (1982) *Research-mindedness and nurse education.* London: Royal College of Nursing

Booklet prepared by the RCN Research Society which outlines ways in which research-mindedness can be encouraged. This is discussed in relation to pre and post registration education, nurse teachers, and library and information services.

3.18.41   Selby, M.L. & Tuttle, D.M. (1985) Teaching research by guided design: a pilot study. *Journal of nursing education* 24(6) 250-252   15 References

Describes a pilot study undertaken on the re-organisation of a Masters level nursing research course. An experiential learning method, guided design, was used. The advantages and disadvantages are discussed. The changes in graduate nurses attitudes towards research knowledge were evaluated.

3.18.42   Sheehan, J. (1982) The research interests of nurse tutor students. *Nursing times* 78(5) February 17 17-20   63 References

The research component of the nurse tutors course in Huddersfield is described. The aim was to give insight into the research process and provide a foundation for teaching research based nursing. An analysis of the projects undertaken is discussed.

3.18.43   Smith, J. & Diekmann, J. (1987) Research fair: a strategy for rekindling research interest in nursing staff. *Western journal of nursing research* 9(4) 631-633   (No references)

Describes a research day organised to re-acquaint staff nurses with the research process. An overview of the process was given from problem identification to publication of findings. Evaluation showed that alternative methods of learning had been offered, there was good interaction, opportunity to share ideas and obtain advice in a non-judgemental environment.

3.18.44   Spector, N.C. & Bleeks, S.L. (1980) Strategies to improve students attitudes to research. *Nursing outlook* 28(5) 300-304   30 References

Resistance to nursing research may be high but it can be changed if teachers are consistent, enthusiastic, are good role models and seen to be applying it themselves to clinical practice.

3.18.45   Swenson, I. & Kleinbaum, A. (1984) Attitudes towards research among undergraduate nursing students. *Journal of nursing education* 23(9) 380-386   14 References

Describes a study whose purpose was to determine if there were attitudinal changes about research among undergraduate students. Pre and post tests were given and the results showed an increased level of confidence in the ability to understand research methods and critically evaluate research studies. There was a lower level of interest in seeking out participation in a research study or actively reading and discussing it.

3.18.46   Thiel, C.A. (1987) The Cookie experiment, a creative teaching strategy. *Nurse educator* 12(3)   6 References

Paper suggests that insufficient attention is paid to how the research component of basic nursing courses is taught. It describes the 'Cookie experiment', a light hearted, non-threatening way of introducing students to some of the important features of research.

3.18.47 VanBree, N.S. (1985) Preparing faculty to teach research. *Journal of nursing education* 24(2) 84-86 6 References

Shortage of appropriately prepared teachers for research programmes is highlighted. A faculty development programme is described which aimed to develop teachers skills and confidence.

3.18.48 Warner, S. & Tenney, J.W. (1985) Strategies for teaching nursing research. *Western journal of nursing research* 7(1) 132-134 4 References

Describes a teaching strategy used in a Masters level course. Students learned research content, participated as both subjects and co-investigators and were exposed to computers and computer assisted instruction. The relative effectiveness of lectures and computer assisted learning were compared.

Suggested textbook reading

	Pages	Cross reference
Hutchinson S.A. & Webb R.B. IN Morse (1989)	285-302	2.36.8

Nursing research abstracts

Bond S.	83/135
Bond S., Stephenson J. & Wallace E.	81/123
Bridge W. & Dunn P.	83/136
Damnosch S.P.	87/323
Davis B.	83/108
Dunn P. & Bridge W.	83/397
Economic & Social Research Council	85/223
Hockey L.	82/424
Hunt M.	82/430
Jones R. & Simmons S.	86/008
Runciman P.	82/294
Salter B.	83/234

3.19 RESEARCH AND HIGHER EDUCATION

The role of institutions of higher education are crucial in teaching nurses how to do research. Opportunities are increasing in the UK for nurses to undertake diplomas and degrees as part of, or after, their initial training, so the number now with research knowledge is increasing.

Annotations
3.19.1 Armstrong-Esther, C.A. & Myco, F. (1987) Higher education: nursings' panacea or Achilles heel? *Recent advances in nursing* 18: 46-75 45 References

Article describes how and why health care and nursing may need to change in the future, and the repercussions this has for nursing education and professional practice.

The British, Canadian and American systems of nurse education, including preparation for basic and higher degrees, are compared and contrasted. It is also noted that there is a gap between academic and professional practice, and that less research is carried out into nursing practice than other areas of nursing.

3.19.2 Butterworth, T. (1991) *Continuity in research and teaching: the role of departments of nursing in higher education.* Paper given at the Royal College of Nursing Research Advisory Group Conference, 13th April 1991 at the University of Manchester

Paper examines the role of nursing departments in universities in relation to research education, the problems of attracting and keeping experienced researchers, government controls on programmes and funding. Also discussed are the position of research units and developing multi-disciplinary programmes. The results of a survey of nursing research units in the United Kingdom are given which identified the broad areas of work being undertaken. Author urges further discussion on how research can find expression in clinical excellence (CR 3.8, 3.13, 3.23).

3.19.3 Copp, L.A. (1984) Deans identify factors which inhibit and facilitate nursing research. *Journal of advanced nursing* 9(5) 513-517   4 References

Discusses the importance of the dean's role in relation to nursing research. Deans in the USA were asked to identify factors which inhibit and facilitate nursing research. The progress of nursing research is outlined.

3.19.4 Hart, S.E. (ed) (1989) *Doctoral education in nursing: history, process and outcome.* New York: National League for Nursing   ISBN 0887374204   References NLN Publication No 15-2238

Text covers several perspectives on doctoral education in nursing. Historical aspects are discussed, variations in degree designations, funding issues, development of doctoral programmes and the environment needed for scholars. Questions which need to be answered when consideration is being given to setting up such programmes, are also included (CR 3.12).

3.19.5 LeLean, S.R. (1981) Nursing research and higher education. *Journal of advanced nursing* 6(3) 240-241   2 References   Janforum

Discusses the place of nursing research in higher education, the achievements to date, problems and further developments.

3.19.6 Mensah, H.H. (1982) Academic espionage: dysfunctional aspects of the publish or perish ethic. *Journal of advanced nursing* 7(6) 577-580   6 References

Author argues that excellence in classroom teaching and success in the clinical field are not highly valued in deliberations to grant tenure and advancement in academic rank. Research and publications are the major yardsticks upon which judgements are made. This places nurses in an invidious position as they have high clinical workloads and have not been socialised for academic survival. Suggestions are made to relieve this pressure and these are: anticipatory planning, balancing the workload and understanding the dimensions of collegiality.

3.19.7 Oldham, G. (ed) (1982) *The future of research.* Guilford: Society for Research into Higher Education, University of Surrey ISBN 0900868864 References SRHE Monograph No 47

Book centres on the research function of higher education in Britain and reports the outcome of a seminar based on specially commissioned papers. These included a framework for analysis, the functions of research, funding and policy for research in the natural sciences and humanities, and the post-graduate training of researchers. Conclusions are drawn and recommendations made for the future.

3.19.8 Roberts, S.A. (ed) (1984) *Academic research in the United Kingdom: its organisation and effectiveness.* London: Taylor Graham ISBN 094756800X Proceedings of a symposium of the Association of Researchers in Medicine and Science

The theme of this symposium was to put the case for research careers in this country to be considerably improved. Papers cover the purposes of academic research and the objectives of polytechnics and universities; the problems encountered; the possibilities of these being eased if there were more research career opportunities, and what other mechanisms could be devised.

Nursing research abstracts
Jupp V.   82/289
LeLean S.R.   82/4

3.20 RESEARCH SUPERVISION/MENTORSHIP

Providing students with appropriate and constructive supervision demands different skills from those of doing research. Teachers may therefore themselves need guidance, and institutions often set up short courses, or arrange for staff to learn from each other by working together.

Annotations
3.20.1 Economic and Social Research Council (1986) *The preparation and supervision of research theses in the social sciences.* London: Economic and Social Research Council ISBN 0862261260

Booklet gives advice to students and supervisors on four phases in preparation of a research thesis: the matching of student and supervisor, preparation of the research outline, research and development of the outline and the writing of the thesis to completion (CR 3.21).

3.20.2 Elton, L. & Pope, M. (1989) Research supervision: the value of collegiality. *Cambridge journal of education* 19(3) 267-276   38 References

Discusses the organisational and interpersonal factors necessary in developing the relationship between staff and students in a research training programme.

3.20.3 Hawthorn, P.J. (1981) Supervision of dissertations of undergraduate nursing students. *Nursing times* 77(8) March 5 29-30   7 References   Occasional Paper

Discusses the role of the supervisor and gives some practical advice.

3.20.4 Jackson, N.E. (1982) Choosing and using a statistical consultant. *Nursing research* 31(4) 248-250

Article gives advice about the preparation needed prior to consulting a statistician, and how to choose and communicate with one. The consultant's point of view is given together with his role in the production of the final study.

3.20.5 National Board for Nursing, Midwifery and Health Visiting for Northern Ireland (1990) *Supervision of students.* Belfast: The National Board   Occasional Paper NB/2/90

Gives guidance on various aspects of supervision over the whole curriculum.

3.20.6 Schlotfeldt, R.M. (1985) Mentorship: a means to desirable ends. IN McCloskey, J.C. & Grace, H.K. (eds) *Current issues in nursing.* 2nd edition Boston: Blackwell Scientific   ISBN 0865420919X   References   Part 2   11 139-148

Chapter discusses the role of mentorship in nursing, the need, its development and potential hazards. Its value in the continuing development of nursing research is explored.

3.20.7 Werley, H.H. & Newcomb, B.J. (1983) The research mentor: a missing element in nursing? IN Chaska, N.L. *The nursing profession: a time to speak.* New York: McGraw Hill   ISBN 0070106967   References   Chapter 16   202-215

Discusses the background to mentor development and relationships, and describes the characteristics of the master-apprentice and mentor-protégé. The lack of available mentors is highlighted and the potential benefits which may take place where good matching has been achieved (CR 3.6.2).

Suggested textbook reading

	Pages	Cross reference
Howard & Sharp	22-25/160-161	
	167-171	3.21.5

3.21 STUDENT GUIDES TO RESEARCH

One of the features not usually included in research texts is guidance to students about some of the more practical aspects of undertaking research. A few books which include such guidance are annotated here.

Annotations

3.21.1 Adamson, A. (1986) *A students guide for projects, field studies and research.* 3rd edition Oxford: Oxford Polytechnic, Thamesman Publication ISSN 01413044 References

Guidebook provides a framework for students when carrying out written assignments. Some of the common practical methods, pitfalls, experiences and conventions are explained. An example report is included which illustrates the principles discussed.

3.21.2 Allen, D. (1982) *The process of doctoral research: constraints and opportunities.* Manchester: Health Services Management Unit, Department of Social Administration, University of Manchester. Working Paper No 65 (No ISBN number)

Paper examines problems of doctoral research from three perspectives − the design of courses, the supervisor and the student. Many questions are posed, the solutions to which require different approaches, and ideas for resolving them are presented for discussion. (Contains list of Working Paper Series, numbers 1-64) (CR 3.20).

3.21.3 Bell, J. (1987) *Doing your research project: a guide for first-time researchers in education and social science.* Milton Keynes: Open University Press ISBN 0335159877 References

Book is a source of reference and guide to good practice for beginning researchers. It is derived partly from course material written for the Open University Advanced Diploma in Educational Management. Pitfalls and false trails are identified and good research habits encouraged.

3.21.4 Dixon, B.R., Bouma, G.D. & Atkinson, G.B.J. (1987) *A handbook of social science research: a comprehensive and practical guide for students.* Oxford: Oxford University Press ISBN 0198780230 References

A text designed for students taking introductory research methods courses or doing small scale projects. It assumes little knowledge of research processes and takes the reader through each step in a clear jargon-free style. Each chapter concludes with a summary and questions for review.

3.21.5 Howard, K., & Sharp, J.A. (1983) *The management of a student research project.* Aldershot: Gower ISBN 0566004623 References

A practical guide for students intending to write up and present for examination the results of research projects.

3.21.6 Madsen, D. (1983) *Successful dissertations and theses.* San Francisco: Jossey-Bass ISBN 0875895557 References

Book gives practical advice on all aspects of writing dissertations and theses. This includes starting and completing the work, working with ones advisers, selecting the topic, preparing the proposal, following research procedures, organising and writing the work, defending it, adapting it for publication and using the library. Two sample proposals are included, one using a historical approach and the other an experimental approach (CR 2.99).

3.21.7 Moore, N. (1983) *How to do research.* London: The Library Association ISBN 0853659052 (No references)

A practical, introductory guide to anyone undertaking research. Examples are taken from library and information work but the principles discussed are generally applicable.

3.21.8 Phillips, E.M. & Pugh, D.S. (1987) *How to get a PhD.* Milton Keynes: Open University Press ISBN 0335155367 References

This practical text provides a realistic understanding of the process of doing research for a doctoral degree. Its main aim is to help students understand and achieve the necessary skills, and assist supervisors in planning and executing appropriate research programmes (CR 3.20).

3.21.9 Smith, R.V. (1984) *Graduate research: a guide for students in the sciences.* Philadelphia: ISI Press ISBN 0894950371 References

This workbook is designed for self-instruction by students in a wide variety of disciplines. Chapters cover the whole process of undertaking research and include: getting started, commitment, making choices, time management, ethics, developing library and writing skills, presenting papers, obtaining funds and getting a job.

3.21.10 Stock, M. (1985) *A practical guide to graduate research.* New York: McGraw Hill ISBN 0070615837 References

Text methodically covers the procedures and aspects essential in graduate research. It includes the graduate programme, getting started, grant proposals, thinking, talking and writing about research (CR 2.99, 2.100, 2.103).

3.22 UNIVERSITIES AND POLYTECHNICS

Nurses have been educated for many years in colleges and universities in the USA, and the number of courses at diploma and degree level in the UK is increasing. As one component within basic degree programmes, students are learning how to undertake research, and this may later be followed by studies at Masters or Doctoral level. Also it is becoming the norm, rather than the exception, for senior posts to be offered to candidates who have gained diplomas and degrees, and the opportunities are increasing all the time.

[This section includes several major directories which will enable appropriate diploma/degree courses to be found. Other UK research courses/workshops/study days are listed in Appendix A]

Annotations

3.22.1 Association of Commonwealth Universities (1990) *British universities guide to graduate study 1990/1991.* London: Association of Commonwealth Universities ISBN 0851431240

Describes all taught courses in British universities. A short description is given of course content, assessment methods, length, title and award qualification. Descriptive notes on universities and colleges are also included.

3.22.2 Association of Commonwealth Universities (1991) *University entrance.* London: Association of Commonwealth Universities ISBN 0851431259

Gives practical information on getting started, universities in outline and course tables covering many subjects including nursing. Book also contains a list of books on higher education, grants and careers.

3.22.3 Baker, J. (1988) *What next: post-basic opportunities for nurses.* Basingstoke: Macmillan Education ISBN 0333447840 References Chapter 8 Higher Education 61-78

Chapter covers diploma and degree courses and lists institutions where degrees in nursing, education and multi-disciplinary subjects may be undertaken. A short general section on research is included.

3.22.4 Carr, J. & Birnbaum, M. (eds) (1989) *Comparative guide to American Colleges: for students, parents and counsellors.* 14th edition. New York: Harper & Row ISBN 0060964804

Comprehensive guide to admissions, costs, scholarships and loans available to students. Each entry includes: name, address, nearest airport, student numbers – full time/part time, description, admission, academic environment, faculty and student body. Also given is information on religious orientation, sports, campus life, annual costs and general institutional data.

3.22.5 Committee of Directors of Polytechnics (1990) *Polytechnic courses handbook 1991 entry.* 20th edition London: Committee of Directors of Polytechnics ISBN 1872007023

Covers first degree, DipHE, HND and other advanced courses, together with post-graduate degrees and diplomas.

3.22.6 CRAC* (1990a) *DOFE 1990/1991: the complete guide to all non-university courses in the UK.* Cambridge: Hobsons Publishing ISBN 1853243434

A comprehensive guide to all institutions offering further and higher education courses. Courses leading to vocational qualifications are also listed.

[* CRAC – Careers Research Advisory Centre]

3.22.7 CRAC (1990b) *Graduate studies 1990/1991: the complete reference source for post-graduate study in the UK.* Cambridge: Hobsons Publishing ISBN 185324340X

A comprehensive guide to post-graduate study in the UK comprising summaries of research facilities and courses, with basic information about each institution. The book is normally updated annually.

3.22.8 Eberhard, F. (ed) (1989) *International handbook of universities and other institutions of higher education.* Paris: M Stockton Press for the International Association of Universities ISBN 0333436423

Information is given for 115 countries and territories. Each entry identifies institutions by name, postal address and includes details on faculties and departments, history and structure, admission requirements, fees, language of institution, degrees and diplomas awarded. The number of volumes in each library is given, the press or publishing house, academic staff and the number of enrolled students.

3.22.9 Mohr, B. & Leibig, I. (eds) (1988) *Higher education in the European Community: student handbook.* 5th edition London: Kogan Page ISBN 1850915016

A source of information on higher education in the European Community which includes its structure in each country, list of institutions and the qualifications offered, admission requirements, application processes, tuition fees, scholarships and grants. Also included are entry and residence regulations and social aspects e.g. health, advisory services, accomodation and other services.

3.22.10 Polytechnics Central Admissions (PCAS) (1990) PCAS Cheltenham, Glos: PCAS ISBN 0948241101

Gives specific information on how to apply for admission to polytechnics.

3.22.11 Rosier, I. & Earnshaw, L. (1989) *Mature students handbook: a survey of courses and career opportunities.* Richmond, Surrey: Trotman ISBN 0856601292

Gives practical information of interest to mature students. It covers access courses, distance learning, credit transfer, the Open University, Open College and the University of the Third Age. First degrees, other higher education courses, further education programmes and courses for professional qualifications are also included.

3.22.12 Tight, T. (1989) *Part-time degrees, diplomas and certificates: a guide to part-time higher education courses at universities, polytechnics and colleges.* Cambridge: Hobsons Publishing ISBN 1853242519

Contains information on all higher education courses which can be studied on a part-time basis or by correspondence.

3.22.13 **Universities Central Council on Admissions** (1990) *UCCA: the UCCA handbook 1991 entry.* Cheltenham, Glos. UCCA ISBN 0900951761

Gives specific information on how to apply for admission to a university or college.

3.22.14 **Wiley, K.** (1989) Focus of research for PhD in nursing. *Journal of nursing education* 28(4) 190-192   2 References

Reports a survey which aimed to investigate the foci for nursing PhDs. Categories included clinical nursing (96%), nursing administration (67%), nurse education (59%) and others.

Note: Degree structure
    Bachelor degree e.g. Bachelor of education/nursing studies
                       Bachelor of philosophy
    Masters degree e.g. Master of science/arts ... taught courses
                       Master of philosophy ... research based
    Doctoral degree e.g. Doctor of philosophy ... PhD/DPhil

3.23 RESEARCH PRIORITIES

There have been several studies which aimed to establish priorities for nursing research in clinical practice and nurse education. Some of those reported here have been undertaken comparatively recently, so there may be a considerable time lag before the chosen areas are described in the literature.

Annotations

3.23.1 Baker, G., Bevan, J.M., McDonnell, L. & Wall, B. (1987) Identifying the priorities for future research. IN Authors *Community nursing: research and recent developments.* London: Croom Helm   ISBN 0709944152   References   Chapter 6 216-234

Results of a postal survey, views of leaders of the professions and professional organisations and an extensive literature review provided the basis for suggesting priorities for research in community nursing. Areas identified were management structures, attachment versus geographical deployment of community nurses, role of community nurses and out of hours services provided by district nurses.

3.23.2 Bond, S. & Bond, J. (1982) *Clinical nursing research priorities: a Delphi survey.* Newcastle upon Tyne: Health Care Research Unit, University of Newcastle upon Tyne and Northern Regional Health Authority   (No ISBN number) References

Purpose of study was to identify research priorities which could form the basis of a nursing research programme in the Northern Region. It also aimed to provide data to inform decision making by government and other funding bodies. The Delphi method of data collection is described (CR 2.68, 3.8).

3.23.3 Butterworth, T. (1990) *Generating research in mental nursing.* (From a lecture first given as the Eileen Skellern Memorial Lecture at the Institute of Psychiatry, London October 1990) (Accepted for publication)

Paper explores some research priorities for mental health nursing in the United Kingdom. Areas identified include historical research, policy related research, the role of the mental health nurse as a provider of a therapeutic milieu, as therapist and teacher. Ways of promoting mental health research are outlined. The author stresses that valuable archival data must not be lost with the closure of psychiatric hospitals.

3.23.4 Dennis, K.E., Howes, D.G. & Zelauskas, B. (1989) Identifying nursing research priorities: a first step in programme development. *Applied nursing research* 2(3) 108-113   13 References

Reports a study which determined nursing research priorities in a single institution. Clinical priorities were prevention and treatment of pressure sores, pain management, nosocomial infections and patient education. Other priorities were staffing and its effects on turnover and patient care, job satisfaction and factors influencing the quality of care.

3.23.5 English National Board for Nursing, Midwifery and Health Visiting (1988) *Annual report 1987-1988.* London: ENB 18

Briefly covers activities of the Research Committee. These included discussing areas of mutual interest with officers of other nursing organisations, establishing research priorities and the allocation of funds, to development of the Board's staff and to teachers to prepare for future changes (CR 3.23.6).

3.23.6 English National Board for Nursing, Midwifery and Health Visiting (1990) Research priorities for 1990/1991. *Feedback* Summer 3

Lists topics identified by each of the Board's committees as priority areas for research. These are grouped under three major headings: the learning environment, examinations and the assessment of competence and teaching and teachers (CR 3.23.5).

3.23.7 Hayward, J. (ed) (1986) Research issues. IN Author *Report of the Nursing Process Evaluation Working Party.* London: Nursing Education Research Unit Report No 5   Chapter 6 34-38

Chapter summarises the need for further research into the nursing process through a series of issues. Each one is presented under a problem statement, associated research questions, possible research methods and a grid reference, which shows the scale and scope of necessary research (CR 2.105.11).

3.23.8 International Council of Nurses (1989) Priority research for health for all. *International nursing review* 36(1) 30-31   24

A review of the 'health for all' targets is given and the research areas needed to achieve them are cited. Five themes given are: health policy and organisational behaviour, inequalities, community participation and intersectorial collaboration, better information systems, indicators for the targets and collaborative studies.

3.23.9 Keighley, T. (1989) And research is always incomplete. *Senior nurse* 10(3) 19-23   4 References

Identifies many priority areas for nursing research and expresses concern that researchers have not yet addressed some current, crucial issues. They are urged to undertake research which is relevant to determining the future of the National Health Service and those areas where it is needed are clearly identified.

3.23.10 Lewandowski, L. & Kositsky, A. (1983) Research priorities for critical care nursing: a study by the American Association of Critical Care Nurses. *Heart and lung* 12(1) 35-44   44 References

The Delphi technique is used to define research priorities for critical care nursing in the USA. The technique is defined and described and detailed information is given about its use in this particular study (CR 2.68).

3.23.11 Macmillan, M. (1989) Priorities in nursing research. *Senior nurse* 9(1) 12   4 References

Range of methods used by researchers to select appropriate subjects for research are identified. A Delphi survey carried out by the Nursing Research Unit in Edinburgh is described (CR 2.68, 3.13.20).

3.23.12 Rodgers, J.M. (1985) An examination of research priorities in nurse education. *Journal of advanced nursing* 10(3) 233-236   20 References

Identifies aspects of nurse education which require study. Specific recommendations made are an examination of curriculum content, particularly the inclusion of research findings, methods of teaching and learning and linking theory and practice. Assessment and support of learners and the role of the nurse teacher are also considered.

3.23.13 Tanner, C.A. & Lindeman, C.A. (1987) Research in nursing education: assumptions and priorities. *Journal of nursing education* 26(2) 50-59   38 References

Study aimed to identify assumptions about the nature of research in nursing education and rank order critical research questions. The Delphi technique was used to generate the data. Findings included that research in nursing education can and should meet criteria for scientific merit; should not be viewed as secondary in importance to practice research; should emphasise the clinical nature of nursing and be less fragmented. Priorities included the integration of findings into nursing curricula, the development of problem-solving skills, approaches to clinical teaching and the level of practice of graduates of different basic preparations (CR 2.68).

3.23.14 Tierney, A.J. (ed) (1989) *Proceedings of the Consensus Development Conference on priorities for nursing research in Scotland.* 26.10.1988 Edinburgh: Nursing Research Unit, Department of Nursing Studies, University of Edinburgh

Contains a report of the conference, together with the papers presented. It includes an account of a Delphi survey undertaken by the unit. The consensus of a panel representing a wide range of interests identified the following themes: the assessment and improvement of quality and standards of nursing practice; the organisation of nursing services which have an impact on nursing practice; manpower planning; nurses' job satisfaction and performance in practice and educational aspects of nursing practice (CR 2.68, 3.26).

Suggested textbook reading

	Pages	*Cross reference*
Bergman R.	195-203	3.27.1

Nursing research abstracts

Pyne R.	84/6	

3.24 RESEARCH REGISTERS/DIRECTORIES

One of the ways of disseminating research findings is the compilation of a register or directory and this is an area where there are comparatively few examples at present.

Annotations
3.24.1 Armitage, S. & Player, L. (1987) The nursing research activity register in Wales. *Senior nurse* 7(3) 30-32   No references

Describes the introduction of a computerised register of nursing research in Wales. Its uses, users and contributors are identified.

3.24.2 Commonwealth Department of Health (1984) *Directory of nursing research in Australia.* 3rd edition Canberra: Australian Government Publishing Service   (ISBN number not found)

Research information is provided in a standard format and the directory is designed to facilitate communication amongst researchers and encourage dissemination of research findings.

3.24.3 Hawthorn, P.J. & McCullough, J.M. (1988) *The Trent Regional Health Authority Register of Nursing Research: projects and innovations.* Nottingham: Nursing Studies Unit, University of Nottingham   (No ISBN number)

A compilation, although incomplete, of nursing research undertaken in the Trent Region. It is hoped to update this annually. Information included for each study is: name and address of researcher, title, summary, reason for study, name of supervisor, ethical clearance, source of funding, if study leave was given, computer assistance, availability of report, willingness to speak at meetings, publications and keywords. Research studies included were sometimes commissioned by the health authority, undertaken as part of an ENB or other advanced course or self-motivated.

3.24.4 Levy, J.E. (ed) (1983) *The medical research directory.* Chichester: Wiley   ISBN 0471103357

Contains both current and recent medical and nursing research in universities, polytechnics, colleges, hospitals and research establishments. A short description is given of each study.

Nursing research abstracts
Berry J.M.   83/105
Chester R.   85/0377

RESEARCH REVIEWS

3.25 RESEARCH REVIEWS

There are comparatively few reviews of research apart from individual studies but the two included in this section provide overviews of many nursing studies.

Annotations

3.25.1 Macleod Clark, J. & Hockey, L. (1979) *Research for nursing: a guide for the enquiring nurse.* Aylesbury, Buckinghamshire: HM + M Publishers ISBN 085602077X References

Book is divided into four major sections, understanding research in which the basic research approach is outlined and an overview of design and methods given. Parts 2 and 3 analyse studies relating to patient care and those relating to nurses, nursing management and education. Each study is examined under the following headings: main research question(s), research design and method, findings and implications. The final section briefly examines training for research, career possibilities, resources, and research as a change agent (CR 3.25.2).

3.25.2 Macleod Clark, J. & Hockey, L. (eds) (1989) *Further research for nursing.* London: Scutari ISBN 1871364140 References

A companion volume to *Research for nursing: a guide for the enquiring nurse*, which aims to help nurses understand the value of research in their practice. A general introduction to research is given, together with its relevance to nursing and an overview of research processes. The remainder of the book contains overviews of research in twelve topic areas. Each is illustrated by a précis of one or two specific studies. Several chapters are devoted to studies about specific patient groups and others to more general nursing issues (CR 3.25.1).

CONFERENCE PROCEEDINGS/REPORTS

3.26 CONFERENCE PROCEEDINGS/REPORTS

Research conferences are one of the major ways in which findings can be made known to a wider audience and proceedings which are subsequently published also provide a link in this vital chain.

Annotations
3.26.1 Altschul, A. (1981) Research, a base for the future. *Nurse education today* 1(5) 6-7 2 References

An overview of a nursing research conference held in Edinburgh in 1981. Papers included bringing researcher and practitioner closer together and the relationships between knowledge and power.

3.26.2 Christensen, E.H. & Lerheim, K. (eds) (1990) *Workgroup of European Nurse-Researchers, 10th Workgroup Meeting: Portugal 1987 and 11th Workgroup Meeting, 4th Open Conference: Israel 1988.* Copenhagen: Danish Nurses Organisation ISBN 8772660635 References

Book includes selected proceedings from meetings entitled 'The role of nursing research in achieving health for all by the year 2000' and 'Collaborative research and its implementation in nursing'. One major paper is included from each meeting, a historical overview of the WENR 1978-1988, statements and annual reports from member countries about developments in nursing research (CR 3.2.7).

3.26.3 Redfern, S.J., Sisson, A.R., Walker, J.F. & Walsh, P.A. (1982) *Issues in nursing research.* London: Macmillan ISBN 0333324501 References

Papers from the 22nd annual'conference of the Royal College of Nursing Research Society Papers are included under the following headings: history of nursing, nurse education and research, nurses, the work of midwives and health visitors, changing behaviour and attitudes in open and closed settings, managing the needs and provision of services for the elderly, nursing practice and methodological issues.

3.26.4 Workgroup of European Nurse-Researchers (1984) *Nursing research — does it make a difference?* London: Royal College of Nursing ISBN 0902606891 References Proceedings of the 7th Workgroup Meeting, 2nd Open Conference London: 10-13th April 1984

Papers are included under the following headings: developments in nursing research, plenary sessions on various aspects of nursing research, primary health care, midwifery, nurse education and training, care of the elderly, nursing history and nursing roles, psychiatry and mental handicap, information giving and patient care, occupational health of nurses, quality of care and care of wounds.

Nursing research abstracts

Abdel-Al H.	84/131
Ashworth P.	89/001
Bond S.	83/135
Davis B.D.	83/108
Fairbrother C.	83/3
Hamrin E.	83/134
Hardy L.K.	83/364
Hunt J.M.	83/352, 84/140
Laing E. & Johnson R.A.	83/354
Lerheim K.	83/357

[Notes: The Royal College of Nursing Research Advisory Group hold an annual conference, the proceedings of which are held by the RCN library in London. The set of these is incomplete so readers are advised to telephone for availability.

Only a very small number of references to conferences are included here. Please see 1.3.1 and 1.9.3 for further information on past and forthcoming conferences.]

3.27 INTERNATIONAL NURSING RESEARCH

There are some differences in meaning of the term international nursing research in the literature and the annotations cited here reflect this.

Definition
The nursing profession in other cultures

Example
Ashworth, P.A. et al (1987) *Peoples' needs for nursing care: a European study.* Copenhagen: WHO Regional Office for Europe   ISBN 928901041X   References

Describes a study undertaken in 11 European countries which aimed to determine people's needs for nursing care and help and to supply information needed for change. Study has enhanced knowledge of nursing research, stimulated the establishment of research groups and provided an educational experience for many researchers (CR 2.15).

Annotations
3.27.1 Bergman, R. (ed) (1990) *Nursing research for nursing practice: an international perspective.* London: Chapman and Hall ISBN 041233500X References

Book includes contributions from researchers around the world. Each chapter gives a brief description of their major health care system, problems which have been encountered, the scope and development of nursing research and research on a selected topic. Chapter 1 discusses the role of international organisations in nursing research (CR 3.1, 3.2, 3.4, 3.23).

3.27.2 Dier, K.A. (1988) International nursing: the global approach. *Recent advances in nursing* 20: 39-60   55 References

Examines the development of international nursing research from World War 2 up to the present, with particular attention being given to third world countries. The evolution, global and country perspectives, social structure, cultural and health care values and a taxonomy of health care systems are all discussed. The functions of health personnel and the scope of international nursing are explored.

3.27.3   International Council of Nurses (1989) Whither ICN on its 90th birthday. *International nursing review* 36(6)   Issue No 288 167-170   (No references)

Article looks back at ICN's history and states its long term objectives. Those relating to research include an increase in scholarly activities, the need for computer facilities, new modes of practice/service/management and new concepts and methods of research.

3.27.4   Manfredi, M., Ailinger, R.L. & Collado, C. (1990) The process, benefits and costs of conducting multi-national nursing research. *International journal of studies* 27(4) 325-332   6 References

Discusses the process, benefits and costs of conducting a six country research study on nursing practice in Latin America. The political, economic and professional outcomes are examined and suggestions offered for further multi-national studies.

3.27.5   Meleis, A.I. (1989) International research: a need or a luxury? *Nursing outlook* 37(3) 138-142   13 References

Author urges the development of cross-national, collaborative studies in order to further nursing science. Policies required and personal considerations are discussed, global priorities given and strategies for achieving these goals.

3.27.6   Skeet, M. (1987) Internationalisation of nursing. IN Hockey, L. (ed) Current Issues *Recent advances in nursing* 18: 109-128   13 References

Discusses internationalism, why nursing has become internationally minded and its activities in clinical practice, management and education. The work of the International Council of Nurses, the Red Cross and other groups of nurses are explored together with the role of the individual nurse (CR 3.27.3).

3.27.7   Stinson, S.M. & Kerr, J.C. (eds) (1986) *International issues in nursing research.* Beckenham: Croom Helm   ISBN 0709944373   References

Book presents a review of specific international themes in nursing research. It includes methodological issues, policy and funding, preparation for nursing research, publication issues and the role of professional associations. Contributors are leading authorities in the UK, USA and Canada (CR 2.102, 3.10, 3.12, 3.15).

3.27.8 to 3.27.12 *Western journal of nursing research* (1987) 9(3) International nursing research, Meleis, A.I. (ed) (selected items)

[Please note the format of this entry differs from previous ones and articles have not been annotated.]

3.27.8   Davis, A.J. Ethical issues in nursing research: international nursing research. 400-402   3 References

3.27.9   Meleis, A.I. International nursing research for knowledge development. Editorial 285-287

3.27.10   Meleis, A.I., Mahidal, V.T., Ju-ying, M.L. & Minami, H. International collaboration in research: forces and constraints, by leaders from Thailand, Peoples' Republic of China, Japan and Brazil. 390-399

3.27.11   Morse, J.M. Technical notes: doing international nursing research. 403-407

3.27.12   Seabrooks, P.A. & Rogers, S. Sources of data: international nursing research. 385-389

RESEARCH AND OTHER DISCIPLINES

3.28   RESEARCH AND OTHER DISCIPLINES

In the past much research into nursing was undertaken by those in other disciplines and they made an important contribution to knowledge. This is now happening less frequently as nurses are developing the necessary skills. There are however still many opportunities where nurses could collaborate with other researchers, as patients' needs span many disciplines.

Annotations

3.28.1   Dingwall, R. (1982) Reflections on sociological aspects of nursing research. *Nursing review* 1(2) 3-5   19 References

The sociologists contribution to nursing is described. It is suggested that nursing research should not become an isolated specialty, but should combine with other disciplines in order to meet the changing needs of society.

3.28.2   Disbrow, M.A. (1983) Conducting interdisciplinary research: gratifications and frustrations. IN Chaska, N.L. *The nursing profession: a time to speak.* New York: McGraw Hill   ISBN 0070106967   References   Chapter 18   225-236

Discusses the value of interdisciplinary research, its processes, methods, stages and the issues involved. Problems are identified and suggestions made for overcoming difficulties (CR 3.6.2).

3.28.3   Kilty, J. (1976) Can nursing research learn from educational research? *International journal of nursing studies* 13(2) 97-102   9 References

Author suggests that research in health care and education are similar and have difficulties common to both. Solutions which have been effective in educational research are discussed. Collaboration is urged between researcher and practitioner so ensuring that findings are relevant to practice.

Nursing research abstracts

Association of Researchers in Medical Science	81/280
Barrett E.	90/115
Lahiffe M.E.	83/353
Melia K.	83/147
Morse J.M.	87/222
Royal College of Nursing	89/001
Stewart G.	84/273

REFERENCES

[Note: these references relate to those books and articles consulted during the development of the book]

Anonymous (1988) Research without consent continues in the UK. *Institute of Medical Ethics Bulletin* 40 July Review 13-16

Bannister, D. (1988) IN A lexicon of psychology, psychiatry and psychoanalysis. Edited by Kuper, J. London: Routledge 298

Bernard, J. (1973) My four revolutions: an autobiographical history of the American Sociological Association. *American journal of sociology* 78: 782

Brandt, A.M. (1978) *Racism and research: the case of the Tuskegee syphilis study.* Hastings Centre Report 6 21-29

Brink, P.J. (ed) (1976) *Transcultural nursing: a book of readings.* New Jersey: Prentice Hall 1-5

Brockopp, D.Y. & Hastings-Tolsma, M.T. (1989) *Fundamentals of nursing research.* Glenview, Illinois: Scott, Foresman & Co. 372

Conway, M.E. (1978) Clinical research: instrument for change. *Journal of nursing administration* 8: 27-32

Dracup, K.A. & Bruce, C.S. (1977) Strengthening practice through research utilisation IN Batey, M. (ed) *Community nursing research.* 10 Boulder, Colorado: Western Interstate Commission for Higher Education

Field, P.A. & Morse, J.M. (1985) *Nursing research: the application of qualitative approaches.* Rockville, Maryland: Aspen 27

Flanagan, J.C. (1947) *The aviation psychology programme in the army air forces.* AAF Psychology Programme Research Report No 1 Washington DC: Government Printing Office

Flanagan, J.C. (1954) The critical incident technique. *Psychological bulletin* 51(4) 327-358

Fox, D. (1982) *Fundamentals of research in nursing.* 4th edition Norwalk, Connecticut: Appleton-Century-Crofts 197

Gray, B.J. (1975) *Human subjects in medical experimentation.* New York: Wiley

Holm, K. & Llewellyn, J.G. (1986) *Nursing research for nursing practice.* Philadelphia: Saunders 92

Horsley, J.A., Crane, J. & Bingle, J.D. (1978) Research utilisation as an organisational process. *Journal of nursing administration* 8:4-6

Johnson, J.E. (1977) Nursing research impact vital for the profession. *American nurse* 9: 15

Krampitz, S.D. & Pavlovich, N. (1981) *Readings for nursing research.* St.Louis: Mosby 43

Krippendorf, K. (1980) *Content analysis: an introduction to its methodology.* Beverly Hills: Sage 117

Krueger, J., Nelson, A. & Wolanin, M.O. (1978) *Nursing research: development, collaboration and utilisation.* Germantown, Md. Aspen Systems

Kuper, L. (ed) (1988) *A lexicon of psychology, psychiatry and psychoanalysis.* London: Routledge

Leininger, M.M. (1985) *Qualitative research methods in nursing.* Orlando: Grune & Stratton 68

Leininger, M.M. (1987) Importance and uses of ethnomethods: ethnography and ethnonursing research. *Recent advances in nursing* 17: 13

Lindeman, C.A. & Krueger, J.C. (1977) Increasing the quality, quantity and use of nursing research. *Nursing outlook* 24(9) 450-456

Linstone, H.A. & Turoff, M. (eds) (1975) *The Delphi method: techniques and applications.* Reading, Massachusetts: Addison-Wesley 10

McFarlane of Llandaff, Baroness J. (1984) Research process in nursing – the future. IN Cormack D.F.S. (ed) *The research process in nursing.* Oxford: Blackwell Scientific x-xi

Miller, P.McC. & Wilson, M.J. (1983) *A dictionary of social science methods.* Chichester: Wiley vii

Nicholson, R. (1987) Sickness of the secret society. *The Mail on Sunday* November 15

Ogier, M.E. (1982) *An ideal sister.* London: Royal College of Nursing

Pappworth, M.H. (1967) *Human guinea pigs.* Boston: Beacon Press

Pappworth, M.H. (1978) Medical ethics committees: a review of their functions. *World medicine* February 22 19-21,57,61,64,67-69,71-72,74,76,78

Patton, M.Q. (1981) *Qualitative evaluation and research methods.* 1st edition Beverly Hills: Sage 18

Penguin Dictionary of Psychology (1985) Edited by Reber, A.S. Harmondsworth: Penguin

Phillips, D.C. (1987) *Philosophy, science and social inquiry: contemporary methodological controversies in social science and related applied fields of research.* Oxford: Pergamon 116

Phillips, L.R.F. (1986) *A clinicians guide to the critique and utilisation of nursing research.* Norwalk, Connecticut: Appleton-Century-Crofts xiii, 87, 364, 463

Polit, D.F. & Hungler, B.P. (1987) *Nursing research: principles and methods.* 3rd edition Philadelphia: Lippincott 3,200,332,507

Psathas, C. (1978) *Phenomenological sociology: issues and applications.* New York: Wiley & Sons

Readers Digest Universal Dictionary (1987) London: Readers Digest Association Ltd.

Reason, P. & Rowan, J. (eds) *Human inquiry: a sourcebook of new paradigm research.* Chichester: Wiley xiii

Rice, V. & Johnson, J. (1984) Pre-admission self instruction booklets, post admission exercise performance and teaching time. *Nursing research* 33(3) 147-151

Roberts, C.A. & Burke, S.O. (1989) *Nursing research: a quantitative and qualitative approach.* Boston: Jones & Bartlett 4-5

Rothman, D.J. (1982) *Were Tuskagee and Willowbrook studies in nature?* Hastings Centre Report 2 5-7

Spender, D. (1978) Notes on the organisation of women's studies. *Women's studies international quarterly* 1(3) 259

Stetler, C.B. & Marram, G. (1976) Evaluating research findings for applicability in practice. *Nursing outlook* 24(9) 559-563

Treece, E.W. & Treece, J.W. Jr. (1986) *Elements of research in nursing.* 4th edition St. Louis: Mosby 208

Waltz, C.F., Strickland, O.L. & Lenz, E.R. (1984) *Measurement in nursing research.* Philadelphia: Davis 255, 285

Websters Third New International Dictionary (1961) London: Bell & Son Ltd.

Woods, N.F. & Catanzaro, M. (1988) *Nursing research: theory and practice.* St. Louis: Mosby 189, 326, 335, 347

Yin, R.K. (1984) *Case study research: design and methods.* Beverly Hills: Sage 99

APPENDIX A

ADDRESSES AND INFORMATION ON RESEARCH COURSES/ WORKSHOPS IN THE UNITED KINGDOM

Note: Most Bachelor and taught Masters courses contain a research component and prospective students are advised to obtain further information from the university or polytechnic of their choice. Please see guides in section 3.22.

Open University — Research Methods in Education and Social Sciences   Course Code: DE 304

This course provides information and skills needed to evaluate research in the Social Sciences and Education.

One assessment option is intended for people in the health care professions who would like to do a small piece of research in their own environment.

Certification — Certificate of satisfactory completion. This is transferable towards a BA degree.

Information may be obtained from: The Open University, Walton Hall, Milton Keynes MK7 6AA

Council for National Academic Awards (CNAA) Postgraduate Diploma in Research Methodology

Diploma in Nursing (University of London)

Please see guides in section 3.22

Diploma in Research Methods for the Caring Professions

Information may be obtained from: Department of Nursing and Applied Social Studies, Bristol Polytechnic, Coldharbour Lane, Frenchay, Bristol BS 16 1QY

Royal College of Nursing of the United Kingdom — Research Units

It is possible for students who wish to develop their knowledge of research to study modules from integrated degree programmes on a 'stand alone' basis. Credit would be given for successful completion of these if students subsequently wish to study for a degree.

Information may be obtained from: Mr A. Myles, Institute of Advanced Nursing Education, Royal College of Nursing, 20 Cavendish Square, London W1M 0AB

English National Board for Nursing, Midwifery and Health Visiting — An Introduction to the Understanding and Application of Research   Course Number 870

Information may be obtained from: English National Board for Nursing, Midwifery and Health Visiting, Resource and Careers Services, Woodseats House, 764a Chesterfield Road, Sheffield, S8 0SE

Nursing Research Unit, Department of Nursing Studies, University of Edinburgh

Nursing Research in Practice — Study Days
Developing a Research Proposal — Study Workshops
Introduction to Nursing Research — Summer School

Information may be obtained from: Nursing Research Unit, Department of Nursing Studies, University of Edinburgh, 12, Buccleuch Place, Edinburgh EH8 9JT

Institute of Advanced Nursing Education — An Introduction to the Understanding and Application of Research

Information may be obtained from: Institute of Advanced Nursing Education, Royal College of Nursing, Northern Ireland Board, 17 Windsor Avenue, Belfast BT9 5QQ

Southern Area College — Research Awareness

Information may be obtained from: Southern Area College, Craigavon Area College, Craigavon, Co. Londonderry BT 63 5QQ

Research Workshops for Nurses

Information may be obtained from: Research Workshops for Nurses, PO Box 162, Cardiff CF5 3RY

For further reference:

Directory of continuing education for nurses, midwives and health visitors (1990) London: Newpoint   ISBN 0862631297 (Endorsed by the Royal College of Nursing)

Directory combines information on continuing education and lists the courses available in the UK. It includes statutory position, professional accreditation and academic awards within higher education. Also contains chapters on nursing education and the role of the statutory bodies, personal and professional responsibility, choosing a course, qualifications and their value, post-registration clinical courses, courses for midwives and other specialist courses. Information is included on higher education, teacher preparation, management and open and distance learning (CR 3.22)

APPENDIX B

COMPUTER PACKAGES FOR STATISTICAL ANALYSIS – a selected list

Purpose, addresses and documentation

GENSTAT

Purpose: A high level language for data manipulation and statistical analysis. Used mainly for analysis of experimental data.

Address: Stats Package Co-ordinator, NAS Central Office, 7 Banbury Road, Oxford OX2 6NN

Documentation: Alvey, N.G. et al (1977) GENSTAT: a general statistical programme. Harpenden, Herts: Statistics Department Rothamstead Experimental Station

---

GLIM

Purpose: An interactive programme designed for the fitting of generalised linear models to data, together with other applications.

Address: The Numerical Algorithms Group Ltd, 7 Banbury Road, Oxford OX2 6NN

Documentation: User manual
Newsletter

MINITAB

Purpose: a general interactive statistical computing system.

Address: MINITAB Inc., 3081 Enterprise Drive, State College, PA 16801, USA

Documentation: Ryan, B.F., Joiner, B.L. & Ryan, T.A. Jr. (1985) MINITAB Handbook. 2nd edition Boston: Duxbury Press   ISBN 0871504707 (CR 2.88.13)

P-STAT

Purpose: A large conversational type system offering file management and data display features, cross-tabulation and numerous statistical procedures.

Address: P-STAT Inc., PO Box 285, Princeton, New Jersey 08540
Documentation: A Pocket Guide to P-STAT 78 (1979)
P-STAT Inc.

SAS

Purpose: Provides tools for data analysis; information storage and retrieval; data modification and programming; report writing; statistical analysis and file handling.
Address: SAS Institute Inc., Box 8000, SAS Circle, Cary NC 27511
Documentation: Helwig, J.T. (1978) SAS Introductory Guide Raleigh NC SAS Institute Inc.

SIR (Scientific Information Retrieval)

Purpose: Integrated, research orientated data base management system which supports hierarchical and network relationships and interfaces directly with SPSS.
Address: SIR Inc., PO Box 1404, Evanston, IL 60204, USA
Documentation: Schulzinger, F.J. (1984) The SIR/DBMS Primer Madison: Wisconsin University of Wisconsin at Madison Academic Computing Centre

---

SPSS (Statistical Package for the Social Sciences)

Purpose: Integrated package for data analysis and file management.
Address: SPSS Inc., 444 N Michigan Avenue, Chicago, IL 60611
Documentation: SPSSX (1986) Users Guide 2nd edition SPSS Inc.

Reference: Francis, I. (1981) Statistical Software: a comparative review. New York: Elsevier, North Holland ISBN 0444006583 (CR 2.88.4).

APPENDIX C

JOURNALS ANNOTATED IN THIS BOOK

Administrative science quarterly
Advances in nursing science
American journal of public health
Annual review of public health
Anthropology and education quarterly
Applied nursing research
Australian journal of advanced nursing
Behaviour therapy
British journal of addiction
British medical journal
Cambridge journal of education
Canadian journal of nursing administration
Canadian journal of nursing research (formerly *Nursing papers*)
Canadian nurse
Character and personality
Communicating nursing research: collaboration and competition
Community medicine
Educational researcher
Feedback − English National Board
Health education journal
Heart and lung
Hospice journal
Hospital topics
Image: the journal of Nursing scholarship
Institute of Medical Ethics bulletin
International journal of nursing studies
International nursing review
Journal of advanced nursing
Journal of clinical oncology
Journal of continuing education in nursing
Journal of family therapy
Journal of medical ethics
Journal of nursing administration
Journal of nursing education
Journal of philosophy and social science
Journal of professional nursing

Medical care
Medical education
Medical Research Council news
Medical teacher
Midwifery
Military medicine
Nature
Nurse education today
Nurse educator
Nursing administration quarterly
Nursing and health care
Nursing economics
Nursing focus
Nursing forum
Nursing mirror (incorporated into *Nursing times*)
Nursing outlook
Nursing papers (now *Canadian journal of nursing research*)
Nursing practice
Nursing research
Nursing review
Nursing science quarterly
Nursing times
Oral history review
Pediatric nursing
Philosophy of the social sciences
Professional nurse
Psychological bulletin
Qualitative sociology
Recent advances in nursing (ceased publication in October 1990)
Research in higher education
Research in nursing and health
Senior nurse
Social history of medicine
Sociology
Sociology of health and illness
Topics in clinical nursing
Urban life
Western journal of nursing research
World medicine

APPENDIX D

RESEARCH AWARENESS SERIES

Distance Learning Centre, Polytechnic of the South Bank, London

List of modules with cross-reference numbers

Module	Title	Cross reference
1	Nursing research in professional development	3.6.4
2	Sources of nursing knowledge	2.6.5
3	What is research?	2.3.2
4	Searching the literature	1.1.9
5	Identifying and defining questions for research	2.18.3
6	Ethics in nursing and midwifery research	2.17.7*
7	The ethnographic perspective	2.43.12
8	The survey perspective	2.55.12
9	The experimental perspective	2.29.5
10	Evaluating research	2.98.4
11	Using research findings: a guide for practitioners	2.105.8

[* Module 6 will be published in 1992

Module numbers 12 and 13, listed in those already published, have been omitted from this book since they were not available at the time of going to press.

APPENDIX E

SOURCES OF DEFINITIONS

'Selection of terms and definitions is difficult because of indistinct lines between methodological issues and philosophical terms and debates' (Miller & Wilson 1983).

Each definition included in this book has been obtained from existing literature, glossaries or dictionaries and readers will note the variety of sources.

There are many different ones which could have been included, but the authors have chosen those which appeared to be most clear and concise. However researchers, teachers and students may wish to use other definitions depending upon their own research perspectives.

	Author(s)	Page in source text	Reference in this volume
2.4	Treece & Treece	510	2.1.65
2.5	Websters Third New International Dictionary	1698	(References)
2.6	Phillips D.C.	203	2.5.12
2.7	Woods & Catanzaro	568	2.1.72
2.8	Phillips L.R.F.	463	2.98.11
	Holm & Llewellyn	12	2.1.26
2.9	Bryman	94	2.9.1
2.10	Spender (adapted)	259	(References)
2.11	Reason & Rowan	Back Cover	2.11.5
2.12	Phillips L.R.F.	149	2.98.11
2.13	Kidder & Judd	26	2.1.30
2.15	Websters Third New International Dictionary	443	(References)
2.17	Wilson H.S.	726	2.1.69
2.18	Woods & Catanzaro	564	2.1.72
	Brockopp & Hastings-Tolma	376	(References)
2.19	Holm & Llewellyn	274	2.1.26
	Phillips L.R.F.	456,458	2.98.11
2.20	Holm & Llewellyn	265,269	2.1.26
	Dixon, Bouma & Atkinson	48	3.21.4
2.21	Castles	55	2.1.15
2.22	Giovanetti IN Williamson	171,172	2.1.67
2.23	Cormack	33	2.1.20
2.24	Leininger	68	2.1.36
	Holm & Llewellyn	270	2.1.26
2.25	Leininger	68	2.1.36

	Author(s)	Page in source text	Reference in this volume
	Field & Morse	139	2.1.24
	Phillips L.R.F.	454,455,457	2.98.11
2.26	Denzin	471-475	2.1.23
2.27	Polit & Hungler	526	2.1.56
2.28	Field & Morse	137	2.1.24
2.29	Holm & Llewellyn	262,263	2.1.26
	Phillips L.R.F.	462	2.98.11
2.34	Polgar & Thomas	84	2.1.55
2.35	Woods & Catanzaro	564	2.1.72
2.36	Abdellah & Levine (adapted)	391	2.1.1
2.37	Cohen & Manion	217	2.1.19
2.38	Phillips L.R.F.	453	2.98.11
2.39	Polit & Hungler	526	2.1.56
2.40	Polit & Hungler	528	2.1.56
2.41	Brink	1-5	(References)
2.42	Cook	469	2.42.5
2.43	Leininger	35,36,237	2.1.36
	Field & Morse	23,24	2.1.24
2.44	Abdellah & Levine	391	2.1.1
2.45	LoBiondo-Wood & Haber	417	2.1.38
2.46	Polit & Hungler	530	2.1.56
2.47	Woods & Catanzaro	558	2.1.72
2.48	Websters Third New		
	International Dictionary	1073,1074	(References)
	Seldon & Pappworth	4	2.48.9
2.49	Phillips L.R.F.	460	2.98.11
2.50	Phillips L.R.F. (adapted)	459	2.98.11
2.51	Polit & Hungler	534	2.1.56
2.52	Woods & Catanzaro	563	2.1.72
2.53	Woods & Catanzaro	563	2.1.72
2.54	Websters Third New		
	International Dictionary	1968,2122	(References)
2.55	Phillips L.R.F.	464	2.98.11
	Treece & Treece	178-181,207	2.1.65
2.56	Woods & Catanzaro	560	2.1.72
2.57	Polit & Hungler	530	2.1.56
2.66	Polit & Hungler	528	2.1.56
	Brockopp & Hastings-Tolma	372	(References)
2.67	Flanagan	327-358	2.67.5
2.68	Linstone & Turoff	3	2.68.6
2.69	Field & Morse	85	2.1.24
2.70	Holm & Llewellyn	267	2.1.26
2.71	Treece & Treece (adapted)	506	2.1.65
2.72	Seaman	433	2.1.62
2.73	Seaman	434	2.1.62
2.74	Abdellah & Levine	390	2.1.1
2.75	Phillips L.R.F.	462	2.98.11
2.76	Holm & Llewellyn	270	2.1.26
2.77	Treece & Treece	318	2.1.65

	Author(s)	Page in source text	Reference in this volume
2.78	Penguin Dictionary of Psychology	532	(References)
	A Lexicon of Psychology, Psychiatry & Psychoanalysis	298	(References)
2.79	Grady & Wallston	112	3.11.2
2.80	Readers Digest Universal Dictionary	347	(References)
2.82	Phillips L.R.F.	455	2.98.11
2.85	Phillips L.R.F.	456	2.98.11
2.86	Phillips L.R.F.	459	2.98.11
2.91	Polit & Hungler	535	2.1.56
2.92	Polit & Hungler	535	2.1.56
2.93	Woods & Catanzaro	563	2.1.72
2.94	Hakim	1	2.94.2
2.95	Glass	3	2.95.3
2.98	Phillips L.R.F.	462	2.98.11
2.99	Abdellah & Levine	392	2.1.1
2.104	Holm & Llewellyn	271	2.1.26
2.105	Phillips L.R.F.	465	2.98.11
3.7	Phillips L.R.F.	463	2.98.11
3.27	Dier IN Morse	40	2.41.6

Notes:

In most instances authors of definitions are listed in the order in which they appear in the book, unless there are several definitions in a particular section.

Items listed under references may be found on pages 333–335.

AUTHOR INDEX

KEY TO AUTHOR INDEX

This author index only gives the cross reference number in the text. Page numbers may be found in the expanded contents list at the beginning of the book.

It includes all authors names together with titles of government and professional bodies, databases and sources.

In some instances authors have chosen not to use all their initials in works included in this book and they are therefore treated separately in the index.

All authors in section 2.1 (Research texts) are normally included once only.

The order of entries in the index is as in the book, i.e. example, major text/article, annotations, suggested textbook readings, *Nursing research abstracts*.

2.38   Section number/example

2.23.1   Individual item/cross reference number

STR   Suggested textbook reading

            Example entry: Aamodt, A.   2.43   STR

            Indicates that this author has contributed part of a book relating to ethnomethods in 2.43. The cross reference number will be found in this section

NRA   Nursing Research Abstracts

            Example entry: Reed, V.   2.88   NRA 86/454

            Indicates that in section 2.88, Reed, V. has an entry in *Nursing research abstracts* of 1986, item number 454

*   Entry has not been annotated

Aamodt, A. M. 2.6 STR, 2.43 STR, 2.43.1
Aaronson, L. S. 2.82 NRA 90/010
Abbott, N. K. 2.17 STR
Abdel-Al, H. 2.101 NRA 84/131, 3.26 NRA 84/131
Abdellah, F. G. 2.1.1
Abraham, I. L. 2.88 NRA 86/456, 2.88 NRA 87/004, 2.88 NRA 90/004, 2.95.1, 3.2.1
Abramson, J. H. 2.42.1
Ackerman, P. G. 2.64.1
Adams, G. R. 2.1.2
Adams, H. E. 2.59.2
Adamson, A. 3.21.1
Adelman, C. 2.39.1, 2.80.1
Adkins, R. T. 1.2.1
Agan, R. D. 3.5.1*
Agar, M. H. 2.43.2
Ager, J. 2.63.19
Aggleton, P. 2.6.1
Ahlbom, A. 2.42.2
Ailinger, R. L. 3.27.4
Akinsanya, J. 1.2.8, 2.91.1, 3.18.1
Alderman, C. 3.13 NRA 82/281
Alderson, P. 2.17 NRA 81/116
Alderton, J. 3.6 NRA 84/263
Alguire, P. C. 2.98.1
Allemang, M. M. 2.48.1
Allen, B. 2.48.2
Allen, D. 3.21.2
Allen, D. G. 3.5.2*, 3.15.1
Allen, L. M. 2.46.5
Allen, M. 3.18.2
Allen, P. A. 2.17 NRA 83/1
Allen, T. H. 3.10.1
Altman, D. G. 2.97 NRA 84/1, 2.102 NRA 84/1
Altschul, A. 2.17 NRA 82/47, 3.3 STR, 3.13 NRA 82/282, 3.18.3, 3.26.1
American Psychological Association 2.102.1
Ammon-Gaberson, K. B. 2.89.1
Amramson, J. H. 2.55 NRA 80/376, 2.55 NRA 85/006
Anderson, A. J. B. 2.96.1
Anderson, B. 2.43.17
Anderson, J. M. 2.52 STR
Anderson, R. 3.6.8
Andersson, G. 2.83.10
Andrew, C. 2.78 NRA 86/469

Andrulis, R. S. 2.59.1
Angerami, E. L. S. 3.1 STR
Anonymous 2.17.1
Applied Social Sciences Index & Abstracts 1.12.1
Arber, S. 2.88.3, 2.94.1
Arkava, M. L. 2.1.3
Armitage, P. 2.35
Armitage, S. 2.105.1, 3.16.1, 3.18.4, 3.24.1
Armstrong, R. L. 2.20 STR
Armstrong-Esther, C. A. 3.19.1
Arnold, R. M. 2.17.17
Aron, M. S. 2.51.1, 2.66.1
Artinian, B. A. 2.36.18*
Arundel, K. F. 1.10.23
Ashworth, P. 3.6.1, 3.26 NRA 89/001
Ashworth, P. A. 3.27
Association for Information Management 1.3.1
Association of American Medical Colleges 2.17.2
Association of Commonwealth Universities 3.22.1, 3.22.2
Association of Researchers in Medical Science 3.12 NRA 81/280, 3.28 NRA 81/280
Athanasiou, R. 2.65.7
Atkins, E. 2.1.53
Atkinson, G. B. J. 3.21.4
Atkinson, I. 2.76 NRA 88/101, 2.76.1
Atkinson, J. 2.56.4
Atkinson, J. M. 2.92.1
Atkinson, P. 2.1.46, 2.1.49, 2.43.10
Atwood, J. 2.15.5
Atwood, J. R. 2.15.1, 2.29.1, 2.46.1, 2.57.1
Austin, J. 2.41.1
Australian Government 2.101 NRA 85/224
Avant, K. C. 2.7.12

Back, K. 2.48.4
Backer, T. E. 2.62.11
Badger, F. 2.16 NRA 84/2
Baer, E. D. 2.39, 3.4.1
Bailey, P. 1.3.3
Baker, G. 3.23.1
Baker, J. 3.22.3
Baldamus, W. 2.18.1
Ball, J. A. 2.63.1

351